# Essentials of Oral and Maxillofacial Surgery: Volume 1

# Essentials of Oral and Maxillofacial Surgery: Volume 1

Bruce Johnson

AMERICAN
MEDICAL PUBLISHERS
www.americanmedicalpublishers.com

AMERICAN
MEDICAL PUBLISHERS
www.americanmedicalpublishers.com

**Cataloging-in-Publication Data**

Essentials of oral and maxillofacial surgery: Volume 1 / Bruce Johnson.
p. cm.
Includes bibliographical references and index.
ISBN 979-8-88740-104-1
1. Mouth--Surgery. 2. Maxilla--Surgery. 3. Dentistry, Operative. 4. Face--Surgery.
5. Jaws--Surgery. I. Johnson, Bruce.
RK529 .E87 2023
617.522 059--dc23



American Medical Publishers,
41 Flatbush Avenue,
1st Floor, New York,
NY 11217, USA

ISBN 979-8-88740-104-1 (Hardback)

# Contents


Preface ..... VII

Part I **Oral and Maxillofacial Surgery: An Overview** ..... 1

Chapter 1 **Status of Oral and Maxillofacial Surgery in India** ..... 3
Kishore Nayak

Part II **Assessment and Preparation of Patients before Operation** ..... 8

Chapter 2 **Preoperative and Preanesthetic Evaluation** ..... 10
B. Krishnan and Satyen Parida

Chapter 3 **Dealing with Medical Comorbidities** ..... 24
Aditya Moorthy and Shreya Krishna

Chapter 4 **Handling Medical Emergencies** ..... 48
Nallamilli V. S. Sekhar Reddy

Part III **Usage of Anesthesia** ..... 58

Chapter 5 **OMS and Local Anesthesia** ..... 60
Reena Rachel John

Chapter 6 **OMS: Office-Based Anesthesia** ..... 77
Payal Verma and Deepak G. Krishnan

Chapter 7 **Maxillofacial Surgery: Application and Issues with Anesthesia** ..... 92
Rebecca Jacob, Subramanyam S. Mahankali, Renita Maria, Suman Ananathanarayana, Garima Sharma and Mary Thomas

Part IV **OMS and Medical Imaging** ..... 115

Chapter 8 **Fundamentals of Radiology in Maxillofacial Surgery** ..... 117
Shyamsundar K. Joshi and Annie I. Kochuveettil

Part V **Maxillofacial Surgery: Essential Concepts** ..... 166

Chapter 9 **Infection Prevention and Surgical Protocols** ..... 168
Rishi Kumar Bali

Chapter 10 **Role of Pharmacology and Pharmacotherapy in OMS** ..... 190
Latha P. Rao

Chapter 11 **Wound Care and Closure: Tools and Techniques** ........ 210
Ravi Veeraraghavan

Chapter 12 **Providing Postoperative Care to Patients** ........ 231
J. Naveen Kumar and Poornima Ravi

**Permissions**

**Index**

# Preface

Surgery is an invasive technique that involves the physical intervention on organs or tissues for diagnostic or therapeutic purposes. The surgical specialty that focuses on the reconstructive surgery of the face, facial trauma surgery, oral cavity, head and neck, mouth and jaw, and facial cosmetic surgery is referred to as oral and maxillofacial surgery. Subspecialties of oral and maxillofacial surgery include cosmetic facial surgery, craniofacial surgery, microvascular reconstruction and maxillofacial regeneration. The purpose of reconstructive surgery is to rebuild the body parts for its proper functioning. Cosmetic surgery is done to improve the natural appearance of a person. Various surgical procedures performed on the craniomaxillofacial complex include dentoalveolar surgery to extract impacted teeth, orthognathic surgery for treatment of dentofacial deformity, cosmetic surgery of the head and neck for browlift, cheek augmentation, and neck liposuction. The topics included in this book on oral and maxillofacial surgery are of utmost significance and bound to provide incredible insights to readers. Through it, we attempt to further enlighten the readers about the new concepts in this area of surgery.

This book is a result of research of several months to collate the most relevant data in the field.

When I was approached with the idea of this book and the proposal to edit it, I was overwhelmed. It gave me an opportunity to reach out to all those who share a common interest with me in this field. I had 3 main parameters for editing this text:

1. Accuracy - The data and information provided in this book should be up-to-date and valuable to the readers.

2. Structure - The data must be presented in a structured format for easy understanding and better grasping of the readers

3. Universal Approach - This book not only targets students but also experts and innovators in the field, thus my aim was to present topics which are of use to all

Thus, it took me a couple of months to finish the editing of this book.

I would like to make a special mention of my publisher who considered me worthy of this opportunity and also supported me throughout the editing process. I would also like to thank the editing team at the back-end who extended their help whenever required.

**Editor**

# Part I

# Oral and Maxillofacial Surgery: An Overview

# 1

# Status of Oral and Maxillofacial Surgery in India

Kishore Nayak

## 1.1 History of Our Missions and Our Challenges

Any discussion about the history of surgery inevitably begins with an invariable reference to *Suśruta* and his contributions to facial surgery, in particular. While the contributions of the sixth-century sage surgeon may somewhat be nebulous in a foggy poorly documented history, they are inevitably (and arguably) numerous but need not be elaborated here in any manner. What is lesser known and not often spoken about is that Suśruta considered surgery the first and foremost branch of medicine and stated, "Surgery has the superior advantage of producing instantaneous effects by means of surgical instruments and appliances. Hence, it is the highest in value of all the medical tantras. It is eternal and a source of infinite piety, imports fame and opens the gates of Heaven to its votaries. It prolongs the duration of human existence on earth and helps men in successfully fulfilling their missions and earning a decent competence in life." [1, 2]

When applied specifically to the context of the specialty of Oral and Maxillofacial surgery (OMS) emerging in India, it raises many important questions on how we have emerged and more importantly what we see ourselves evolving into in the years to come. Perhaps all those debates that we labored along numerous times were all a part of our coming of age!

Like elsewhere in the world, in the mid-twentieth century, we were probably practitioners of dentoalveolar surgery working under very trying circumstances moving on to where we are today. The specialty in India today, is truly all encompassing in its scope. It embraces the entire and extended spectrum of the practice of oral and maxillofacial surgery, and as the Association of Oral and Maxillofacial Surgeons of India (AOMSI) approaches its 50th year in 2019, there is no better time to look back and reflect on the past and contemplate where we are heading. The changes that we have witnessed have been rapid and hopefully progressive. From being oral surgeons, we transitioned and added maxillofacial surgery and to our quiver and perhaps to the chagrin competing specialties treaded into areas, once considered "gray" and broadened the scope of our practices.

Mino S Ginwalla is regarded as the pioneer of oral and maxillofacial surgery in India. In the 1950s, Dr. Ginwalla arrived in Mumbai following surgical training in Montreal, Canada, and set up his practice at Nair Hospital. He was a part of the founding group of surgeons of the AOMSI in 1969. By the mid-70s, training programs were established in most of the major dental colleges throughout India. Today, there are numerous OMS training programs in India.

The dental qualified persons are governed by the statutes of the Dental Council of India [3]. Currently, the Dental Council of India provides for a comprehensive 3-year program that includes a syllabus and curriculum that exposes trainees to standard procedures covering the full spectrum of oral and maxillofacial surgery [4]. This provides a legal framework for the OMS to function. This qualification itself is only permission to practice the specialty. In today's system, competence and eventual ownership of key surgical domains often only come from structured post-qualification training.

Thus, traditionally, the specialty in India continues to be predominately a dental subspecialty that leans toward the idea of a surgical branch of dentistry. While many arguments have been made for and against the need for a medical degree to augment the specialty, it is safe to postulate that for the near future, we will remain a dental specialty for a variety of reasons. North Americans seem to have found a middle ground and of the 101 OMS training programs in the US, 55 are single-degree programs (dental degree only) and 43 are dual-degree (dental and medical) programs, and three offer both options.

Drawing comparisons to the international scenario, the specialty has always been on a pendulous path remaining undecided on the idea of whether it wants to stay a dental

K. Nayak (✉)
Bhagwan Mahaveer Jain Hospital, Bangalore, India

specialty or whether it wants to incorporate the medical degree. In the USA where this trend initially started, the practice of the specialty is protected by national, regional, and local legislature as a dental specialty. In reality, there is no perceivable practical difference in the scope of practice between single- or double-degree practitioners in the States. In the UK and many parts of Europe, the specialty has taken leaps and bounds toward the medical path of training and it could very well be only a matter of time before the Specialty remains only remotely associated with Dentistry. The primary challenge was a lack of understanding, which centered on the debate of whether a medical as well as a dental qualification was required prior to surgical training [5].

Oral and maxillofacial surgery remains a specialty of dentistry in India and most training programs involve a graduate study and thesis to obtain the Masters in Dental Surgery (MDS) degree. The dental practice act allows all qualified dentally trained oral and maxillofacial surgeons to practice the unrestricted and full scope of the specialty, similar to what occurs in the European nations that require a medical degree. In most of Europe, OMS has become a medical subspecialty.

Public perception of the scope of practice of the specialty remains below par. The specialty gets confused with other surgical domains within both dentistry and medicine that we share a scope.

## 1.2 Expertise, Familiarity, and Competence

"Innovation is the combination of different ideas and contribution of the different minds."

Laskin [6] attempts to address this problem by dividing the scope of oral and maxillofacial surgery into three parts: areas of expertise, competence, and familiarity.

- Areas of expertise include oral pathology/oral medicine, dentoalveolar surgery, preprosthetic surgery (including implantology), and maxillofacial traumatology.
- Areas of competence involve orthognathic surgery, temporomandibular joint surgery, and local reconstructive surgery.
- Areas of familiarity are cleft lip and palate surgery, regional reconstructive surgery, oncologic surgery, craniofacial surgery, and cosmetic surgery.

Laskin's system of classification, while seemingly appearing comprehensive, opens itself to a lot of debate and question. While there is no doubt that the areas of "expertise" are unique to our specialty, it is our foray into those areas of competence and familiarity that has led to the expansion of the scope of our specialty. This expansion and contraction of our scope may also be fundamental to continual evolution. A large majority of our colleagues in India and worldwide operate within the boundaries of that scope of practice defined as "expertise." However, to turn areas of familiarity into competence and expertise will require that the training units and staff have the required skills and volume of cases to ensure hands-on experience and documentation. Only under these circumstances can we be assured that the skill sets and competencies will be transferred and become enduring.

It is ideal that all trainees are trained to achieve competence in craniomaxillofacial trauma, orthognathic surgery, and TMJ surgery (i.e., maxillofacial surgery). This and only this can provide the transition from Oral to Maxillofacial surgery. There, however, is a clear and present reality that not all training programs are equipped to achieve this goal. Even though training standards and syllabi exist, these standards are so broad that even programs with a very limited scope of training will meet accreditation standards by reporting a narrow set of hospital-based procedures that are not representative of the scope of practice required of modern OMS. Further, the interest of the trainee in training in the full scope of surgery is a factor that leads to mediocre training. The system of choosing a postgraduate training in OMS in India is severely handicapped and primitive. The factors that decide a trainee's choice of an advanced training program have nothing to do with their aptitude or interest in a specialty. It is purely based on their standing in a national entrance examination or their affordability of a position in a private institution. This leads to complete neglect of the student's natural aptitudes leading to prosthodontists becoming orthodontists and endodontists doomed into the world of oral and maxillofacial surgery. A disinterested trainee will be barely motivated to improve the scope of their practice following completion of their training, often limiting their practice to general dentistry and minimal indulgence in areas of "expertise."

Bell [7], when contemplating the future of education and training in the specialty, raises some very valid concerns, which seem to reflect the issues that affect the specialty and its future worldwide. Many reasons for the training disparities exist today—including training program location, the presence or absence of a trauma center, limited head and neck surgery experience, and local politics—but regardless, the goal should be the same: to train oral and maxillofacial surgeons to competence in the core areas of the specialty that they will eventually practice.

The key point is that we, as a specialty, should ensure that we train to competence and expertise based on geographic location, years in practice, fellowship training, and academic involvement. In years past, if an OMS graduate wished to obtain training in any areas beyond basics, then he or she often sought it outside of the specialty, in either otolaryngology or plastic surgery. With the emergence of several teaching hospitals and colleges as well as standalone independent centers of excellence, this scenario has drastically transformed in India. Further, the development of a number of fellowships that have been facilitated by the AOMSI has resulted in a robust system within the specialty that caters to the trainee's desire, merit, and quite often desire to embrace technique and technology. The rapid and natural advent of OMS into areas of oncology and reconstruction, cleft lip and palate, craniofacial surgery, and aesthetic surgery has been unprecedented and the critical mass of those who now fit in comfortably with these are their areas of expertise is on the rise.

This has been a radical transformation. A few decades ago, wandering beyond the realms of dentoalveolar surgery and facial trauma inevitably encountered a glass ceiling. Today this has been most certainly breached. Moreover, while the majority of the specialty holds itself within the original areas of expertise, there is no doubt that the Big Bang Moment for OMS in India has happened and it is a great time to contemplate where we are heading. What does the future hold for the specialty as we drift on our very own Starship Enterprise?

## 1.3 Predicting the Future

"Look back over the past, with its changing empires that rose and fell, and you can foresee the future, too." Marcus Aurelius.

Are we truly at a threshold or are we pieces in some continuum? What factors will drive our evolution as a specialty in India and our extended regions? What trends can we predictably follow to predict our future? Can we perhaps take a page from other fields in medicine to learn about ourselves? Will changing attitudes and aptitude of a new generation have a powerful impact on our profession or will we forever remain loyal to the vestiges of the legacy left behind for us?

Technology will undoubtedly play an important role in our future. Not just technology in patient care, but technology in our lives. Telemedicine and teleconsults will become a part of our everyday practice allowing us to practice beyond geographic limitations. Teleconferencing will make biannual AOMSI face-to-face conferences obsolete. In 2018, the American Association of Oral and Maxillofacial Surgeons (AAOMS) simulcasted their Dental Implant Conference, as did the American Society of Anesthesiologists. Their experience is that the while their total registration at these meetings went up, the number of in-person registrants did not dissipate. Consultant oral and maxillofacial surgeons all over the world have embraced telemedicine naturally, whether they realized it or not. Mobile technology allows the transfer of patient images and radiographs easily both for opinions and treatment planning. Such ease of access to patient images and documents has become a routine tool in emergency room triages of patients in the evaluation of the priority of care.

While technology in its current form is often perceived, as interruptive to one's lifestyle choices, the advent and immersion of artificial intelligence (AI) will make today's technology ubiquitous without being intrusive. Operating theaters of the future are likely to be guarded by artificial intelligence. Imagine an operating theater that prepares itself based on the radiofrequency identification (RFID) of the surgeon who swipes her/his badge at the door—that surgeon's preference cards get read by the system and a central core will prepare the instruments and supplies based on that surgeon's choices for that particular case booked for him.

Anesthesiology, radiology, and pathology are low-hanging fruits in the AI world. Radiologists in large tertiary-care centers in China, today, do not read radiographs anymore; they simply look at false positives read the previous night by their AI system. The system then learns from such mistakes and makes corrections forever. Computer systems today have the capacity of a thousand human brains to process data. The more data we feed these AI systems, the smarter they get. Google's AI product called LYNA or LymphNode Assistant is a trained algorithm that is capable of spotting the features of tumors that have metastasized, which are notoriously difficult to detect. Self-teaching algorithm systems will likely replace monitoring duties of the anesthesiologists and critical care nurses in the hospital.

Surgical robots are also constantly evolving incorporating precision haptics and AI. Robotic arms can already perform tasks independent of a surgeon yielding it. Imperfections and errors that a surgeon may cause in an operation are avoided in robotic surgery by consistent movements, angles, and access that can only be achieved by that robot. Imagine a robotic arm that can be programed to remove a mesioangular impacted mandibular third molar? The robot surgeon can assess the angulation of the impacted tooth based on the patient's radiograph, adjust its angulation and access, make a buccal trough, and split the tooth precisely. Less error and more precision, perhaps?

The day is not far before a robotic arm can obtain a tissue sample from our patients at a mall kiosk. Algorithms can then diagnose that tissue and their radiographs distancing the patient further away from the conventional practice of medicine. What is the future of our practices and our education in these scenarios? A well-informed patient with access to information and technology may surpass the traditional medicine man for their healthcare. Direct to consumer marketing of healthcare tools such as genetic testing is already prevalent in many countries. Several patients are aware of which chemotherapy may be best effective for the management of their cancers even before they see their doctor, today. Where does that place a specialist in the future?

In a keynote address at the Royal College of Surgeons in London at the 50th anniversary of the IAOMS, Brian Schmidt DDS, MD, PhD, Director, Bluestone Center for Clinical Research, and Professor of Oral and Maxillofacial Surgery at New York University pondered about the future of OMS internationally. He emphasized three units of care that oral and maxillofacial surgeons provide universally—

1. Management of maxillofacial trauma.
2. Management of oral cancer.
3. Management of craniofacial anomalies.

His views suggested that the advent of seatbelts, airbags, and safer road conditions in most countries is diminishing our total volume of trauma. Further, patterns of wars have changed from the bayonets of World War I to drone-controlled annihilation that ensures death! While bar fights and interpersonal violence continue to create left-sided ZMC and mandibular fractures, the world of facial trauma is most certainly changing.

He recognized examples of how personalized medicine is influencing the care of cancer patients. With our ability to map genomes and mutations, our ability to interpret cancer biology has had a meteoric rise even in the last decade. This leads to personalizing management via either chemotherapy or radiotherapy with predictable success making most cancers chronically manageable diseases rather than a death sentence. The future of personalized medicine will most likely put the cancer surgeon out of an occupation.

He introduced a study that demonstrated how a serendipitous finding in mice with Treacher-Collin's syndrome treated for endometrial cancer with a chemotherapeutic agent knocked out the gene causing the craniofacial anomaly in the following generation. This suggested that we could potentially be looking at gene therapy for craniofacial anomalies, including cleft lip and palate.

Schmidt's observations and predictions suggest that the diseases and conditions that are the mainstay to our profession will alter significantly in the future. Laboratories in Boston are very close to creating a template stem cells construct that will replace dental implants with naturally grown teeth. A dental caries vaccine is pending worldwide use.

How will these fundamental changes alter the practice of our specialty in the future?

Super specialization within the specialty is bound to happen. Attendees of the annual sessions of the British Association of Oral and Maxillofacial Surgeons will be struck by the design of the sessions. There are sessions designed for oral surgeons, implantologists, educators, deformities surgeons, ablative surgeons, and separately for reconstructive surgeons, as there are for minimally invasive surgery, aesthetic surgeons, and lab research. Larger sister specialties like ENT-Otolaryngology have also separated themselves into subspecialties. In the US, Pediatric otolaryngology, head and neck Surgery, facial plastic surgery, otology, skull-based surgery and surgery for sleep disorders are all recognized subspecialties within ENT in the US, for which fellowship training is offered. The pediatric otolaryngologist who specializes in airway surgery is unlikely to attend a conference organized for the otologists.

Similarly, domains within oral and maxillofacial surgery are already starting to branch out into subspecialty pods and practices are being limited to the practice of such subspecialties. That focus on a specific area within the specialty is also likely to be influenced by reimbursement for services. The subspecialties that rake in more money for the provider will thrive quicker and heftier than the latter. Changes in reimbursement strategies by hospitals will also evolve in this equation. For instance, in the US, where a large third-party payer system exists, clinical production for a practitioner is often not measured in actual dollars, but in revenue value units (RVUs). Complex longer cases like a head and neck disease ablation and reconstruction may not be related to a large reimbursement of dollars for the surgery alone; but the fact that the operating facility was used for several hours with the utilization of other resources such as nursing care, critical care, specialists like physical therapists, speech therapists, nutritionists, and a follow-up rehabilitation facility, all add up value to the health system ensuring reimbursement.

While this model seems to be working for now, the practice of medicine in the future unfortunately will be largely devised by the market and economics. The educational debt for training our future generation is getting out of hand. In a world where access to information is undoubtedly easier, the cost of a formal education is skyrocketing. Alternate models of education may arise disrupting this traditional model. Apprenticeships of the Osler era may be aft. Centers of excellence are likely to develop that allows a pathway of nontraditional training to an interested and talented trainee. Validation agencies like the International Board of Certification of Oral and Maxillofacial Surgeons (IBSCOMS) will have a bigger role in providing bonafide certification outside of the current commercialized and often-diluted education system.

The millennial and the gen Z student will also play a large role in the evolution of the specialty. Today's trainee learns differently, synthesizes information differently. They grew up on smartphones and Google searches and not in libraries or poring over Encyclopedia Britannica. They are visual learners with a panache for hand-eye coordination. They are multitaskers. No doubt that there will exist friction between a generation of older teachers and this generation of learners. And, that too will only be momentary. The new trainee is focused on lifestyle choices and is not unabatingly focused on education and patient care. The new trainee values life outside of work just as much as work. This will bring a new kind of diversity to the workplace. To make things worse, they will be treating a generation of aging patients who are used to a different kind of doctor from their times. The average patient is older and healthier and has demands that may have been considered unreasonable at one time. They are likely to be tech-savvy themselves. They will seek many opinions before they commit to the recommendations of their provider. They are likely to choose a surgeon based on the reviews on social media and the internet. Globalization of the medical industry and technology means that they might be willing to travel to have the same procedure and product used elsewhere than their hometown hospital.

Surgeons are working longer than they ever did as well. What impact does that have in a crowded marketplace? Will aging populations of patients and surgeons see an impact on the way we work? Will longevity and increased career years keep the younger ambitious surgeon from getting to the top? The retirement age of surgeons differs all over the world. Surgery is mentally and physically demanding. What effects does that chronic stress have on both the cognitive and physical decline in surgeons? Bhatt et al. did a narrative review on the topics of "ageing" and "surgeon" in Medline in 2016 [8]. They could not find any common ground in these studies. A surgeon who has to hang up his knife at 40 because of severe carpal tunnel in his hands is very different from one that has excellent physical health but severe cognitive decline. The variables were too many for them to consider any consensus on their research question—"when should surgeons retire?" They concluded that," Competence should be assessed at an individual level, focusing on functional ability over chronological age; this should inform retirement policies for surgeons."

OMS is like no other branch of medicine or dentistry. It has innovated, expanded, and usurped. It has replicated the old kingdoms, which created vast expanses as it rolled along. Eventually though, experience tells us that it can collapse under its own weight and might. As we look into the future, we must not ignore our past. Empires end for two reasons… problems from within and failure to protect their borders. As for empires, so for OMS. Our mistakes and pettiness must be acknowledged, accounted for, and learned so as not to repeat them.

We might have the ability as a specialty to control most of our destiny, but some of it may be adapted based on our environments. At the end of it all, if the specialty takes heed of three fundamental principles—patient care, education, and meaningful research, we will continue to justify our existence in the future.

## References

1. Suśruta Samhita. English translation by Kaviraj Kunja Lal Bhishagratna, Calcutta, 1907, Chapter 16, 152–154.
2. Raju VK. Suśruta of ancient India. Indian J Ophthalmol. 2003;51:119–22.
3. Paul G. The future of maxillofacial surgery as a specialty of dentistry. J Maxillofac Oral Surg. 2017;16(1):1–2. Published online 2017 Jan 16.
4. Revised 2007 regulation of the Dental Council of India, Gazette of India Extraordinary No DE 22–2007, Government of India, dated 20th November 2007, pp 56–68.
5. Nayak K. Oral and maxillofacial surgery: It's future as a specialty. J Maxillofac Oral Surg. 2011;10(4):281–2.
6. Laskin M. The past, present, and future of oral and maxillofacial surgery. J Oral Maxillofac Surg. 2008;66:1037–40.
7. Bryan Bell R. Infinite cornucopia: the future of education and training in oral and maxillofacial surgery. Oral Surg Oral Med Oral Pathol Oral Radiol. 2016;121(5):447–9.
8. Bhatt NR, Morris M, O'Neil A, Gillis A, Ridgway PF. When should surgeons retire? Br J Surg. 2016;103(1):35–42.

# Part II
# Assessment and Preparation of Patients before Operation

# 2

# Preoperative and Preanesthetic Evaluation

B. Krishnan and Satyen Parida

## 2.1 Introduction

A meticulous preoperative evaluation with the intention of identifying modifiable clinical conditions and understanding the risk stratification is imperative for all patients being subjected to any invasive procedure, inclusive of oral and maxillofacial surgery. Preoperative evaluation of such patients would of course differ, often dictated by age and the overall health condition that they present with. The choice of anesthesia may vary depending on the surgical procedure intended: general anesthesia, conscious sedation, regional blocks, local anesthesia, or various combinations of all of these. The current chapter focuses on the preoperative evaluation of patients posted for maxillofacial surgery under a general anesthetic in a formal operating room setting. Nevertheless, it is essential to realize that a preoperative evaluation is more or less standardized, irrespective of the type of surgery and practice (office-based dentoalveolar surgery, trauma, orthognathic surgery, elective esthetic surgery, craniofacial surgery, etc.) and anesthesia being planned. The goals of preoperative evaluation are summarized in Fig. 2.1 [1]. The intention is to minimize perioperative morbidity and mortality, to the best possible extent. The major step toward this goal requires the surgeon to be conscientiously aware of the general condition and clinical state of the patient so that in the eventuality of a critical event, he can intervene effectively and pertinently. This would involve modifying and customization of the patient's overall management to ensure that perioperative adverse events are avoided.

B. Krishnan (✉)
Department of Dentistry, Jawaharlal Institute of Postgraduate Medical Education and Research (JIPMER), Puducherry, India

S. Parida
Department of Anesthesiology and Critical Care, Jawaharlal Institute of Postgraduate Medical Education and Research (JIPMER), Puducherry, India

## 2.2 Preoperative Evaluation

The process of preoperative evaluation often begins with a standard history-taking and physical examination for the particular patient. A detailed history of prior medical problems, any previous surgical procedures, family, personal, and social history, any chronic medications and allergies or addictions needs to be obtained. In addition, it is worthwhile obtaining details about the patient's family physician if any, whether he has health insurance, the employer's details if the patient is employed, contact details of relatives, and any other information that may be deemed appropriate. The maxillofacial surgeon has to judge how the medical problems of the patient will affect perioperative care, and conversely, how perioperative events would influence the management of the patient's medical conditions. The patient's comorbidities could result in a significant physiologic decompensation due to myriad factors such as stress of the surgical procedure, original goals of the surgical intervention not being adequately met, and potential interactions between the regular medications that a patient may be on or with drugs that may be required to be instituted as part of the perioperative protocol. The maxillofacial surgeon should, therefore, be cognizant of what could possibly go wrong, and how those situations could be remedied. Also, it is critical that the surgeon be aware of all the medications (antidiabetic drugs, anticoagulants, antiplatelets, etc.) and medical comorbidities (cardiopulmonary, central nervous system, hepatic and renal disease, etc.) that the patient may be exposed to that could threaten the safe performance of the surgical procedure and have an adverse impact during the postoperative period. It is essential that every member of the perioperative team must be able to perform an independent assessment of the patient. This does not imply being ignorant of the other person's assessment since information needs to be shared by all components of the team, but each member should have his own way of assimilating such information by adding to it by his own independent assessment. This is important because

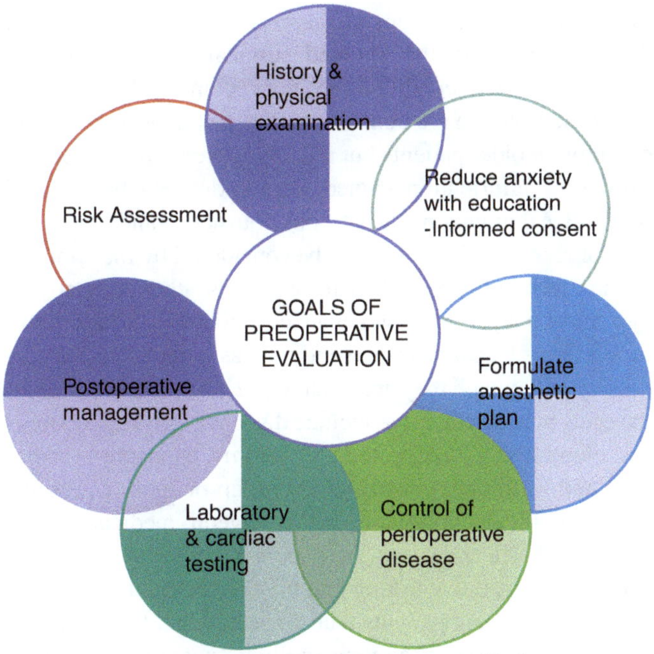




**Fig. 2.1** Goals of preoperative evaluation

every specialty would have its independent perspective, about the patient, although they would all be in the latter's best interests. For example, the surgeon might look upon older age in terms of postoperative functional recovery, while the anesthesiologist would be contemplating the various comorbidities that could be associated. Accordingly, each specialist would have his own concerns regarding the state of the patient, and therefore, the preoperative assessment provides a meeting ground for all these concerns after everyone has performed his own independent assessment. The use of a medical history questionnaire provides the maxillofacial surgeon with valuable information about the physical and psychological condition of the patient. Any medical history questionnaire can either be extremely useful or totally worthless and its ultimate value depends upon the ability of the surgeon to interpret the significance of the answers and to elicit additional information through physical examination and dialogue history. A prototype of a health history questionnaire is seen in Table 2.1 [2].

A preoperative physical examination begins with a recording of the patient's vital signs. The oral and maxillofacial system, by virtue, of the proposed surgical site, receives close attention by the surgeon. Of particular interest for the surgeon would be recognizing potential difficulties in surgical access and the need for alternative strategies and additional surgeries (e.g., bone grafting/skin grating). The cardiopulmonary examination assesses the rate and rhythm, murmurs, wheezing, rhonchi, and stridor. The musculoskeletal examination will include a range of neck motion and potential donor site evaluation. Finally, a neurological examination would assess the patient's mental status and any signs of pre-existing nerve or head injuries. A detailed description of the examination of all systems is beyond the scope of this chapter and the reader is advised to consult the references at the end of this chapter [1, 3–5].

**Table 2.1** Preoperative medical evaluation questions for a healthy patient

| Questions |
|---|
| 1. Do you usually get chest pain or breathlessness when you climb up two flights of stairs at normal speed? |
| 2. Do you have kidney disease? |
| 3. Has anyone in your family (blood relatives) had a problem following an anesthetic? |
| 4. Have you ever had a heart attack? |
| 5. Have you ever been diagnosed with an irregular heartbeat? |
| 6. Have you ever had a stroke? |
| 7. If you have been put to sleep for an operation, were there any anesthetic problems? |
| 8. Do you suffer from epilepsy or seizures? |
| 9. Do you have any problems with pain, stiffness, or arthritis in your neck or jaw? |
| 10. Do you have thyroid disease? |
| 11. Do you suffer from angina? |
| 12. Do you have liver disease? |
| 13. Have you ever been diagnosed with heart failure? |
| 14. Do you suffer from asthma? |
| 15. Do you have diabetes that requires insulin? |
| 16. Do you have diabetes that requires tablets only? |
| 17. Do you take any regular medications like antiplatelet or anticoagulants? |
| 18. Are you taking any over-the-counter medications, psychiatric medications, natural remedies? |
| 19. Do you have habits like smoking, alcohol, or use of recreational drugs? |

Once the history and physical examination are complete, the clinician would be in a situation to risk stratifying the patient according to the American Society of Anesthesiologists' (ASA) classification system (please see chapter on Ambulatory anesthesia for ASA table). Further investigations or specialist consultation is determined by the ASA status. This is especially imperative in patients with ASA Class III or IV who need to be further evaluated for their ability to withstand the proposed surgical procedure. Such patients, almost always, require inpatient admission due to a higher risk of perioperative adverse events. Patients of ASA Class V are extremely moribund and would therefore invariably require admission irrespective of the surgical procedure involved. It is extremely uncommon for a patient in this category to undergo any maxillofacial surgical procedure.

Preoperative risk stratification can also include a surgical classification system [6] (Table 2.2). This classification is quite useful for healthy patients undergoing a surgical procedure, as risk assessment in these patients is now determined solely by the nature of the procedure rather than the ASA

**Table 2.2** Cardiac Risk Stratification for Noncardiac Surgical procedures

| Cardiac risk stratification | Procedure examples |
|---|---|
| High Risk (>5%) | Aortic, Major vascular Surgery, Peripheral vascular Surgery |
| Intermediate Risk (1–5%) | Intraperitoneal and Intrathoracic Surgery, Carotid endarterectomy, Head and neck surgery, Orthopedic Surgery, Prostate Surgery. |
| Low Risk (<1%) | Endoscopic procedures, Superficial procedures, Cataract surgery, Breast surgery, Ambulatory surgery |

classification [7]. A similar surgical severity classification for oral and maxillofacial procedures has also been offered [8].

The preoperative assessment for oral and maxillofacial surgery will also require appropriate radiologic imaging for diagnostic information and treatment planning. These include panoramic, periapical, and occlusal radiographs, ultrasound, CT and MRI imaging. The clinical evaluation and imaging studies should help in the formation of a surgical plan, as to whether the surgery is going to be a simple or a complex one, what kind of instrumentation will be required for the same, or whether it would require the expertise of other surgical specialties such as Ophthalmology, ENT, and Plastic Surgery. The anesthesia team can also examine these imaging modalities to identify potential difficulties that may be encountered while intubating and securing the airway.

## 2.3 Laboratory Investigations

Preoperative patient assessment, ASA physical status, and severity of the proposed oral and maxillofacial surgical procedure guide the clinician to select the appropriate adjunctive studies for treatment planning. The ordering of adjunctive laboratory and radiological investigations is often determined by a complex interplay of pre-existing attitudes, practice patterns learnt during training, ease of ordering, fear of medicolegal consequences, and patient requests. When ordering a test, clinicians are attempting to discriminate between patients who have normal values and those who have abnormal ones. This is used to determine the possibility of the existence of a pathological condition that could impact the proposed surgical and anesthetic plan. The "normal" reference range for many clinical lab tests excludes the upper and lower 2.5% of results, and therefore 5% of normal individuals will obtain an "abnormal" result. While these "abnormal results" can be ignored, sometimes they are not and the result is an additional unnecessary investigation. Clinicians must be confident that there is a clinical justification for the actual need for the test. Studies indicate that less than 0.25% of all "abnormal" results of preoperative tests before an elective surgery influences the perioperative management [9]. "Routine" investigations, viz., those carried out preoperatively on all patients, and not directly related to the planned surgical procedure or the patient's physical condition, are not recommended [10, 11]. Age-based criteria are controversial as test abnormalities are common in older patients but are not as predictive of complications as information gained from a detailed history and physical examination. "Cost consciousness" and "stewardship of resources" also have to be considered by the clinician as the commonly ordered "battery of tests," though relatively inexpensive by themselves, can contribute to a significant proportion of healthcare expenditure as a result of the frequency with which they are ordered [12]. Beyond economics, the costs borne by patients include discomfort of needle sticks and blood loss with repeated phlebotomy, exposure to radiation, and additional unnecessary workup of spurious results. Good communication between the surgeon, medical consultant, anesthesia team, and the patient is essential when considering preoperative testing that may affect the timing of the surgery. Fit, young patients who are scheduled for outpatient surgery or low-risk surgery generally do not require any routine preoperative testing and, in the pediatric age group, a thorough clinical examination has been found to be of greater value [13, 14]. Routine urine or blood testing of the pediatric patient is not clinically warranted without a specific indication [15]. In general, test results within the past 6 months are acceptable if the patient's history has not changed. If the patient's condition has changed in the interim, adjunctive tests within the past 2 weeks are more favored [1].

The American Association of Oral and Maxillofacial Surgeons (AAOMS) recommendations on adjunctive studies prior to oral and maxillofacial surgery include, but are not limited to, both laboratory and imaging investigations [16] (Table 2.3). Similarly, algorithms based on the ASA classification, surgical procedure, and age of the patient are also available to assist the clinician to choose the appropriate adjunctive preoperative tests [17, 18].

While most standard texts would lead one to believe that extensive investigations in patients who are supposedly normal on history and clinical appraisal are not instrumental in improving outcomes or economically justified, it must be remembered that these perceptions are built upon data accumulated from the West, where regular health checkups and assessments are the norms. In contrast, in countries like India, a patient's first visit to a hospital may be for the surgery he is being posted for. Patients may also not be aware of existing comorbidities or details of any earlier interventions. This often leaves the clinician with no other option than to do order a "battery" of the so-called routine investigations to screen out potential pathological conditions. Ultimately, the choice of what laboratory investigations a patient may be subjected to is decided by the particular operating unit. It is important that such practices be customized to the population that the hospital caters to, and must be based on reasonable risk-benefit and cost analysis.

**Table 2.3** Indications for commonly ordered preoperative laboratory tests based on specific findings during history and physical examination (independent of patient age, American Society of Anesthesiologists' classification, or surgical procedure)

| Investigations | Indications |
|---|---|
| *Laboratory investigations* | |
| 1. Complete Blood Counts: | |
| WBC count | Patients with infection/fever<br>On chemotherapy<br>Myeloproliferative disorders<br>Immune-compromised states (HIV)<br>History of cancer, chemotherapy, or radiation treatment |
| Platelet count | History of low platelets<br>Bleeding history<br>Thrombopathy<br>Pregnancy<br>Autoimmune disease<br>Splenectomy<br>Liver disease |
| Hemoglobin/Hematocrit | Anticipated blood loss greater than 500 ml<br>Suspicion of anemia<br>Recent chemotherapy/Radiotherapy (within 2 months)<br>Renal disease<br>Active cardiac symptoms<br>Recent blood loss<br>Sickle cell anemia/thalassemia<br>Recent autologous blood transfusion<br>Older patients undergoing major surgery |
| 2. Chemistry: | |
| Electrolytes/BUN/Creatinine | Chronic Kidney Disease<br>Liver cirrhosis<br>Medications (diuretics, ACE inhibitor, digoxin)<br>Diabetes mellitus<br>Malnutrition<br>Dehydration<br>Infections<br>On renal dialysis—$K^+$ tested immediately prior to surgery |
| Creatinine | Older patients undergoing intermediate-or-high-risk surgery<br>Patient for whom nephrotoxins will be used<br>When large fluid shifts or hypotension is likely |
| Glucose-(Fasting/Random/ Postprandial/Glucose Tolerance Test (GTT) /HbA1C) | Diabetes mellitus<br>Long-term steroid medications<br>Liver cirrhosis<br>Pregnancy<br>Infections<br>Pancreatic disease<br>Adrenal disease<br>Pituitary disease<br>>45 Years of age with no prior history of diabetes mellitus |
| 3. Coagulation profile | |
| Prothrombin Time (PT)<br>International Normalized Ration (INR)<br>Partial Thromboplastin Time (PTT) | Personal/ family history of bleeding diathesis or clotting disorders<br>Evidence of purpura or petechiae<br>On current or recent anticoagulation medications (warfarin/heparin)<br>Liver disease<br>Abnormal liver function (jaundice)<br>Alcoholism<br>Severe malnutrition<br>Chronic renal failure<br>History of stroke<br>Autoimmune disorders |
| PT (for warfarin)<br>PTT (for heparin) | Repeated on the evening before/morning of the surgery to document normal coagulation parameters after stopping these medications, if indicated. |
| Bleeding Time (BT) | Not a reliable preoperative indicator of platelet function. Not recommended for presurgical workup |
| Clotting Time (CT) | Time consuming, poor reproducibility, insensitive to high doses of heparin, and sensitive in only extreme factor deficiencies<br>Not of much value in modern laboratory settings |

**Table 2.3** (continued)

| Investigations | Indications |
|---|---|
| 4. Liver function tests | Cirrhosis<br>Hepatitis<br>Jaundice<br>Hepatomegaly<br>Alcohol abuse<br>Pancreatic disease<br>History of cancer<br>Easy bleeding and bruising<br>Malnutrition |
| 5. Type, screen, and cross-sensitivity | Patients with bleeding or coagulation disorders<br>Surgeries with a potential for blood loss (>500 ml) even if transfusion is not expected.<br>*This may help minimize the risk of later transfusion reaction.* |
| 6. Pregnancy testing (Serum/Urine) | Premenopausal women of child-bearing age who have not had tubal ligation or hysterectomy (Urine Human Chorionic Gonadotropin—HCG).<br>*History and physical examination are insufficient to determine early pregnancy, and patients are often unreliable in suspecting that they may be pregnant. Management protocols often change if it is discovered that the patient is pregnant.* |
| 7. Arterial blood gases (ABG) | Only if suspicion for hypoxemia or $CO_2$ retention that would affect postoperative management. |
| 8. Pulmonary function tests | Previously unknown obstructive lung disease<br>Severe asthma<br>Symptomatic COPD<br>Scoliosis |
| 9. Urinalysis | Active symptoms of Urinary tract infection (UTI), dysuria<br>*No good evidence that preoperative abnormal urinalysis is associated with any postoperative complication in nonurinary tract surgery.* |
| 10. Blood cultures | Only if clinical suspicion of septicemia. |
| *Imaging* | |
| 1. Chest X Ray | Significant risk factors for postoperative pulmonary complications (severe/uncontrolled COPD, active pulmonary disease/symptoms, abnormal lung sounds on physical examination, recent pneumonia) with no previous chest X-ray for past 1 year may warrant preoperative chest X-ray irrespective of age.<br>Asymptomatic patients older than 50 years with no risk factors—insufficient evidence for ordering a chest X-ray.<br>Should not be considered as an unequivocal indication for extremes of age, smoking, COPD, stable cardiac disease, and recent resolved upper Respiratory Tract Infection (RTI).<br>*Without symptoms or pertinent medical history, abnormal chest X rays do not predict a worse clinical outcome.* |
| 2. 12 Lead ECG | History of cardiac disease (coronary artery disease, significant arrhythmia, structural heart disease, compensated or prior heart failure)<br>Peripheral artery disease<br>Chest pains<br>Lung disease<br>Morbid obesity<br>History of stroke/cerebrovascular disease<br>Diabetes mellitus<br>Renal insufficiency<br>Patient is having an intermediate- or high-risk surgery<br>*Consider in high-risk group based on epidemiology (males >40 years and females >50 years of age)* |
| 3. Echocardiogram | Recent myocardial infarction<br>Congestive heart failure<br>Abnormal ECG<br>Unstable angina<br>Significant arrhythmias<br>Severe valvular heart disease<br>Previous history of coronary artery disease<br>Dyspnea of unknown origin<br>History of heart failure with progressive symptoms<br>Unstable cardiomyopathy |

## 2.4 Preanesthetic Evaluation

The preanesthetic evaluation aims at getting a favorable outcome, from the points of view of both the surgeon and the anesthesiologist by focusing on risk stratification and modification, and by developing a plan that appropriately addresses the risk-benefit ratio from the procedure, and also explores the other options available. It involves putting together all the elements of the patient's history, physical examination, medications, allergies, laboratory studies, and certain examinations of interest to the anesthesiologist (e.g., airway). This information is assimilated, and decisions are made regarding the plan for anesthetizing the patient once the full picture emerges. This, however, is a dynamic process, and hence accommodates changes in the plan, if new information surfaces, in the best interests of the patient and surgeon. It is also important to be aware of the strengths and limitations of the set-up in which the particular surgical intervention is being undertaken. Further, the preanesthetic evaluation also attempts to allay patient anxiety regarding the procedure, takes necessary steps for risk reduction and to get informed consent. Finally, it leads to the choice of the anesthetic plan to be followed, guided by the risk factors uncovered by the medical history, which covers the entire perioperative period, inclusive of a plan as to where the patient will be cared for postoperatively, and what kind of pain relief he/she should receive after surgery.

## 2.5 Aspects of Evaluation Unique to Anesthesia

The perspective of each specialty also drives the way physical examination is conducted by each of them. All clinicians learn early as part of their training that relevant positive and negative points not only direct the elicitation of history but also examination. Airway examination is something that is uniquely specific to anesthesiologists with the intention of predicting a difficult airway, that is, one that might result in difficulty in ventilating or intubating the patient, or both. The ASA task force on the management of the difficult airway stresses importance on the physical examination of the airway [19]. While no single method can be deemed to be fool proof in this regard, the anesthesiologist is trained to examine different aspects as well as scoring systems to be able to make the assessment of a difficult airway [20–22]. The mnemonic **LEMON** is a helpful tool for assessing the potential for difficult intubation [23, 24] (Fig. 2.2). The Mallampati classification, which relates tongue size to pharyngeal size, is a common component of a thorough airway examination [25]. The examination is performed with the patient in the sitting position, the head held in a neutral position, the mouth wide open, and the tongue protruding to the maximum. The subsequent classification is assigned according to the pharyngeal structures that are visible: (Fig. 2.3).

Class I: visualization of the soft palate, fauces, uvula, and anterior and posterior pillars.
Class II: visualization of the soft palate, fauces, and uvula.
Class III: visualization of the soft palate and the base of the uvula.
Class IV: soft palate not visible at all.

The important aspects of the airway, which can affect intubation, include the degree of mouth opening, the size of the tongue in relation to other oral structures, and the capability to align the oral, pharyngeal, and laryngeal axes in more or less one straight line, with the patient's head and neck in the sniffing position. While the Mallampati classification relates to soft-tissue sizes and their relationships with each other, apart from mouth opening, there are several other anatomical features that need to be considered in the evaluation of the airway (Table 2.4). Examination of systems, other than the cardiopulmonary system, is dependent upon the proposed surgical procedure and planned anesthesia, along with the clinical features of the patient. For example, a patient with a Le Fort II or III fracture may require a careful neurological and ophthalmological examination. Documentation of the findings of history and physical examination must focus on the positive and negative findings after integrating information from the surgeon, patient, and other sources.

## 2.6 Assessment of the Pediatric Patient

The objective of preoperative assessment in the apparently healthy child is to discover medical or anatomic issues, hitherto not acknowledged, that will escalate the risk of surgery and anesthesia. Special attention is warranted by virtue of specific anatomical and physiological differences from the adult patient. Additional risk factors in pediatric patients, apart from the surgery-specific and patient-specific risks,

**Fig. 2.2** LEMON Assessment for difficult intubation

| Physical Signs | Less difficult airway | More difficult airway |
|---|---|---|
| Look externally | Normalface and neck<br>No face or neck pathology | Abnormally face shape<br>Sunken cheeks<br>Edentulous<br>Buck teeth<br>Receding mandible<br>Narrow mouth<br>Obesity<br>Face or neck pathology |
| Evaluate 3-3-2 rule | Mouth opening> 3 fingers<br>Hyoid-chin distance > 3 fingers<br>Thyroid cartilage to mouth floor distance> 2 fingers | Mouth opening < 3 fingers<br>Hyoid-chin distance < 3 fingers<br>Thyroid cartilage to mouth floor distance < 2 fingers |
| Mallampatti scale | Class I and II (Can see the soft palate, uvula, fauces, ± facial pillars) | Class III and IV (Can only see the hard palate ± soft palate ± base of uvula) |
| Obstruction | None | Pathology within or surrounding the upper airway (e.g., peritonsillar adscess, epiglottis, retropharyngeal abscess) |
| Neck mobility | Can flex and extend the neck normally | Limited range of motion of the neck |



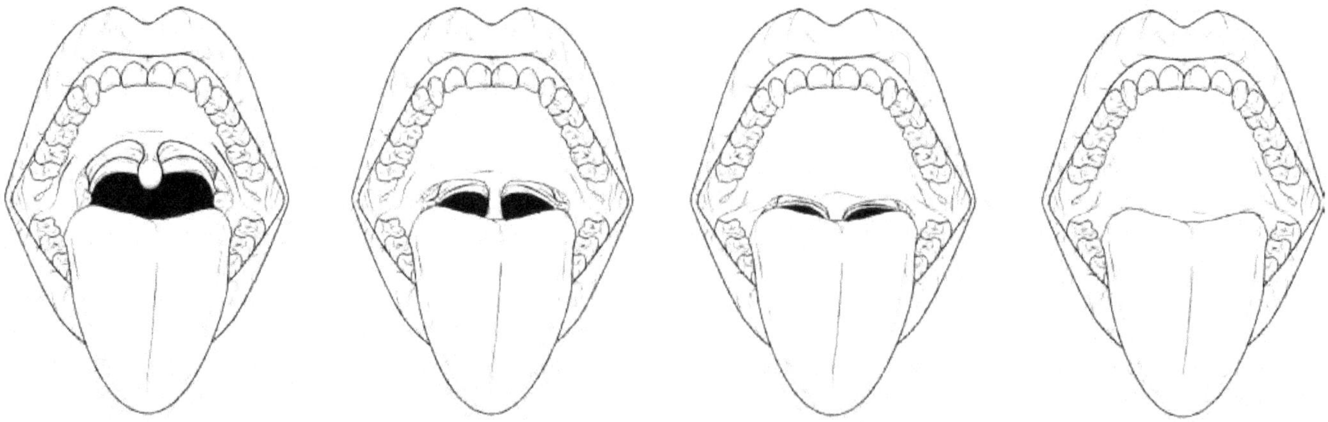

I II III IV

**Fig. 2.3** Mallampati Classification for assessment for intubation. Class I: Cmplete visualization of the soft palate. No additional difficulty. Class II: Complete visualizatin of the uvula. No additional difficulty. Class III: Visualization f only the base of the uvula. Moderate difficulty. Class IV: Soft palate is not visible at all. Severe difficulty

**Table 2.4** Airway compromising conditions

- *Congenital*
  - Pierre-Robin syndrome: micrognathia, macroglossia, cleft soft palate
  - Treacher-Collins syndrome: auricular and ocular defects, malar and mandibular hypoplasia
  - Goldenhar's syndrome: auricular and ocular defects, malar and mandibular hypolasia
  - Down's syndrome: poorly developed or absent bridge of the nose, macroglossia
  - Kippel-Feil syndrome: congenital fusion of a variable number of cervical vertebrae, restriction of neck movement
  - Goiter: compression of trachea, deviation of larynx/trachea
- *Infections*
  - Supraglottis: laryngeal edema
  - Croup: laryngeal edema
  - Abscess (intraoral, retropharygeal): distortion of the airway and trismus
  - Ludwig's angina: distortion of the airway and trismus
- *Arthritis*
  - Rheumatoid arthritis: temporomandibular joint ankylosis, cricoarytenoid arthritis, deviation of laynrx, restricted mobility of cervical spine
  - Ankylosing spondylitis: ankylosis of cervical spine, less commonly ankylosis of temporomandibular joints, lack of mobility of cervical spine
- *Benign tumors*
  - Cystic hygroma, lipoma, adenoma, goiter: stenosis or distortion of the airway, fixation of larynx or adjacent tissues secondary to infiltration or fibrosis from irradiation
- *Malignant tumor, facial injury, cervical spine injury, laryngeal or tracheal trauma*: edema of the airway, hematoma, unstable fracture(s) of the maxillae, mandible and cervical vertebrae
- *Obesity*: short thick neck, redundant tissue in the oropharynx, sleep apnea
- *Acromegaly*: macroglossia, prognathism
- *Acute burns*: edema of airway

include the clinician-related risks; an acknowledgment that superior skills are called for in managing this extremely vulnerable patient population. Children with chronic medical problems require appropriate management and prediction of possible difficulties in management, which the preoperative assessment needs to focus on. Especially for infants, enquiries about prematurity, developmental milestones, and medical background check probing for possible congenital diseases of the cardiac and respiratory systems need to be made. Congenital cardiovascular malformations are frequently associated with many facial malformations, which require a thorough preoperative assessment. Another challenge that pediatric patients present, especially for the anesthesiologist, is the pediatric airway management due to a difference in the airway anatomy vis-a-vis adults. The relatively larger soft tissues in the oropharynx, a more cephalad and anterior position of the vocal cords and the larynx, and a shorter length of the trachea are among the few differences between an adult and pediatric airway anatomy [26]. These unique variations can result in airway management issues, including difficulties in sustaining a patent airway, mask ventilation, insertion of supraglottic airway devices, and endotracheal intubation.

## 2.7 Assessment of the Elderly Patient

Another vulnerable population is the geriatric age group. This is because older age is associated not only with dwindling functions of almost all organ systems but also an increase in the incidence of comorbidities. Further, as life expectancy increases, clinicians are likely to encounter a substantial number of elderly people in their practice, and it is conceivable that a large proportion of these may present for surgery. It is therefore vital that clinicians dealing with patients of this age group should be able to comprehend the alterations in physiology and pathophysiology that occur with aging. A diminished cardiopulmonary reserve puts this patient population under a higher risk of perioperative adverse events. Incidence of coronary artery disease is also prevalent in the geriatric population. Further, there is an increased risk of cognitive dysfunction such as dementia, delirium, and depression, which may be exacerbated in the acute postoperative phase. Elderly patients have impaired hepatic and renal metabolism and delayed clearance of drugs in the systemic circulation, which can cause increased sensitivity to intravenous anesthetics. Also important in relation to the elderly patient are several anatomical alterations, which can affect management. Predominant among these are changes in airway anatomy, such as nasopharyngeal fragility, macroglossia, microstomia, etc. [27]. These can result in difficulty in mask ventilation and placement of supraglottic airway devices and endotracheal tube.

## 2.8 Specialist Consultation and Work-up

The initial evaluation of the patient then leads to subsequent work-up, including obtaining consultations from other specialties if deemed necessary, re-evaluating the need for any additional investigations, taking steps to limit perioperative risks as deemed necessary, evolving an anesthetic plan, and getting informed consent from the patient. As more and more areas of concern may develop, further testing, specialist consultation, and varied approaches to risk management strategies may become imperative. As this dynamic process of comprehensive patient assessment evolves, revision of the anesthetic plan and eliciting additional specific terms of consent from the patient may also become inevitable.

Specialist consultations are needed when the particular condition being evaluated does not come under the purview of the training of the anesthesiologist or surgeon. Such consultations must be specific and try to elicit whether the patient is in the best possible condition with regard to his particular comorbidity to undergo the proposed intervention, or whether the malady for which consultation is being sought, can be further optimized and at what stage of the particular ailment the patient is at. When consultations are merely sent without stating specific objectives of such request, they might meet with a similarly nonspecific response from the consultant that the referral is being sent to, and hence proving to be of not much help for the clarification sought for. Thus, referrals to other disciplines need to be very specific, as to the expectations that the referring unit has of the evaluation and the advice that they should receive. The consultant to whom the referral goes now becomes an important component of the perioperative team. It is essential that this consultant must also appreciate his role in the assessment of the patient, and this would be possible by building support networks among disciplines. This will also save time in the perioperative period, since a few investigations that the consultant being referred to would advise, may be carried out prior to the referral itself. An example would be getting an ECG and echocardiogram done prior to referring a patient with significant coronary artery disease to the cardiologist. Thus, the requirement for circulation of information, among disciplines, is vital and is especially true with regard to communication between consultants. Often, communicating personally with the consultant to whom the patient is being referred to, can expedite the evaluation to a very great extent.

## 2.9 The Process of Risk Assessment

Following a thorough evaluation and perusal of the results of the investigations, the patient-specific risks are evident, while the surgery-specific risks need to be considered upon, the summation of both of which contribute to the overall risk to the patient. Technical factors such as fluid shifts, total blood loss, as well as the site of the surgical intervention, are components of the surgery-specific factors that contribute to the total risk assessment [28]. Oral and maxillofacial surgery being classified as head and neck surgery, would normally be considered as an intermediate risk surgery, unless undertaken as emergency or anticipated to have a risk of excessive blood loss, wherein it would be classified as a high-risk procedure. The correlation between expected blood loss and specific maxillofacial surgeries has been demonstrated [29]. With improving the safety of anesthesia equipment and medications, the historical dangers of anesthesia administration are quite low, and patient- and surgery-specific risk factors almost completely determine the overall risk to the patient [30, 31].

Once the overall risk of the patient is known and calculated, the next step would be to devise a strategy for risk management.

## 2.10 Risk Reduction Strategies

Risk reduction blueprints must be assessed and a risk-benefit ratio evaluated in performing any elective oral or maxillofacial surgical procedure. Alternative procedures and occasionally even avoiding any intervention could be considered when the overall risks in terms of morbidity and mortality to the patient are substantial. Obviously, the most critical step in risk reduction would be to get the patient in the best physical condition to undergo an interventional procedure. To this effect, modifiable risk factors should be addressed (e.g., anemia, hyperglycemia, hypertension) always ensuring that the risk-benefit ratio stays in the patient's favor. As an example, in a smoker who is to undergo an intermediate- or high-risk surgery, the obvious risk reduction strategy would be to quit smoking [32, 33].

This then allows the patient's body to reap the benefits of a simple risk reduction maneuver with the risk now decreasing to a degree that might cause a favorable impact on the morbidity and mortality otherwise expected. Appropriate medical management of the comorbidities might be successful in optimizing patients to a state where they can withstand the rigors of the surgical procedure. The particular anesthetic technique apart, there are at least five other areas that may be targeted as part of overall risk reduction strategies, namely: (a) premedication, (b) antiaspiration prophylaxis, (c) perioperative beta-blockade, (d) postoperative nausea and vomiting (PONV) prophylaxis and (e) effective postoperative pain management.

### 2.10.1 Premedication [4]

An increase in heart rate is the major factor increasing myocardial oxygen demand in the perioperative period. This makes appropriate anxiolysis and management of postoperative pain absolute vital cogs in the overall care of the patient undergoing surgery since anxiety and/or pain can set off a noxious cycle of events starting with tachycardia and hypertension, which could, in turn, result in perioperative myocardial infarction, the incidence of which is highest in the first 72 h. Benzodiazepines induce anterograde amnesia, anxiolysis with mild sedation. Opiates were previously believed to be a vital part of preemptive analgesia, but later they were found to sensitize patients to pain. Clonidine may also be considered preemptive analgesia, especially when administered epidurally. However, the entire concept of pre-emptive analgesia, or antinociceptive treatment prior to initiation of the pain stimulus that prevents the establishment of altered processing of afferent input, that amplifies postoperative pain, is currently mired in controversy. Clonidine has a cardioprotective effect and also decreases the minimum alveolar concentration (MAC). Antihistamines may be used for their sedative and antiemetic properties. However, the clinician needs to know that promethazine, the most commonly prescribed antihistaminic, now carries an FDA warning for apnea and death in children. Anticholinergics are no longer used routinely, but rather to produce an antisialagogue effect when desirable (endoscopic procedures), sedation/amnesia, or to prevent reflex bradycardia.

### 2.10.2 Fasting Guidelines

Patients with a full stomach at the time of induction of anesthesia are perceived to be at high risk of aspiration of gastric contents into their respiratory tract, and also present difficulty with intubation if gastric contents are regurgitated at the time of airway manipulation. This may lead to acute lung injury manifested as pneumonitis, aspiration pneumonia, respiratory failure, or acute respiratory distress syndrome [34]. Following administration of a general anesthetic, patients can no longer have the ability to maintain a patent airway, respiration, or protective reflexes like gagging or coughing. The driving force for inducing aspiration is the barrier pressure, which is the difference between the gastroesophageal sphincter tone that opposes aspiration and the hydrostatic pressure within the stomach. In the presence of a negative barrier pressure, the possibility of regurgitation, vomiting, and aspiration is increased. One of the ways to maintain the barrier pressure positive during the vulnerable period of anesthesia is to instruct the patient to be "nil per oral" prior to surgery, such that the gastric hydrostatic pressure is kept low. What constitutes an appropriate period of fasting before anesthesia has been the subject of substantial research over several years, and current guidelines are based both on the nature of oral intake and the age of the patient [35, 36, 37] (Table 2.5). These recommendations, however, need to be viewed as guidelines, rather than a set of inviolable instructions. The reason why these rules should not be looked upon as impregnable is because these were intended for normal patients. Individual situations may sometimes prevent these nil-per-oral guidelines from providing foolproof safety from aspiration. Conditions that inhibit gastric emptying, including diabetes, morbid obesity (body mass index [BMI] >35), pregnancy, bowel obstruction, previous upper gastrointestinal surgery, and gastrointestinal disease such as gastric ulcer, scleroderma, etc. will all escalate the risk of aspiration and deserve as much attention that a full stomach does [38–40]. Another group of patients who are believed to be at high risk for aspiration comprises those with difficult airways, as these patients will require more prolonged airway manipulation and thus a greater time to intubation [41]. The airway remains unprotected and unsecured for a longer time and hence these patients may benefit from prophylaxis against aspiration. The preanesthetic evaluation needs to identify this special category of patients who appear to be at higher risk of aspiration, despite adhering faithfully to standard nil per oral guidelines and premedicate them for elective surgery. A prokinetic drug and an alkalinizing agent could reduce the complications from gastric aspiration by combating the corrosive acidic nature of gastric juice, even if aspiration does occur [3].

**Table 2.5** Preoperative fasting recommendations for healthy patients undergoing elective surgery

| Liquid and food intake | Minimum fasting period |
|---|---|
| Clear liquids (Water, tea, black coffee, fruit juice without pulp, carbonated beverages) | 2 h |
| Breast milk | 4 h |
| Nonhuman milk, including infant milk formula | 6 h |
| Light meal (e.g., toast and clear liquids) | 6 h |
| Regular or heavy meal (may include fried or fatty food, meat) | 8 h |

The most widely prescribed prokinetic in this regard is the dopamine-antagonist metoclopramide (10 mg orally/IV). However, this drug has the potential to cause extrapyramidal symptoms and should be used cautiously. The other pharmacological agent that increases the pH of gastric juice and makes it less acidic is a Histamine 2 (H2) receptor blocker, viz., ranitidine (150 mg orally; 50 mg IV) or famotidine (20 mg IV). Cimetidine is no longer used due to its ability to induce hepatic enzymes and influence the metabolism of several anesthetic agents. Usually, the prokinetic along with the H2 blocker is administered both on the night before and on the morning of the surgery. Administration of two doses each of both the medications guarantees adequate plasma levels required for an effective action. Lastly, the use of particulate antacids such as citric acid/sodium citrate (30 ml) typically within 2 h prior to the anticipated induction of anesthesia also can neutralize the gastric acid, and reduce the incidence of chemical pneumonitis even if the aspiration occurs. However, its bitter taste and propensity to induce emesis necessitates that it be administered a substantial period prior to intubation.

### 2.10.3 Perioperative Beta-Blocker Therapy

Organ ischemia is a result of an imbalance between the oxygen supply and demand. The heart is especially vulnerable since myocardial work and oxygen demand are very tightly coupled. However, the precise level of myocardial demand at which it outstrips the supply is unclear. Hence, a patient who is susceptible to the development of myocardial ischemia needs to be managed perioperatively in a manner that keeps the demand lowest, while at the same time maximizing supply. Pharmacological manipulation of the myocardial demand is probably effected easier than a significant manipulation of the supply. Physiologically, tachycardia is the most important parameter that increases myocardial demand, with increases in systemic vascular resistance being the second most important [42–44]. Patients having a significant cardiovascular risk need a cardiologist's opinion for an evaluation of the extent of risk and preoperative optimization [6] (Table 2.6). Obviously, modifiable risk factors and reversible disorders need to be addressed and managed. The ACC recommends perioperative beta-blocker therapy for patients with two or more intermediate risk factors or a single major risk factor, especially if being posted for an intermediate-to-high-risk surgical procedure [6]. The evaluating physician can be requested to assess the benefits of beta-blockade in the patient scheduled for maxillofacial surgery. The commonest way of introducing beta-blockade is with the drug metoprolol for a target basal heart rate of 60–65 beats per minute (bpm), and to sustain the rates at no more than 85 bpm during the perioperative period. Beta-blockade should, however, be started well before the surgery so that ample time is available to adjust the dose to the target heart rate and address any side effects that may develop. The administration of a beta-blocker just prior to an emergency surgery is controversial as this has been observed to be associated with a greater risk of perioperative strokes [45, 46]. More research is needed to clearly identify which patient subsets might benefit most from the beta-blockade, and in whom the side effects may be substantial.

**Table 2.6** Clinical predictors of increased perioperative cardiovascular risk

*Major clinical predictors (markers of unstable coronary artery disease)*
- Myocardial infarction <6 weeks: Delay elective surgery, consultation with cardiologist
- Unstable or severe angina (Canadian Cardiovascular Society class III or IV)
- Decompensated heart failure
- Significant arrhythmias (e.g., causing hemodynamic instability)
- Severe valvular heart disease (e.g., aortic or mitral valve stenosis with valve area < 1 cm$^2$)
- CABG or PTCA <6 weeks

*Intermediate clinical predictors (markers of stable coronary artery disease)*
- Previous Myocardial infarction >6 weeks but <3 months (> 3 months if complicated) based on the history or presence of pathologic Q waves on the Electrocardiogram
- Mild angina (Canadian Cardiovascular Society class I to II)
- Silent ischemia (Holter monitoring)
- Compensated heart failure, ejection fraction <0.35
- Post CABG or PTCA >6 weeks and < 3 months, or > 6 years, or on antianginal therapy
- Diabetes mellitus
- Renal insufficiency

*Mild clinical predictors (increased probability of coronary artery disease)*
- Familial history of coronary artery disease
- Age > 70 years
- ECG abnormalities (arrhythmias, LVH, Left bundle branch block)
- Low functional capacity
- History of stroke
- Uncontrolled systemic hypertension
- Hypercholesterolemia
- Smoking
- Post infarction (> 3 months, asymptomatic without treatment
- Post CABG or PTCA (> 3 months and < 6 years, and no symptoms of angina nor on antianginal therapy)

*Major clinical predictors*: All elective operations should be postponed and the patients properly investigated and treated.
*Intermediate clinical predictors*: Proof of well-established but controlled coronary artery disease. Further risk stratification and optimization in consultation with cardiologist.
*Minor clinical predictors*: Increased probability of coronary artery disease, but not of an increased perioperative risk. Further risk stratification and optimization in consultation with cardiologist.
*Emergency procedures*: Proceed for surgery with perioperative surveillance and postoperative risk stratification and risk factor management.

*CABG* Coronary Artery Bypass Grafting, *PTCA* Percutaneous Transluminal Coronary Angioplasty, *LVH* Left Ventricular Hypertrophy

### 2.10.4 PONV Prophylaxis [47]

Oral and Maxillofacial surgeries are generally not considered as high risk for the incidence of postoperative nausea and vomiting (PONV) [48]. Risk factors, including female gender, previous history of PONV or motion sickness, nonsmoking status, and younger age patients, have been associated with an increased incidence and severity of PONV [49]. Therefore, the preoperative assessment should be sensitive to the presence of these indicators and must devise a plan for offering pharmacological prophylaxis to this patient population. The plan for anesthesia devised preoperatively should also take into consideration that use of volatile anesthetics, opioids, and nitrous oxide may be associated with higher PONV incidence, and thus influence the choice of anesthetic agents used. The choices for PONV prophylaxis are between 5HT3 antagonists (ondansetron, granisetron, palonosetron, etc.), dexamethasone, subanesthetic doses of propofol, scopolamine patches, etc. [50]. Generally, a combination of agents seems to work much better than a single agent.

### 2.10.5 Plan for Postoperative Analgesia [51]

Regional anesthesia techniques, including peripheral nerve blocks, are excellent in terms of providing quality analgesia postoperatively, but they do have their own set of risks and may cause discomfort from the ensuing numbness. Hence, it is important that the patient is taken into confidence about the risks and benefits of this modality of pain relief, while also offering alternative approaches that could be opted for. Local anesthesia in adequate concentrations and volume is essential for a pain-free postoperative period. Contrary to earlier practices, the mixing of local anesthetic solutions to apparently harness the best pharmacological effects of both is an approach, which is currently being discouraged. In fact, a successful preoperative nerve block may also be used so as to minimize the incidence of tachycardia during the intraoperative noxious stimuli, and then repeated at the culmination of the procedure, so that the effect can extend into the postprocedure period. This option can be employed by the maxillofacial surgeon resultant to their expertise in regional nerve blocks of the orofacial region. Opioids have traditionally been the workhorse for postoperative analgesia. Intravenous patient-controlled analgesia is an attractive option for the postoperative pain control for the inpatient in whom the effects of the nerve blocks are expected to wane after a few hours. However, there is accumulating evidence that a multimodal approach to pain management works best, with the intent of reducing the side effects of opioids and improving pain scores. Enhanced recovery after surgery (ERAS) protocols to minimize postsurgery hospital stay are gaining wider acceptance, and an important part of such protocols is the inclusion of multimodal opioid-sparing pain management protocols [52].

## 2.11 Preoperative Decision Making and Obtaining Informed Consent: The Team Concept [53]

The preoperative plan blends the patient's requirements, the competence of the perioperative team, and the infrastructure provided by the hospital to get the particular intervention done. This, it is expected, would help achieve the favorable outcome of the intervention. Quite often, the optimization of all of these conditions may not always be possible. The onus then is upon both the patient and the operating team to take a decision on what may be the acceptable course of action. Whether to pursue the performance of a particular intervention or not is, therefore, also an integral part of the preoperative decision-making process.

The final element of a comprehensive preoperative assessment is the process of obtaining a valid, written, and informed consent. Obviously, this process can be initiated, only after a thorough risk estimation has been made, based on the preceding evaluation of the patient, and a tentative anesthetic and surgical plan have been evolved, including strategies for management of postoperative pain. For all practical purposes, an informed consent necessitates presentation of the final residual risk that the patient has, which cannot be further optimized, and its expected interaction with the proposed surgical intervention. The main players in the process of obtaining informed are obviously the surgeon, anesthesiologist, and the patient. Typically, any of them has the autonomy to reject or to suggest modifications to the proposed sequence for the intervention. It is important to note that informed consent is a process of ensuring the patient understands the risks and benefits of the available surgical and anesthetic options. It is not merely signing a consent form. The capacity of a patient refers to the ability to make decisions about their care, and to decide whether to agree to, or refuse, an examination, investigation, or treatment. To have the capacity, a patient must be able to understand and retain information regarding the treatment, evaluate the risks and benefits of treatment, reach a decision regarding their course of treatment, and communicate their decision to the clinician [54]. A patient undergoing surgery is understandably apprehensive, and hence the process of imparting information to him while taking consent must be handled professionally, yet with the utmost sensitivity [55]. It is important that the anesthesiologist and the surgeon should have thrashed out issues relating to perioperative care and broken common ground on all aspects before involving the patient (Table 2.7).

Following discussion and concordance between the surgeon and the anesthesiologist on the course of action, the patient is taken into confidence, informed about the procedure, and his/her consent for the same, sought. The information provided to the patient includes the nature of the risk involved, the benefits, and the alternatives to the proposed plan. If the proposal or any particular element of it is unacceptable to the patient, the operating team must be ready for course correction and should be able to come up with alternatives, which would be acceptable to the patient. However, if no substitute plan can be offered, and the patient is resolute in not accepting the proposed one, there is no option than to abort the proposed surgery. Options, such as referrals to other surgical teams, with different expertise or set-ups that may address the patient's concerns better and satisfy his expectations can be considered. Consequently, acquiring informed consent is a highly interactive process, with the patient being the pivot, to whom the risk-benefit ratio is projected taking into consideration his/her wishes and needs. The Association of Oral and Maxillofacial Surgeons of India consent forms can serve as a useful template for consent taking in one's clinical practice [56].

**Table 2.7** Points of concurrence between surgeon and anesthesiologist before seeking informed consent from the patient

- Diagnosis
- Nature and purpose of the proposed treatment or procedure
- Risks, complications, and consequences of the proposed treatment or procedure
- Alternatives to proposed treatment or procedure
- The consequences if the proposed treatment or procedure is refused
- Benefits and expected results if the proposed treatment or procedure is accepted
- Conflicts of interest
- Who will be providing the treatment or procedure

## 2.12 Conclusion

"Do not operate on a stranger" is the most important mantra to be followed by any surgeon. The preoperative evaluation of oral and maxillofacial surgery patient comprises a critical part of the perioperative period and hence requires a watchful and staged outlook to risk identification and management, putting in place a plan for anesthesia, surgery, and postsurgical pain management. There is no substitute for a properly performed and detailed history and physical examination. Literature suggests that most clinically relevant conditions are recognized during the history and physical examination without the need for further laboratory testing. The surgical team needs to ascertain the risks involved with the comorbidities that the patient may be suffering from, and be able to juxtapose this against the procedure-specific risks to identify the overall risk of the procedure in that particular patient. Risk management and optimization strategies involve the rational use of adjunctive laboratory and imaging studies and professional opinions of consultants of other specialties. This helps evaluate the degree of physiological decompensation a patient might be having due to his comorbidities, and whether this could be either reversed or ameliorated. Acquiring informed consent from the patient involves the development of consensus between the surgeon and anesthesiologist first, with regard to the perioperative plan, irrespective of whether the consent forms for anesthesia and surgery are the same or different documents. This proposed plan, which has the concurrence of both the surgeon and the anesthesiologist, is then presented to the patient along with clear information about the risks and benefits of different clinical strategies, such that the patient can make his up his/her mind, or else request refinement of the proposed plan. This thorough process of preoperative evaluation, it is expected, would be able to keep morbidity and mortality related to the maxillofacial surgery, to an absolute minimum.

## References


1. Galway UA. Preoperative evaluation. In: Sikka PK, Beaman ST, Street JA, editors. Basic clinical anesthesia. New York: Springer; 2015. p. 7–15.
2. Hilditch WG, Asbury AJ, Jack E, McGrane S. Validation of a pre-anaesthetic screening questionnaire. Anaesthesia. 2003;58:874.
3. Wijeysundera DN, Sweitzer BJ. Preoperative evaluation. In: Miller RD, editor. Miller's anesthesia. 8th ed. Philadelphia: Elsevier Saunders; 2015. p. 1085–155.
4. Hata TM, Hata JS. Preoperative patient assessment and management. In: Barash PG, Cullen BF, Stoelting RK, Cahalan MK, Stock MC, Ortega R, Sharar SR, Holt NF, editors. Clinical anesthesia. 8th ed. Philadelphia: Wolters Kluwer; 2017. p. 1479–544.
5. Gupta A, Shiveley T. The preoperative patient evaluation. In: Ehrenfeld JM, Urman RD, Segal S, editors. Anesthesia student survival guide-a case based approach. 2nd ed. New York: Springer; 2016. p. 89–106.
6. Fleisher LA, Beckman JA, Brown KA, Calkins H, Chaikpf E, Fleischmann K, et al. ACC/AHA 2007 Guidelines on Perioperative Cardiovascular Evaluation and Care for Noncardiac Surgery: a Report of the American College of Cardiology/American Heart Association Task Force on Practice Guidelines (Writing Committee to Revise the 2002 Guidelines on Perioperative Cardiovascular Evaluation for Noncardiac Surgery). Circulation. 2007;116:e418–99.
7. Owens WD. American Society of Anesthesiologist physical classification system is not a risk classification system. Anesthesiology. 2001;94:378.
8. Henry A, Dewi F, Atan R, Patel N, Bhatia S. Pre-operative investigations in patients undergoing oral and maxillofacial procedures. Oral Surg. 2016;9:155–9.
9. Tasse JL, Janzen ML, Ahmed NA, Chung RS. Screening laboratory and radiology panels for trauma patients have low utility and arenot cost effective. J Trauma. 2008;65:1114–6.
10. Bryson GL, Wyand A, Bragg PR. Preoperative testing is inconsistent with published guidelines and rarely changes management. Can J Anaesth. 2006;53:236–41.
11. Smetana GW, Macpherson DS. The case against routine preoperative laboratory testing. Med Clin North Am. 2003;87:7–40.
12. Weinberger SE. Providing high-value, cost-conscious care: a critical seventh general competency for physicians. Ann Intern Med. 2011;155:386–8.
13. Benarroch-Gampel J, Riall TS. What laboratory tests are required for ambulatory surgery? Adv Surg. 2013;47:81–98.
14. Feely MA, Collins CS, Daniels PR, Kebede EB, Jatoi A, Mauck KF. Preoperative testing before noncardiac surgery: guidelines and recommendations. Am Fam Physician. 2013;87(6):414–8.
15. Czoski-Murray C, Lloyd Jones M, McCabe C, Claxton K, Oluboyede Y, Roberts J, et al. What is the value of routinely testing full blood count, electrolytes and urea, and pulmonary function tests before elective surgery in patients with no apparent clinical indication and in subgroups of patients with common comorbidities: a systematic review of the clinical and cost-effective literature? Health Technol Assess. 2012;16(i–xvi):1–159.
16. Parameters of Care; AAOMS clinical practice guidelines for oral and maxillofacial surgery (AAOMS ParCare), 6th ed; 2017; J Oral Maxillofac Surg 75:Suppl 1e12-1e33.
17. Fattahi T. Perioperative laboratory and diagnostic testing-what is needed and when? Oral Maxillofac Surg Clins North Am. 2006;18:1–6.
18. National Institute for Health and Care Excellence (NICE) guidelines. Routine pre-operative tests for elective surgery 2016. www.nice.org.uk/guidance/ng45.
19. Apfelbaum JL, Hagberg CA, Caplan RA, Blitt CD, Connis RT, Nickinovich DG, et al. Practice guidelines for management of the difficult airway: an updated report by the American Society of Anesthesiologists Task Force on Management of the Difficult Airway. Anesthesiology. 2013;118:251–70.
20. Prakash S, Mullick P, Bhandari S, Kumar A, Gogia AR, Singh R. Sternomental distance and sternomental displacement as predictors of difficult laryngoscopy and intubation in adult patients. Saudi J Anaesth. 2017;11:273–8.
21. O'Dell K. Predictors of difficult intubation and the otolaryngology perioperative consult. Anesthesiol Clin. 2015;33:279–90.
22. Reed MJ, Dunn MJG, McKeown DW. Can an airway assessment score predict difficulty at intubation in the emergency department? Emerg Med. 2005;22:99–102.
23. Murphy Michael F, Walls RM. Identification of the difficult and failed airway. In: Walls RM, Michael F, editors. Emergency airway management. 3rd ed. Philadelphia: Lippincott Williams & Wilkins; 2008. p. 82–93.
24. Advanced Trauma Life Support (ATLS) Student course manual. Airway and ventilatory management. 9th ed. Chicago IL, 2012. American College of Surgeons Committee on Trauma: 36.

25. Mallampati SR, Gatt SP, Gugino LD, Desai SP, Waraksa B, Freiberger D, et al. A clinical sign to predict difficult tracheal intubation: a prospective study. Can Anaesth Soc J. 1985;32:429–34.
26. Advanced Trauma Life Support (ATLS) student course manual. Pediatric trauma. 9th ed. Chicago IL, 2012. American College of Surgeons Committee on Trauma: 251.
27. Advanced Trauma Life Support (ATLS) student course manual. Geriatric trauma. 9th ed. Chicago IL, 2012. American College of Surgeons Committee on Trauma: 275.
28. Glance LG, Lustik SJ, Hannan EL, Osler TM, Mukamel DB, Qian F, et al. The Surgical Mortality Probability Model: derivation and validation of a simple risk prediction rule for noncardiac surgery. Ann Surg. 2012;255:696–702.
29. Akinbami BO, Onajin-Obembe B. Assessment of intraoperative blood loss during oral and maxillofacial surgical procedures in a Nigerian tertiary health care center. J Blood Transfus. 2014;2014:301467.
30. Lanier WL. A three-decade perspective on anesthesia safety. Am Surg. 2006;72:985–9.
31. Botney R. Improving patient safety in anesthesia: a success story? Int J Radiat Oncol Biol Phys. 2008;71:S182–6.
32. Rodrigo C. The effects of cigarette smoking on anesthesia. Anesth Prog. 2000;47:143–50.
33. Warner DO. Perioperative abstinence from cigarettes: physiologic and clinical consequences. Anesthesiology. 2006;104:356–67.
34. Warner MA, Warner ME, Weber JG. Clinical significance of pulmonary aspiration during the perioperative period. Anesthesiology. 1993;78:56–62.
35. Apfelbaum JL, Caplan RA, Connis RT, Epstein BS, Nickinovich DG, Warner MA. American Society of Anesthesiologists Committee. Practice guidelines for preoperative fasting and the use of pharmacologic agents to reduce the risk of pulmonary aspiration: application to healthy patients undergoing elective procedures: an updated report by the American Society of Anesthesiologists Committee on Standards and Practice Parameters. Anesthesiology. 2011;114:495–511.
36. Brady M, Kinn S, Stuart P. Preoperative fasting for adults to prevent perioperative complications. Cochrane Database Syst Rev. 2003;4:CD004423.
37. Stuart PC. The evidence base behind modern fasting guidelines. Best Pract Res Clin Anaesthesiol. 2006;20:457–69.
38. Fleisher LA, Mythen M. Anesthetic implications of concurrent diseases. In: Miller RD, editor. Miller's anesthesia. 8th ed. Philadelphia: Elsevier Saunders; 2015. p. 1156–225.
39. Krishnan B. Obese oral and maxillofacial surgical patient. J Craniofac Surg. 2009;20:53–7.
40. Hoefnagel A, Yu A, Kaminski A. Anesthetic complications in pregnancy. Crit Care Clin. 2016;32:1–28.
41. Neuman MD, Fleisher LA. Risk of anesthesia. In: Miller RD, editor. Miller's anesthesia. 8th ed. Philadelphia: Elsevier Saunders; 2015. p. 1056–84.
42. Fox KM, Ferrari R. Heart rate: a forgotten link in coronary artery disease? Nat Rev Cardiol. 2011;8:369–79.
43. Tardif JC. Heart rate as a treatable cardiovascular risk factor. Br Med Bull. 2009;90:71–84.
44. Braunwald E. Control of myocardial oxygen consumption: physiologic and clinical considerations. Am J Cardiol. 1971;27:416–32.
45. Lindholm LH, Carlberg B, Samuelsson O. Should beta blockers remain first choice in the treatment of primary hypertension? A meta-analysis. Lancet. 2005;366:1545–53.
46. Bangalore S, Messerli FH, Kostis JB, Pepine CJ. Cardiovascular protection using betablockers: a critical review of the evidence. J Am Coll Cardiol. 2007;50:563–72.
47. Fowler MA, Spiess BD. Postanesthesia recovery. In: Barash PG, Cullen BF, Stoelting RK, Cahalan MK, Stock MC, Ortega R, Sharar SR, Holt NF, editors. Clinical anesthesia. 8th ed. Philadelphia: Wolters Kluwer; 2017. p. 3854–918.
48. Alexander M, Krishnan B, Yuvraj V. Prophylactic antiemetics in oral and maxillofacial surgery: a requiem? J Oral Maxillofac Surg. 2009;67:1873–7.
49. Habib AS, Gan TJ. Evidence-based management of postoperative nausea and vomiting: a review. Can J Anaesth. 2004;51:326–41.
50. Cao X, White PF, Ma H. An update on the management of postoperative nausea and vomiting. J Anesth. 2017;31:617–26.
51. White PF, Kehlet H, Neal JM, Schricker T, Carr DB, Carli F, et al. The role of the anesthesiologist in fast-track surgery: from multimodal analgesia to perioperative medical care. Anesth Analg. 2007;104:1380–96.
52. Misiołek H, Cettler M, Woroń J, Wordliczek J, Dobrogowski J, Mayzner-Zawadzka E. The 2014 guidelines for post-operative pain management. Anaesthesiol Intensive Ther. 2014;46:221–44.
53. Barry MJ, Edgman-Levitan S. Shared decision making–pinnacle of patient-centered care. N Engl J Med. 2012;366:780–1.
54. General Medical Council (GMC). Consent: patients and doctors making decisions together [online]. GMC, 2008. Available: http://www.gmc-uk.org/static/documents/content/Consent-English0414.pdf
55. Sjöling M, Nordahl G, Olofsson N, Asplund K. The impact of preoperative information on state anxiety, postoperative pain and satisfaction with pain management. Patient Educ Couns. 2003;51:169–76.
56. Association of Oral and Maxillofacial Surgeons of India (AOMSI): https://www.aomsi.com/WebPages/downloads.aspx

3

# Dealing with Medical Comorbidities

Aditya Moorthy and Shreya Krishna

## 3.1 Introduction

The management of the medically compromised patient is a topic that has received a great deal of attention in recent times. Unfortunately, most of the literature available discusses this topic from a western context. While the human species and the physiology remains unchanged, challenges in South Asia, especially India, stem from a vastly different social structure, a massive urban-rural socioeconomic divide, and social variables that have a major impact on the practice of medicine. In addition, a mixture of patient ignorance, poor training in soft skills of doctors, and an irresponsible fourth estate has vitiated a hitherto-friendly doctor-patient relationship.

While this chapter is not designed to provide a comprehensive guide to the medical management of a maxillofacial patient (which deserves a textbook in its own right), it attempts to provide an insight into the management of medically compromised patients requiring maxillofacial surgery.

## 3.2 Changing Demographics in India

India encompasses almost a fifth of the world's population with a population estimate of about 1.34 billion [1]. The life expectancy at birth in India has improved from 59.7 years in 1990 to 70.3 years in 2016 for females, and from 58.3 years to 66.9 years for males [1]. In short, the average life span of an Indian has increased by 11 years in the last decade leading to an increase in the geriatric population of the country. The crude death rate has also steadily declined in the last decade from 7.5 to 6.4 per 1000 population [2]. The population continues to grow, as the birth rate has superseded the death rate. This change, while an indicator of improved healthcare delivery, adds to the health burden of the country, and creates a different spectrum of diseases—particularly lifestyle diseases.

There has also been a shift in the societal patterns. We see an increase in urban nuclear families resulting in unattended elderly parents whose medical conditions stay undiagnosed and uncontrolled.

## 3.3 Lifestyle Changes in India

There has been a sea of change in the lifestyle of today's population compared to a couple of decades ago. Sedentary lifestyle, processed food, industrialization, occupational hazards, etc. have led India to a "dual disease burden" scenario. So, even as the incidence of lifestyle diseases is steadily on the rise, a vast majority of rural and poor patients still suffer from infectious and acute diseases.

As recently as 2016, cardiovascular diseases like Ischaemic Heart Disease (IHD) and stroke contributed 28.1% toward mortality in India. This was a 34.3% increase over 16 years, suggesting the impact of lifestyle disease on society. The major contributors for this change are rapidly aging population, pollution, high blood pressure, dyslipidemia, high fasting plasma glucose, and an increased BMI (body-mass index) [3]. Respiratory diseases like chronic obstructive pulmonary disease (COPD) and bronchial asthma—are the second-largest contributors to the total mortality burden of India—at 10.9%. Diabetes analysis shows that it contributes 3.1% toward the total mortality burden.

Air pollution is a major risk factor for both cardiovascular and respiratory illness and increases the risks for acute respiratory infections and exacerbates asthma [4]. Such unique challenges raise questions of following treatment protocols based on western studies. A preoperative chest X-Ray may

A. Moorthy (✉)
Rangadore Memorial Hospital, Apollo Hospitals, Bangalore, Karnataka, India

S. Krishna
Oral and Maxillofacial Surgery, Rangadore Memorial Hospital, Bangalore, India

find an indication in an apparently fit and healthy 28-year-old living in New Delhi (with record levels of pollution) when it would be considered unnecessary for a similar patient from rural Yorkshire.

With the rise of urbanization and urban migration, the problems of air pollution, inadequate sanitation, and an unhealthy diet are accentuated. Population residing in urban areas in India, according to 1901 census, was 11.4%. This count increased to 28.53% by 2001, and the numbers increased to 34% in 2017 [5].

"Cyberchondria" has become a challenge with patients tending to diagnose and treat their problems themselves, and unsurprisingly getting it wrong. India is also among one of the most depressed countries in the world. A World Health Organization (WHO) study states that at least 6.5% of the Indian population suffers from some form of serious mental disorder. The average suicide rate in India is 10.9 for every hundred thousand people with the majority of victims being less than 44 years of age [6]. Diminished mental health is associated with a host of consequences like lack of participation in social activities, odd eating habits, and withdrawal from income generation and employment opportunities—all of which can cascade onto other serious illnesses and even death.

## 3.4 The Changing Face of Oral and Maxillofacial Surgery

As always, training is struggling to keep up with the changing trends in medicine. Trainees are often unaware of new protocols and the changed scenario of medical comorbidities of the population. Surgery has become heavily technology oriented, sometimes at the cost of clinical expertise. Furthermore, there is improved awareness among medical professionals for crossreferral to review dentition, seen mostly by maxillofacial surgeons rather than general dentists. Referrals are required now before radiotherapy, chemotherapy, cardiac surgery, transplants, etc.

Furthermore, maxillofacial surgery as a specialty has blazed a trail hitherto unimagined with successful foray into head and neck surgery, craniofacial reconstruction, and microvascular surgery. This now has put the onus on the surgeon to educate himself enough to be able to manage a sick patient on the ward to the extent of preventing complications and making appropriate referrals. Gone are the days when a physician could be asked to do the job for us and we could enjoy the comfort of being surgical technicians!

### 3.4.1 Medical History and India

While veritable treatises about the science and art of history taking, this part of clinical medicine is a unique investigative effort in the Indian context. The challenges to the maxillofacial surgeon are multifold. The first difficulty is encountered with the patient who may deny illness (often hypertension or diabetes) because he/she is adequately treated and all parameters are within normal limits. The next hurdle is when the patient decides to withhold information wantonly due to social taboos or plain ignorance of its importance to the treating doctor. Dentists and maxillofacial surgeons who question their patients seated on dental chairs in an outpatient setting often experience the latter. This stems from the patients' assumption that the information is inconsequential to their treatment. The last situation is the uneducated patient who is truly unaware of his medical condition.

With these intricacies, the oral surgeon needs to employ several out-of-the-box techniques to extract the history. This includes the much-derided leading questions, questioning relatives, sometimes in private, and playing Sherlock by asking them to bring in their medication and working backwards. But this effort is still of paramount importance in this technology-driven age and the modern oral and maxillofacial surgeon will do well to assimilate all the conventional history-taking skills and learn a few new ones as well.

## 3.5 Cardiovascular System

### 3.5.1 Hypertension

Hypertension is an extremely common condition and often undiagnosed. Since it is mostly asymptomatic, the oral surgeon has the unique opportunity to be the first healthcare professional to identify the condition. Hence, it is imperative that every procedure should begin with recording the patients' vital signs. The following table offers a guideline for the diagnosis and risk stratification of hypertension (Table 3.1).

The authors stress that aneroid manometers are more accurate than digital ones. Like any delicate instrument, these too need frequent calibration [8].

The long-term effects of hypertension have far-reaching implications on maxillofacial surgery, especially under general anesthesia (Fig. 3.1).

**Table 3.1** Guidelines for diagnosis of hypertension [7]

| Category | Systolic (mmHg) | Diastolic (mmHg) |
|---|---|---|
| Optimal | <120 | <80 |
| Normal | 120–129 | And/or 80–84 |
| High normal | 130–139 | And/or 85–89 |
| Grade 1 hypertension | 140–159 | And/or 90–99 |
| Grade 2 hypertension | 160–179 | And/or 100–109 |
| Grade 3 hypertension | >180 | And/or >110 |
| Isolated systolic hypertension | >140 | And <90 |

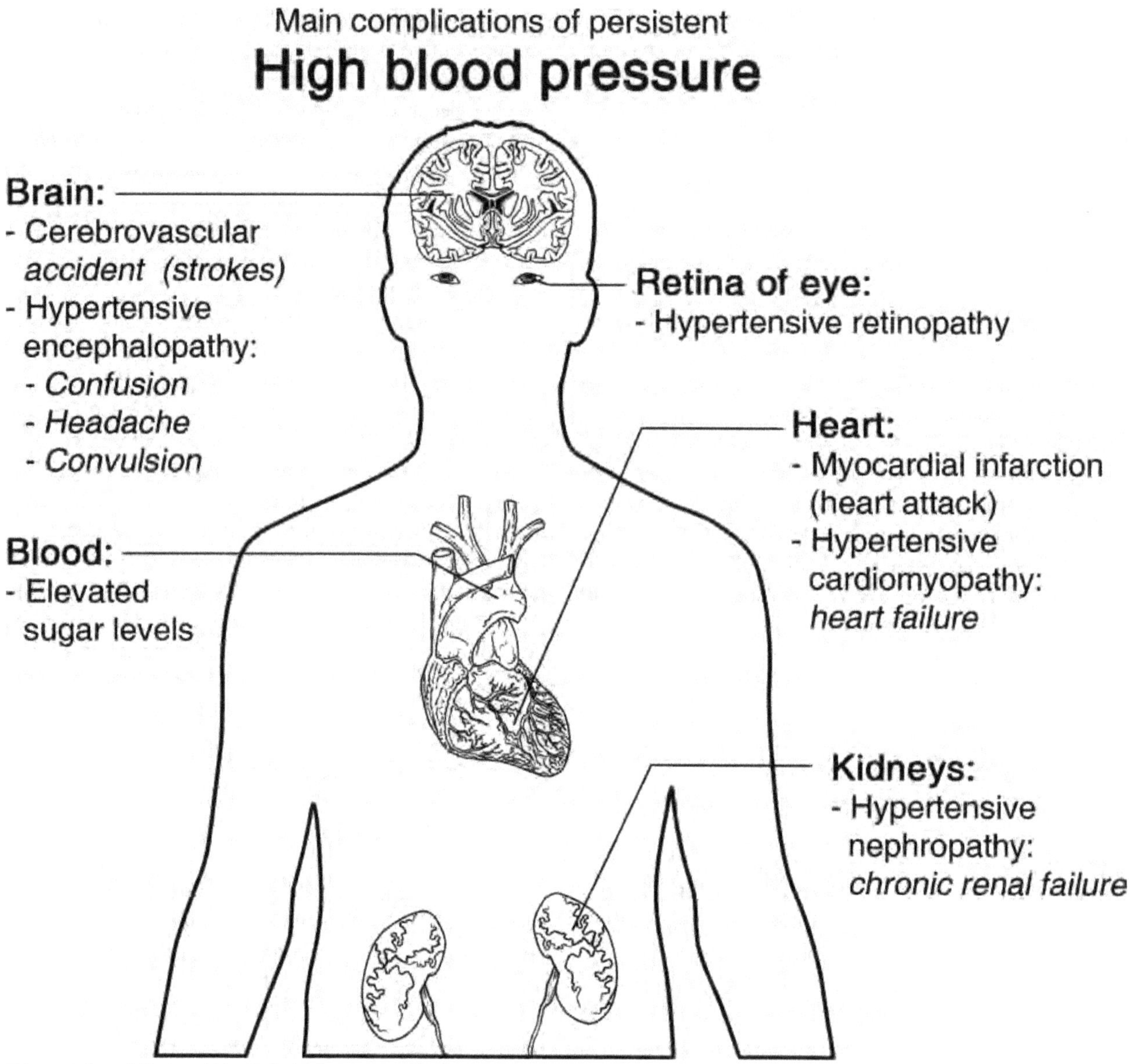




**Fig. 3.1** Long-term effects of hypertension

#### 3.5.1.1 Minor Oral Surgery

A thorough history will elicit symptoms of poor blood pressure control and symptoms of end-organ damage in a known hypertensive.

Conversely, end-organ damage points to poor blood pressure control. If such symptoms exist, elective procedures are to be deferred until good control is achieved. The absolute cut off of blood pressure is supposed to be 180/110 mmHg [9]. However, it is the author's experience that this is too high a cut off in the Indian context with social and logistic challenges. This is especially true for an out-of-hospital standalone dental clinic where the average oral surgeon performs his outpatient procedures. This is because there is a lack of clarity on the effect of stress-induced hypertension (white coat hypertension) and the effect it can have in an already-hypertensive patient. Hence, it is advisable to limit elective extractions to stage 2 hypertension [10] (SBP < 160 mmHg and DBP < 100 mmHg). When minor oral surgery is performed within these parameters, excessive bleeding is an unlikely complication.

#### 3.5.1.2 Major Maxillofacial Surgery

Major surgery introduces two important variables into the mix. First is the procedure itself with surgical trauma and the attendant physiologic response (Table 3.2). The second is the requirement of a general anesthetic. While the anesthesiologist takes the final call on the safety of administering general anesthesia, the surgeon is the one who needs to provide the input regarding the intensity of the surgery. For example, fixing a fractured zygomatic bone can wait while operating on a patient with stridor from Ludwig's angina cannot.

Additionally, perioperative hypotension can also be of significant concern, both systemically and surgically (microvascular flaps need excellent perfusion and hypotension with peripheral vasoconstriction can lead to a flap loss). The surgeon and the anesthetist need to walk a tightrope, especially in a hypertensive patient.

**Table 3.2** Causes of hemodynamic changes [7]

| Hemodynamic changes | Causes |
|---|---|
| Hypotension | Systemic vasodilatation (GA) |
| | Sympathetic blockade (spinal/epidural anesthesia) |
| | Hypovolemia |
| | Blood loss |
| | Mechanical ventilation |
| | Drugs (angiotensin receptor blockers) |
| | Arrhythmias |
| | Acute coronary events |
| | Pulmonary thromboembolism (high-risk surgery for pulmonary thromboembolism and/or patient predisposing factors) |
| Hypertension | Laryngoscopy and intubation |
| | Surgical stimulus |
| | Inadequate plane of anesthesia/analgesia |
| | Hypothermia |
| | Hypervolemia |
| | Reversal and recovery |
| | Hypoxia (post-op) |
| | Inadequate analgesia (post-op) |
| | Full bladder (post-op) |

#### 3.5.1.3 Vasoconstrictors and Hypertension

Vasoconstrictors are routinely used in conjunction with a local anesthetic to reduce bleeding, increase the duration of action, and reduce the requirement of the total volume of the anesthetic. The most commonly used vasoconstrictor is adrenaline. Felypressin (Octapressin) is also available as a vasoconstrictor with Prilocaine—but only in a cartridge. The concentration of adrenaline as a vasoconstrictor ranges from 1:80,000 to 1:200,000.

Physiologic effects of adrenaline in varying concentration [11]:

- 1:80,000 significantly increase in systolic blood pressure (SBP), diastolic blood pressure (DBP), and heart rate;
- 1:100,000 concentrations can increase SBP and heart rate; and
- 1:200,000 is limited to an increase in heart rate, but less significant

Pain itself has a significant effect on SBP, DBP on heart rate and adrenaline, even in the concentration of 1:200,000 significantly increases the duration and depth of local anesthetic. Adrenalin has a beneficial effect in this concentration without negative cardiovascular implications [11].

### 3.5.2 Ischemic Heart Disease (IHD)

Atherosclerosis is a progressive disease involving medium-to-large caliber arteries. It may result in ischemic lesions of the brain, heart or extremities leading to thrombosis, infarction of affected vessels, and end-organ damage.

Ischemic heart disease could present as angina or myocardial infarction (Figs. 3.2 and 3.3). Both conditions are caused

**Fig. 3.2** Types of Angina

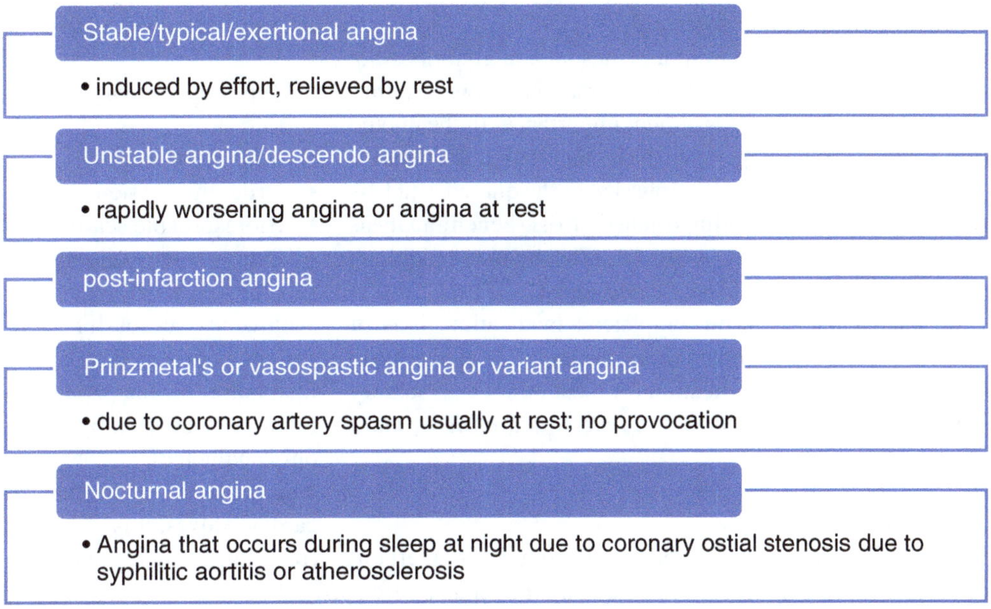

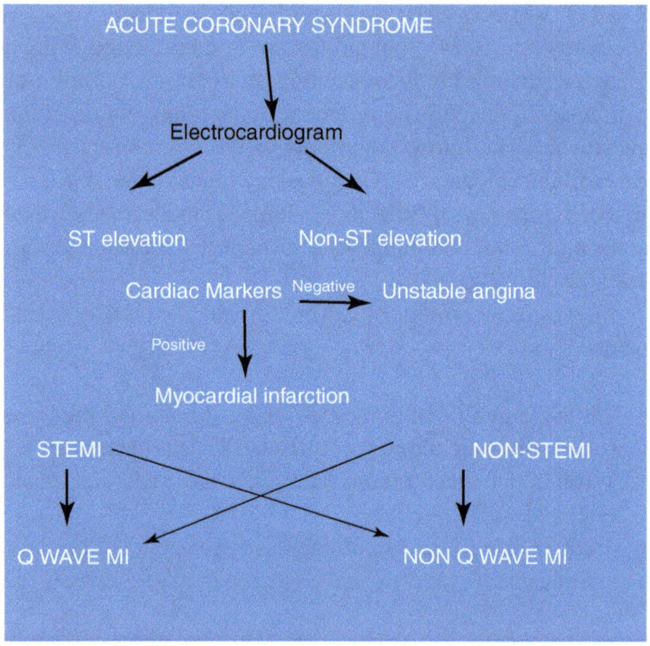




**Fig. 3.3** Types of Acute Coronary Syndrome

by decreased coronary blood flow, increased myocardial oxygen demand, and form two ends of a spectrum with several subclassifications.

Oral surgical procedures cause significant surgical, physiological, and psychological stress. It is imperative that the patient is assessed thoroughly prior to any intervention. Patients with IHD are susceptible for another cardiac event within 6 months [12]. With changing management strategies in cardiac patients and medicolegal aspects in mind, it is prudent to liaise with the cardiologist for all but the most straightforward of situations.

#### 3.5.2.1 Minor Oral Surgery

Previous myocardial infarction or unstable angina does not form a contraindication for dental extractions. However, timing and planning are of paramount importance. In the quoted study, about 10% of patients have reported postoperative chest pain [12]. While the sample size of the quoted article is small, it underscores the importance of risk-benefit analysis before undertaking these procedures. The treatment planning may need further input from a cardiologist.

If such patients are on antiplatelet medication, it is of extreme importance to note that single antiplatelet agents do not constitute a contraindication for most minor oral surgery [13]. *Refer to the section on antiplatelet and anticoagulant drugs and surgery.*

#### 3.5.2.2 Major Surgery

Since most surgery considered in this context is emergent or urgent in nature (trauma, oncosurgery, space infections), the benefit of the life-saving procedure by far outweighs the risk of a further cardiac episode. Such procedures are ideally done in a center equipped to deal with any adverse cardiac event. In a country like India, the onus of keeping the appropriate specialty appraised of the situation before starting the procedure is on the operating surgeon.

### 3.5.3 Postintervention Cardiac Patients

#### 3.5.3.1 Percutaneous Coronary Angioplasty (PTCA) and Coronary Artery Bypass Graft (CABG) and Valve Replacement Procedures

With access to healthcare improving, it is becoming more common for the surgeon to encounter patients with IHD who have had interventions. These range from conventional CABG to Percutaneous angioplasties with stents in place and minimal access CABGs. In our context, the clinician needs to know what these are not only to analyze the impact these procedures have on the maxillofacial procedure but also to tease the information out of the reluctant historian.

**PTCA/PCA**

Percutaneous transluminal coronary angioplasty has become the intervention of choice for coronary artery disease. This procedure involves the insertion of a stent in the narrowed portion of the artery (Fig. 3.4). This stent intimately hugs the endothelium of the vessel and is reliably and completely endothilized in 6 months to a year. The patient is susceptible to stent thrombosis in this period and hence the antiplatelets. There are many varieties of stents and the design and features are always in a state of flux. Therefore, any changes to antiplatelet therapy are to be made in consultation with the treating cardiologist [14].

Types of coronary stents:

- Bare metal stents
- Drug-eluting stents
- Bioresorbable scaffold system
- Drug-eluting balloons

Following successful revascularization procedures, the patient is expected to be in a far better hemodynamic state than before. If the patient remains symptomatic, then he/she requires to be seen by the cardiothoracic surgery team. The only challenge in these patients is the antiplatelet/anticoagulant medication. In the case of patients with prosthetic cardiac valves, it is vital to provide endocarditis prophylaxis (read following content).

**Fig. 3.4** Mechanism of PTCA

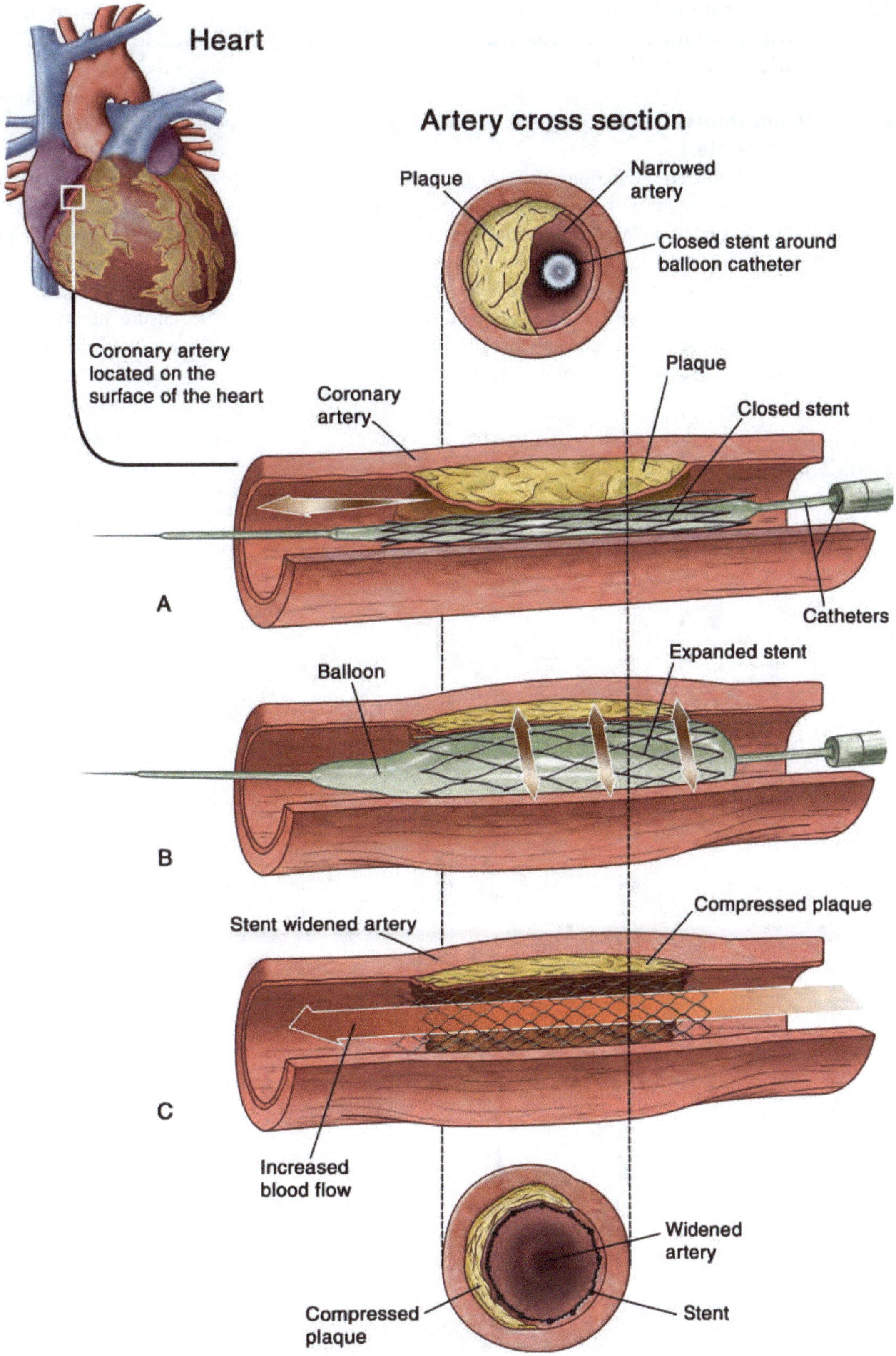

### 3.5.4 Conventional Antiplatelets, Anticoagulants, and Novel Oral Anticoagulants (NOAC)

#### 3.5.4.1 Minor Dentoalveolar Surgery: Antiplatelets

There are several concerns regarding the risk of excessive bleeding following minor oral surgery in anticoagulated patients and those on antiplatelet medication. Most of these are unfounded for dentoalveolar procedures. In most dentoalveolar procedures, we have the advantage of a bony cavity where physical pressure can be effectively applied to obtain hemostasis. This can be further augmented with other local hemostatic measures (sutures, surgical R, AbgelR, etc.). This obviates the need to stop antiplatelet drugs (read following content). However, in patients on dual antiplatelet therapy, the authors suggest caution when operating in critical areas like the floor of the mouth as hematomas can cause airway embarrassment.

Conventional antiplatelets bind irreversibly to platelets and the normal clotting process is restored only with the production of new, unaffected platelets (Fig. 3.5, Table 3.3). It takes 5–10 days for platelets to be produced in the quantity required to produce a clinically normal platelet action. In the interim, if a procedure causes excessive bleeding, the only reliable way to ensure hemostasis is platelet transfusion. However, the newer ones are reversible and can be stopped for 24 h prior to the procedure as a "switch on-switch off"

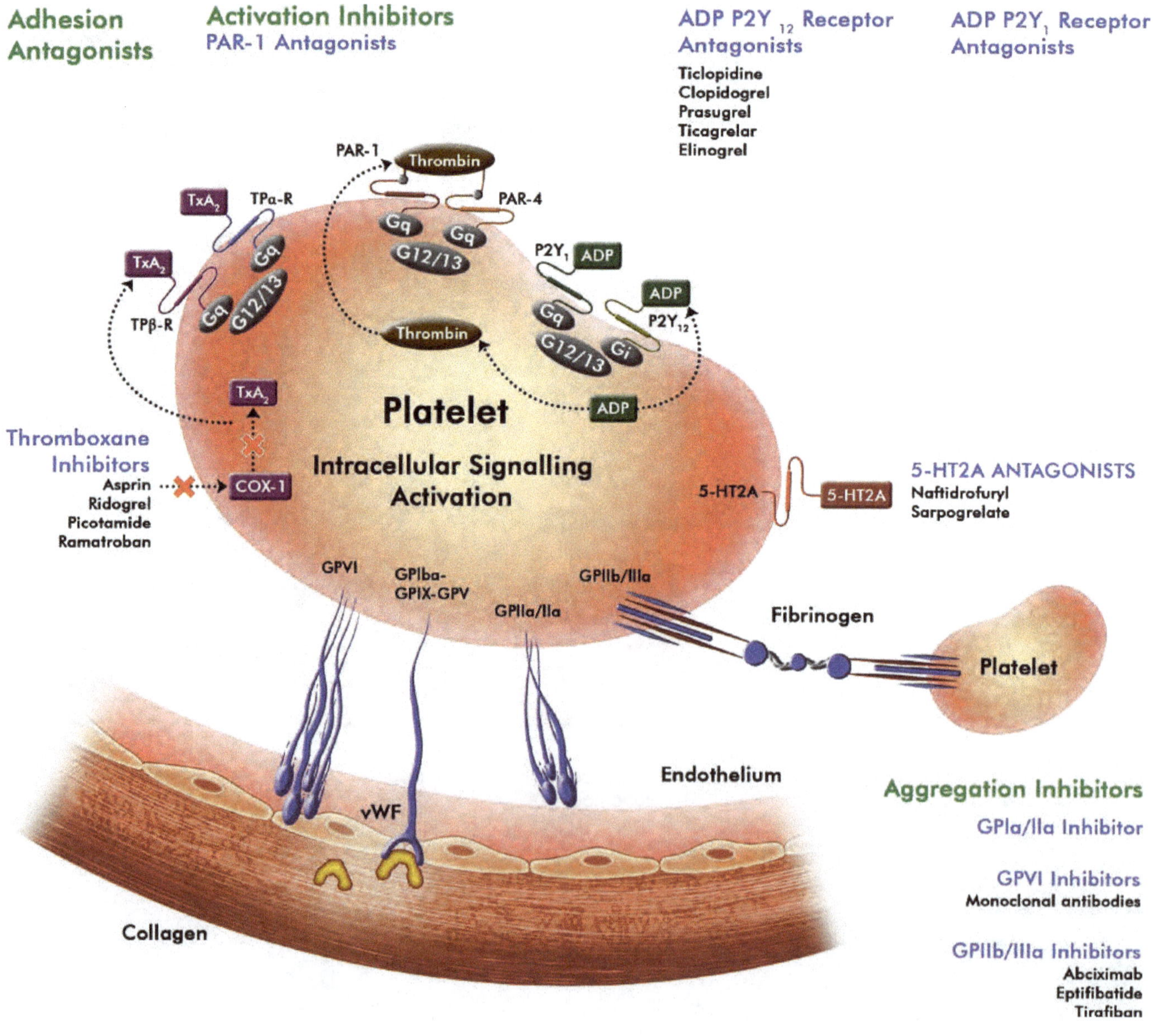


**Fig. 3.5** Mechanism of action of commonly used antiplatelet drugs

**Table 3.3** Commonly used antiplatelet agents and their characteristics [15]

| Drug | Mechanism of action | Loading dose | Maintenance dose | Half-life | Time to recover platelet function after drug withdrawal | Platelet inhibition | Administration route |
|---|---|---|---|---|---|---|---|
| Aspirin | COX-1 inhibition | 325 mg | 75–325 mg daily | 15–20 min | 30% at 48 h | Irreversible inhibition | Oral |
| Clopidogrel | P2Y12 receptor inhibition | 30–600 mg | 75 mg daily | 7–9 h | 40% at 3 days | Irreversible inhibition | Oral |
| Prasugrel | P2Y12 receptor inhibition | 60 mg | 10 mg daily | 7 h | 2–3 days | Irreversible inhibition | Oral |
| Ticagrelor | P2Y12 and Partly P2Y1 receptor inhibition | 180 mg | 90 mg twice a day | 7–9 h | 57% at 24 h | Reversible inhibition | Oral |
| Cangrelor | Adenosine triphosphate analogue with a high affinity for the P2Y12 receptor | 30 μg/kg | 2–4 μg/kg/min | 3–6 min | Rapid (mins–hours) | Reversible inhibition | i.v |
| Abciximab | Glycoprotein IIb/IIIa receptor inhibitor | 0.25 μg/kg | 0.125 μg/kg/min | 10–15 min | 12 h | Reversible inhibition | i.v |
| Eptifibatide | Glycoprotein IIb/IIIa receptor inhibitor | 180 μg/kg | 2 μg/kg/min | 2.5 h | 2–4 h | Reversible inhibition | i.v |
| Tirofiban | Glycoprotein IIb/IIIa receptor inhibitor | 0.4 μg/kg | 0.1 μg/kg/min | 2 h | 2–4 h | Reversible inhibition | i.v |

drug. But these are very expensive and most of the below-poverty-line patients are likely to be on older antiplatelets for some time to come.

#### 3.5.4.2 Maxillofacial Surgery

Patients who need procedures with low risk of bleeding (e.g., fixation of fracture of the parasymphysis) may continue oral antiplatelet/anticoagulation therapy. This applies especially to high-risk patients (e.g., mechanical heart valves). However, when the risk of bleeding is obvious, it outweighs the benefit of continuing antiplatelet/anticoagulant therapy. In such cases, heparin is used as bridge therapy.

#### 3.5.4.3 Bridging with Heparin

In cases where the patient is at high risk for a thromboembolic episode, a "bridge"—a balance between surgical bleed and risk of thrombosis may be achieved either with intravenous unfractionated heparin or with subcutaneous low-molecular-weight heparin [16].

#### 3.5.4.4 Anticoagulants and Oral/Maxillofacial Surgery

While several indications exist for the use of anticoagulants, the authors have noted that there is significant resistance in the medical community to prescribe anticoagulants in these cases and they are often replaced by antiplatelets in India. This is especially true for the rural patient who may not have regular access to monitor his anticoagulation status. However, in urban centers, NOAC are in regular use.

Common indications for anticoagulation—prevention of thrombotic events in:

Mechanical Heart Valves.
Atrial Fibrillation.
Deep Vein Thrombosis and Pulmonary Embolism.
Myocardial infarction.
Acute Ischemic Stroke

The target International Normalized Ratio (INR) range for most conditions is between 2.5 and 3.5.

#### 3.5.4.5 Minor Oral Surgery

It is beyond doubt that warfarin/acetrom therapy need not be discontinued and INR need not be normalized prior to dento-alveolar surgery. The risk of a thrombotic episode does not justify the risk of a minor bleed that can be controlled by local measures [17]. Simple dentoalveolar surgery (e.g., three simple extractions) can be safely performed with an INR of 3.5 or less with appropriate local hemostatic measures [18]. However, it is imperative that the patient is closely followed. It is sensible to schedule these procedures in the morning.

#### 3.5.4.6 Major Maxillofacial Surgery

Depending on the indication for anticoagulant therapy and the drug used, the decision regarding the control of anticoagulation is made. Ideally the prescribing physician is involved in decision making (Fig. 3.6) (read following content).

### 3.5.5 Infective Endocarditis Prophylaxis

Much has changed over the years with regard to infective endocarditis (IE) and antibiotic prophylaxis. Since the guidelines change by the year, the authors strongly recommend that the surgeon takes recourse to his smartphone to keep abreast of the changing scenery (Tables 3.4 and 3.5).

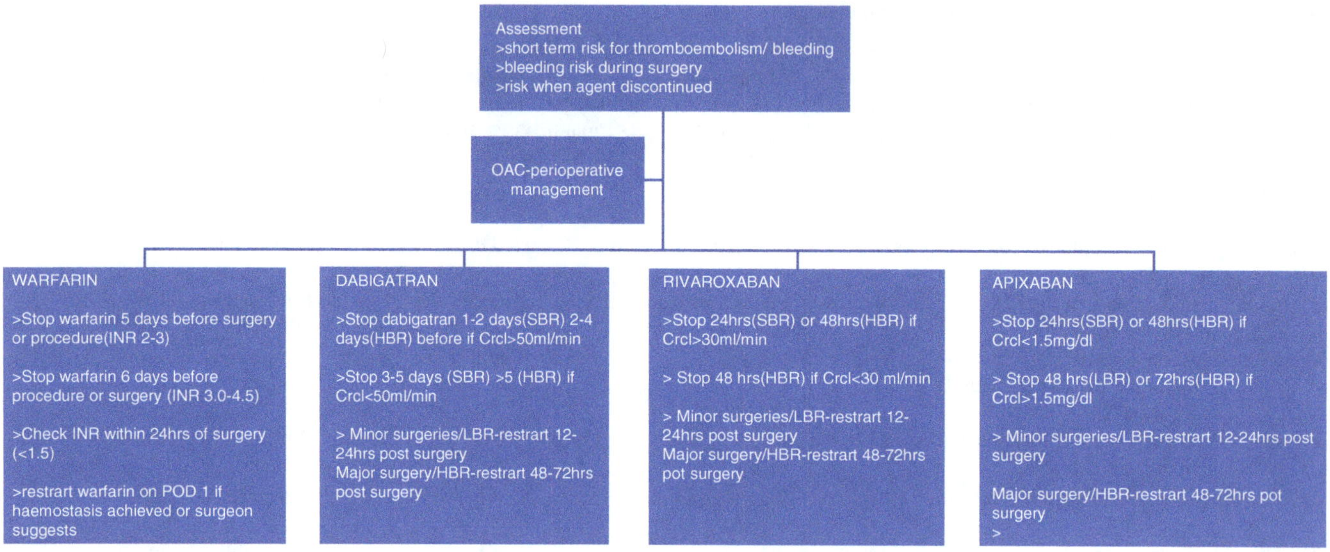


*OAC; Oral anticoagulant,POD; Post-operative day, INR; International normalized ratio, LBR; Low bleeding risk, SBR; Standard bleeding risk, HBR; High bleeding risk, CrCl; Creatinine clearance



**Fig. 3.6** Perioperative management of oral anticoagulants [19]

### 3.5.6 Implantable Cardioverter Defibrillators (ICD)

An ICD is a battery-powered device implanted in a patient that generates a small electrical impulse. Indications are patients at risk of sudden cardiac death—ventricular fibrillation/ventricular tachycardia, malignant ventricular tachyarrhythmias. ICDs are also used to treat Brugada syndrome [21].

#### 3.5.6.1 Implications

Bleeding: patients may either be on antiplatelets or anticoagulated. (read earlier content).

Devices: Electrocautery, especially monopolar diathermy, may interfere with the device and this may have to be turned to a "safe mode" by the electrophysiology technician. The concerned cardiologist should be able to assist with the technical details.

Infective endocarditis prophylaxis: Risk being low, current guidelines DO NOT recommend prophylaxis for these patients.

## 3.6 Impact of Central Nervous System Disorders in Maxillofacial Surgery

Of the many conditions which affect this system, the effects of epilepsy and stroke are most commonly encountered in maxillofacial surgical practice.

**Table 3.4** AHA, ESC, and NICE guidelines for infective endocarditis prophylaxis

| 2007 AHA guidelines | 2015 ESC guidelines | 2016 NICE guidelines |
|---|---|---|
| Highest risk of adverse outcomes:<br>• Previous IE<br>• Prosthetic valve<br>• Unrepaired cyanotic congenital heart disease (CHD)<br>• 6-month period postprosthetic repair of CHD<br>• Repaired CHD with residual defects<br>• Cardiac transplant with valvulopathy | Highest risk of IE:<br>• Previous IE<br>• Prosthetic valve/ Prosthetic material for valve repair<br>• Any cyanotic CHD<br>• 6-month period postprosthetic repair of CHD<br>Intermediate risk of IE:<br>• History of rheumatic fever<br>• Any form of native valve disease<br>• Unrepaired noncyanotic CHD | Risk of developing IE:<br>• Previous IE<br>• Valve replacement<br>• Acquired valvular heart disease<br>• Structural Congenital heart disease<br>• Hypertrophic cardiomyopathy |
| Antibiotic prophylaxis:<br>• All dental procedures involving gingival tissue manipulation or periapical region of teeth or oral mucosa perforation<br>• Procedures on respiratory tract or infected skin/ musculoskeletal tissue. | Antibiotic prophylaxis: Considered for dental procedures involving gingival tissue manipulation or periapical region of teeth or oral mucosa perforation | Antibiotic prophylaxis: Not routinely recommended |

**Table 3.5** Revised AHA guidelines for infective endocarditis prophylaxis [20]

| Patient group | Antibiotic | Dose (30–60 min before procedure) | |
|---|---|---|---|
| | | Adults | Children |
| Able to take oral medicine | Amoxicillin | 2 g | 50 mg/kg |
| Unable to take oral medication | Ampicillin | 2 g i.m/i.v | 50 mg/kg i.m/i.v |
| | or | | |
| | Cefazolin/ ceftriaxone | 1 g i.m/i.v | 50 mg/kg i.m/i.v |
| Allergic to penicillin or ampicillin and able to take oral medication | Cephalexin[a,b] | 2 g | 50 mg/kg |
| | or | | |
| | Clindamycin | 600 mg | 20 mg/kg |
| | or | | |
| | Azithromycin/ clarithromycin | 500 mg | 15 mg/kg |
| Allergic to penicillins or ampicillin and unable to take oral medication | Cefazolin/ ceftriaxone[b] | 1 g i.m/i.v | 50 mg/kg i.m/i.v |
| | or | | |
| | Clindamycin | 600 mg | 20 mg/kg |

Note: *i.m* intramuscular; *i.v* intravenous

[a]Or other first- or second-generation cephalosporins at equivalent adult and pediatric dose

[b]Cephalosporins should not be given to a patient with a history of anaphylaxis, angioedema, or urticaria with penicillin or ampicillin

## 3.6.1 Epilepsy

A seizure is a result of excessive electrical discharges in a group of brain cells, whereas epilepsy is described as a disease characterized by recurrent seizures. A single seizure does not constitute epilepsy, which is defined as having at least two or more unprovoked seizures. The incidence worldwide is approximately 0.5–0.9%, affecting over 50 million individuals [22].

Etiology of epilepsy can be divided as primary or idiopathic, where the cause is unknown and this constitutes the vast majority of cases. In secondary or acquired epilepsy, the cause can be determined and these include metabolic, genetic, structural, and functional abnormalities.

An increase in the incidence in the elderly can be attributed to conditions such as stroke, tumors, trauma, and Alzheimer's disease. Systemic conditions include diabetes, hypertension, infections, electrolyte imbalances and dehydration, or lack of oxygen. Withdrawal from high-dose, long-term use of drugs such as cocaine, heroin, barbiturates, amphetamines, and alcohol can also precipitate seizures [23]. Seizures generally last for a few seconds to minutes. Although many types exist, they are broadly divided into two groups (Fig. 3.7).

Primary generalized seizures—which begin with involvement both sides of the cerebral hemispheres.

Partial seizures—start in a localized area [25].

### 3.6.1.1 Basic considerations

While recording history, the duration, type, frequency of the seizure as well as the most recent episode must be recorded as well as the type of medication taken, if any. If the patient is aware of how the seizure starts, if there is any warning or "aura," this too must be noted [23].

Several factors are capable of provoking seizures. These include improper use of medication, lack of sleep, drug abuse, drug interactions, hypoglycemia, electrolyte imbalance among others. Antiepileptic drugs should generally be continued without alteration.

### 3.6.1.2 Outpatient maxillofacial considerations

If seizures are predictable, then appointments should be scheduled accordingly. Frequency of seizures determines the urgency of treatment. Procedures, unless emergent, should be postponed if frequency of seizures is high. The clinician must reduce anxiety to the patient. Short morning appointments are ideal. Sudden bright lights, noise, or movements must be avoided as these may trigger a seizure [23].

### 3.6.1.3 Major Surgical Considerations

Trauma is a common consequence of seizures and may result in lacerations of the face or oral cavity and fractures of the maxillofacial skeleton. Other injuries include hematomas, dislocation of temporomandibular joint (TMJ) fracture/loss of teeth. An electroencephalogram (EEG) along with imaging such as CT/MRI is recommended if there is no previous seizure history. Open reduction should be preferred over closed for treatment of facial fractures, as further episodes of seizures might lead to aspiration if intermaxillary fixation (IMF) is attempted [25].

Local anesthetic is considered safe in well-controlled epileptics, as is sedation. General anesthesia is preferred in uncontrolled epileptics, especially if coupled with a mental deficit, as a seizure might be triggered due to stress from difficulties in communication. One drawback of general anesthetic is temporary anoxia to the brain, which itself might trigger a seizure [26].

### 3.6.1.4 Precautions, complications, & management

As mentioned earlier, appropriate recording of history gives an insight into planning the procedure, particularly for elective surgeries. Objects with the potential to cause harm must be kept away from the vicinity of the patient. Antiepileptics such as phenytoin have been known to cause gingival enlargement, which can be managed either by surgery or by a change in medication. Aspirin, antifungal azoles, metronidazole can interfere with phenytoin. Propoxyphene and erythromycin can interfere with carbemezepine. Contraindicated drugs are chlorpromazine, flumazenil, ketamine, lignocaine in large doses and quinolones, tramadol, and tricyclic antidepressants [25].

### 3.6.1.5 Management of an acute episode on the dental chair

If possible, all foreign body/material should be removed from the oral cavity. The chair should be reclined to a supine position with the patient turned onto their side to minimize the

**Fig. 3.7** ILAE 2017 classifications of seizure types basic version [24]

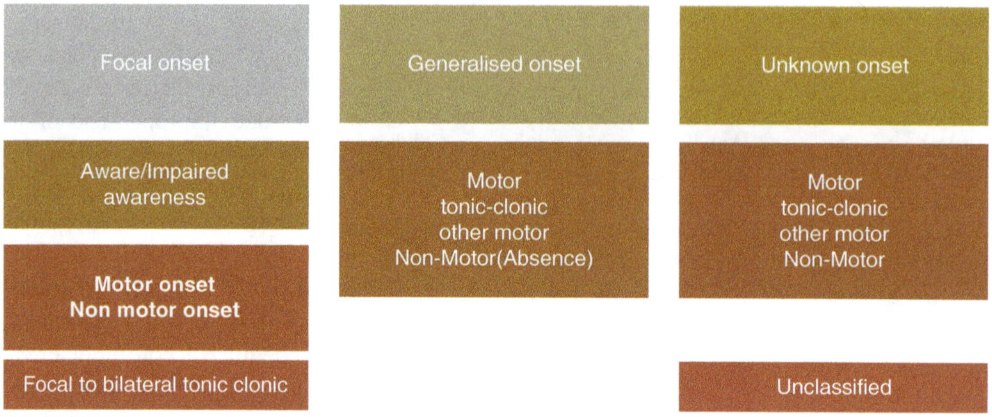




risk of aspiration. Passive restraint is used only to prevent them from falling out of the chair. A recurrent seizure or a seizure of more than 3 min requires drug administration. The patient should be monitored to prevent airway obstruction. After the patient recovers, appropriate medical consults should be arranged. Elective treatment should be postponed [23]. However, prolonged seizures, which continue in spite of medication, may lead to status epilepticus, which may be fatal if untreated. Airway patency and peripheral venous access are first line of management. If seizures persist even after administration of drugs such as lorazepam or diazepam, the patient must be shifted to the hospital for further management.

## 3.6.2 Stroke

Stroke (cerebrovascular accident) is a serious, occasionally fatal neurologic event characterized by the rapid appearance of a focal deficit of brain function. It is estimated that 85% of patients presenting with stroke would have sustained a cerebral infarction because of inadequate blood flow to a part of the brain, with the remainder suffering from an intracerebral hemorrhage. Often, survivors of cerebrovascular accidents are left debilitated in motor function and/or speech [27].

A stroke may be a result of hemorrhage or ischemia as given later (Fig. 3.8).

The initial presentation of stroke includes loss of combination of sensory and motor functions with occasional loss of consciousness. The presenting features include hemiparesis or paraparesis, dysphagia, ataxia, aphasia, dysarthria, loss of vision. Early detection is by assessing facial and arm weakness and any slurring of speech. Mechanism of stroke may be ischemic, primary intracerebral hemorrhage, and subarachnoid hemorrhage. The oral impact of stroke includes facial weakness, dysphagia, and speech impairment [29].

### 3.6.2.1 Basic Considerations

At the outset, it is paramount to assess the extent of disability of the patient—both physical and mental, as this is vital in determining whether performing the procedure is safe in the outpatient setting. There may be a dependence on others for basic needs. History of past strokes needs to be elicited: including dates, severity and current neurological deficit. Treatment is performed in consultation with the neurologist and precautions according to the specific characteristics of the stroke.

### 3.6.2.2 Maxillofacial considerations

Outpatient appointments must be ideally scheduled in the morning and must be of short duration. Patients must be treated in an upright position as much as possible, as they are more prone to aspiration due to impaired protective reflexes. Another important consideration is difficulty in oral hygiene maintenance due to facial weakness and xerostomia, which may be observed as a side effect of medications prescribed [24]. Although procedures must be deferred for as long as possible, in unavoidable circumstances such as trauma or progressing head and neck cancers, general anesthesia is reasonably safe. Shorter duration surgery, intraoperative monitoring and maintaining cerebral perfusion, anticoagulation status, and precaution all aid in reducing the incidence of a further episode.

Antiplatelets and anticoagulation: Ref previous section.

### 3.6.2.3 Precautions

Monitoring of Blood pressure pre- and postprocedure is vital, procedures should be deferred if systolic is >180 mmHg or diastolic is >110 mmHg. Poststroke patients are usually on antiplatelet or anticoagulant medications; hence, coagulation status must be ascertained prior to any procedure. Vasoconstrictors are to be used cautiously as they can increase the risk of adverse outcomes like cerebral hemorrhage due to acute hypertension [29].

Opiods are best avoided as they may result in severe hypotension and benzodiazepines may cause respiratory depression. The practitioner must be mindful that sudden loss of consciousness could result from stroke, and emergency management is the protection of airway and shift to hospital [24].

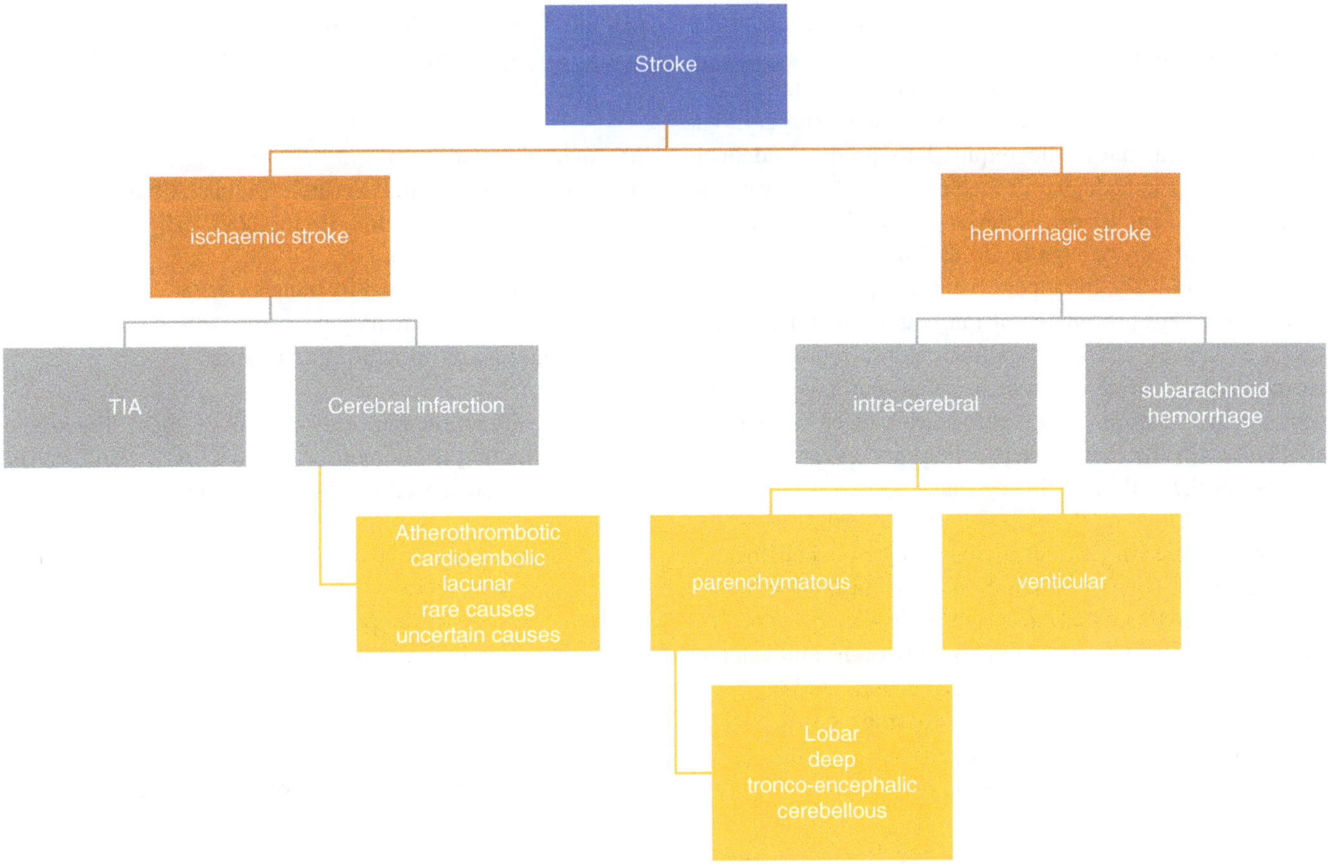




**Fig. 3.8** Common causes of stroke [28]

## 3.7 Impact of Psychiatric Disorders in Maxillofacial Surgery

Psychiatric and psychological disorders are of rising concern in modern society, affecting all aspects of a patient's life, including oral health. Poor oral hygiene is usually due to a combination of lethargy, side effect of medications, and possibly fear of treatment [30]. Common disorders encountered in practice are related to mood, anxiety, substance dependence, eating, or somatoform in nature [31].

Occasionally, oral symptoms may be the initial or single manifestations of the underlying issue. Patients who present with atypical facial pain with vague symptoms, oral dysesthesia, abnormal sensation or movement, salivation often with no identifiable physical cause could be suffering from undiagnosed underlying emotional disturbances. Early detection in such cases benefits both the patient and the practitioner [32, 33].

### 3.7.1 Maxillofacial Considerations

Pain related to the TMJ and associated structures seems to be another condition, which fits into the previous category, commonly seen and treated by the maxillofacial surgeon. In the absence of an identifiable organic cause, there must be a low threshold for considering an underlying emotional disturbance.

Patients with diagnosed psychiatric conditions and on medication present with obvious oral symptoms. Most common among these are dental caries and periodontal disease. The primary cause of these is due to decreased salivary flow or xerostomia, which is a side effect of medications, including tricyclic antidepressants, lithium carbonate, phenothiazines, and benzodiazepines. Sialorrhea or excessive salivation is a well-known side effect of clozapine and reduction in dose may be of use [32]. Candidiasis is another condition, which may manifest due to xerostomia, especially in denture wearers. Fear of dental treatment is well known. However, recognition of the nature and extent of this fear is important to prevent noncompliance. Anxiety disorders and phobia often stem from two types of experiences, a painful or traumatic procedure, usually at a young age, or a negative interaction with healthcare professional [32]. A specific maxillofacial consideration in this respect is suturing of facial wounds under local anesthetic, in young children. The authors recommend sedation if not a general anesthetic, particularly in extremely young children, where such procedures are required.

Alcohol, tobacco, and drug abusers are particularly tricky to treat, be it minor or major maxillofacial surgery. The amount of local anesthetic required to produce adequate analgesia tends to be higher in such patients. These groups of patients are at a higher risk of developing oral cancer. Effects of withdrawal can be significant and this must be kept in mind preoperatively, intraoperatively, and postoperatively—especially where procedures of long duration and extended stay are planned. Use of drugs like chlordiazepoxide might be required to offset delirium tremens, particularly in the postoperative period. Head and neck cancer particularly affects the psyche, making a psychologist a very important member of the multidisciplinary team.

Patients suffering from clefts of the orofacial region require multiple surgeries at various stages of their life and the effects of surgery and rehabilitation can be debilitating on both the child and the parents. Timing of surgeries is vital as they disrupt the life of the entire family of the child and for this parental counselling is extremely important [33].

While management of trauma might be comparatively straightforward, one must not underestimate the effect on the psyche in the recovery phase, especially if this is coupled with post-traumatic stress disorder (PTSD). Although these injuries are among the most common treated, these can lead to depression, drug abuse, antisocial behavior, especially in those with a post-traumatic residual defect [34].

Orthognathic surgery, while primarily carried out for cosmetic reasons, occasionally may be performed for functional reasons, as in obstructive sleep apnea. Counselling prior to surgery is useful and the entire process can take up to 3 years. Serious psychological and psychosocial problems have been reported [33].

While awareness of maxillofacial surgery and its benefits is gradually growing in our country, with most centers providing information about technical aspects of surgery, the psychological aspect is often ignored. Communication needs to improve and an assessment of patients' emotional state before and after surgery could help in improving patient satisfaction [33].

## 3.8 Dental and Maxillofacial Implications in Liver Disease

### 3.8.1 Introduction

At approximate of 1.4 kg, this reddish, rubbery structure forms an important organ system. Along with the Gall Bladder and Pancreas, the liver works to digest, process, and absorb food. Liver aids in detoxification in the body and is the primary organ of drug metabolism. It also helps in the production and transport of bile [35].

#### 3.8.1.1 The Function of the Liver [36]

Detoxification—Removal of ammonia, exogenous hormones

(a) Alcohol metabolism
(b) Synthesis of essential Serum Proteins (Albumin)
(c) Synthesis—coagulation Factors (V, VII, IX, X), prothrombin, fibrinogen.
(d) Production of Bile and its transporters
(e) Regulation of nutrients
(f) Conjugation of lipophilic compounds

Liver dysfunction hence alters all of these functions, thereby disrupting the homeostasis in the body, which has to be taken into consideration when providing dental and maxillofacial therapy.

Vitamin K levels are significantly lowered in advanced liver disease hampering the production of coagulation factors. This, along with portal hypertension, results in thrombocytopenia, thus resulting in excessive bleeding, which is of consideration during dental and maxillofacial management [37].

### 3.8.2 Classification of Liver Dysfunctions [35]

Acute or Chronic

(a) Infective (Hepatitis) & Noninfective (Substance abuse)
(b) Extent of damage—steatosis (fatty liver), fibrosis, cirrhosis, hepatocellular carcinoma

#### 3.8.2.1 Viral Hepatitis

Hepatitis A—caused due to Hepatitis A virus, spreads via the orofecal route. It is endemic in nature and is self-limiting.

Hepatitis B—caused by (HBV) that replicates within the hepatocyte; it is a dangerous form of viral disease with high risk to healthcare workers. The surface antigen is routinely detected in the saliva of infected individuals, and hence transmission through the saliva is of concern to the Oral Surgeon [38]. Prevalence of HBV infection is three to five times more in dentists than the general population. Younger individuals with chronic HBV infections have a greater prevalence of developing hepatocellular carcinoma.

Hepatitis C—Caused by a bloodborne virus, it is the most common cause for chronic hepatitis, which over long term could lead to cirrhosis or hepatocellular carcinoma.

#### 3.8.2.2 Autoimmune Hepatitis

It is a chronic liver inflammatory disease as a result of IgG Hypergammaglobinemia as a result of environmental or viral factors inciting an autoimmune response leading to cirrhosis [39].

#### 3.8.2.3 Fulminant Hepatitis

A sudden acute and severe dysfunction of the liver with resulting hepatocellular necrosis and encephalopathy with a very poor prognosis. These patients require liver transplant.

#### 3.8.2.4 Cirrhosis

It is the irreversible damage to the hepatic architecture due to long-term fibrous scarring. A rise in the production of total liver collagen and matrix protein that is troublesome to the function and form of the liver [40].

#### 3.8.2.5 Hepatocellular Carcinoma

It is the fifth most common cancer and a life-threatening malignancy with poor survival rates. HBV and HCV are the most common causes of it.

#### 3.8.2.6 Alcoholic Liver Disease

It is the 10th most common cause of death with 3% of fatalities in the industrialized world [35]. Alcoholism results in varied disruption of the hepatic system ranging from simple fatty liver to complicated life-threatening cirrhosis.

### 3.8.3 Oral Manifestations of Liver Disease

Foetor hepaticus (Breath of the dead odor of rotten eggs with garlic) is a characteristic late feature of liver dysfunction [36]. Evidence of liver diseases has been noted in the oral cavity as icteric mucosal alteration with gingival bleeding and also associated hemorrhagic changes like hematoma, petechiae [37]. HCV-associated hepatitis is noted as a common cause for Sjogren's syndrome and lichen planus in the oral cavity [41]. Alcoholic hepatitis in association with nutritional deficiencies could cause glossitis along with delayed healing post surgery [37]. Occasionally, parotid enlargement is also noted. These oral manifestations are associated with concomitant general symptoms of liver disease such as hepatomegaly, malaise, confusion, fatigue, weight loss, nausea, and altering the well being of the person [37].

### 3.8.4 Implications of Liver Disease

1. Hepatic metabolism of drugs is Unpredictable
2. Defective hemostatic cascade and poor coagulation
3. Increased risk of infection

#### 3.8.4.1 Liver Disease and Maxillofacial Surgery

Risk of viral contagion and crossinfection is one of the implications of viral hepatic disease. Hep C viruses are found to be stable at room temperatures for approximately 5 days. The virus is also detected at different surfaces in the clinic after the patient is treated. It is vital to maintain adequate sterilization and observe strict universal protection when treating such patients. Needlestick injury precautions must be adhered to.

Detailed history taking is important to identify any indications of liver disease, including that of hepatitis, jaundice, alcohol intake, recreational drugs, or rank abuse. Abnormal bleeding patterns are elicited in history [42]. Past surgical history provides a valuable indicator for any doubts regarding the adequate functioning of the liver system. Additional information of identifying the etiology for cirrhosis and any continued risk factors like alcohol consumption should be noted [35]. Review of blood investigations such as serum bilirubin, albumin, alanine aminotransferase (ALT), Aspartate aminotransferase (AST), complete blood counts, and coagulation profile must be performed prior to any surgical planning [43].

Elective surgery is contraindicated in acute phases of viral hepatitis and acute liver failure. Patients who present with hepatitis due to alcohol/drug abuse are poor candidates for elective surgery due to liver dysfunction and psychological impact of withdrawal during their hospital stay.

Plasma level of coagulation factors is depressed in liver disease and can potentially alter the hemostasis. Complete blood counts, PT, PTT, INR, and liver functions tests are mandatory in all patients with any signs/symptoms of liver dysfunctions. The goal of surgical therapy is to minimize trauma to the tissues. It is also advisable to involve the hematologist if required. Any dental or minor oral surgical procedure must terminate with the use of local hemostatic agents or antifibrinolytic agents to aid in hemostasis. Maxillofacial surgical work and major invasive oral surgery are ideally performed in the hospital. Fresh Frozen Plasma and Vitamin K infusions to optimize the coagulating process might be required to offset intraoperative bleeding.

Patients with liver disease are more susceptible to infection with a greater risk post invasive dental or maxillofacial procedure. Antibiotic prophylaxis is recommended.

Drug metabolism is altered in these patients (Table 3.6). Unlike serum creatinine, which is an indicator of renal function, the liver function test is more of an indicator for liver damage. Hence, it is difficult to obtain exact dose modification formulae when medicating patients with liver disease. Drug usage, dosage, and interactions must be consulted with the specialist prior to their usage.

The metabolism of these drugs is well tolerated in mild liver dysfunctions but is impaired in severe dysfunction and hence requires modifications and contraindications. The beta lactams mainly utilized in maxillofacial surgery are quite safe. NSAIDS are to be used with caution to avoid gastric bleedings [35]. Hepatotoxic drugs should be avoided eg. erythromycin, ketoconazole, halothane, phenytoin etc. Prilocaine or articaine is preferred over lidocaine. Sedatives,

**Table 3.6** Drugs metabolized in the liver [37]

| | |
|---|---|
| Local anesthetics | Lidocaide, Bupivacaine, Prilocaine, |
| Sedatives | Barbiturates, Diazepam |
| Analgesics | Paracetamol, Aspirin, Ibuprofen, Codiene |
| Antibiotics | Erythromycin, Clindamycin, Tetracyclin |
| Antifungal | Ketaconozol, Fluconozol |

hypnotics or opiods should be used with caution. A balance has to be struck constantly to maintain the anesthesia and concern is of the depressive action of alcohol and central nervous system depressors. Postoperative care in view of alcohol withdrawal must be noted. Ensure alcohol-based mouth rinses are avoided.

## 3.9 Maxillofacial Implications in GI Disorders

### 3.9.1 Perioperative Maxillofacial Implications

#### 3.9.1.1 GERD

Extraesophageal symptoms of GERD must be identified to prevent any airway issues primarily. Due to delayed gastric emptying, preoperative fasting hours must be prolonged. In high-risk patients, Proton pump inhibitors and H2 receptor antagonists are potent drugs to increase gastric pH and reduce secretions. Nasogastric suctioning through nasogastric tube aids in protecting the airway from gastric secretions during surgery. It is important to manage nausea and vomiting postoperatively effectively.

#### 3.9.1.2 Peptic Ulcers

Stress reduction protocol is vital. GI symptoms from NSAIDS are delayed and identified when the ulcers are in an advanced stage with a greater risk of bleeding. Corticosteroids must be avoided in these patients along with NSAIDS. GI bleeding due to ulceration could cause anemia and has to be managed prior to any surgery. Surgery is contraindicated in active peptic ulcers. Ranitidine, when used over a long phase for management, could cause thrombocytopenia [44].

#### 3.9.1.3 Ulcerative Colitis

One must rule out anemia in these patients and assess the effect of long-term steroid therapy. Antibiotics such as clindamycin, ampicillin, and cephalosporins are implicated in aggravation of colitis and are hence avoided. If the patient has undergone Vitamin K malabsorption, its effects are considered.

Postoperative nausea and vomiting, though not a complication, is still detrimental in patient management perioperatively. Volatile inhalation anesthetic agents and opiod analgesics are emetogenic and need to be used with caution. Postoperative anxiety, dehydration, and pain could result in nausea and vomiting. Scarred ulcers in the duodenum delay gastric emptying resulting in vomitus. Antiemetics in these patients must be prescribed at the end of the surgery and dexamethasone 1 h prior to the surgery is helpful if not contraindicated. In high-risk patients, antiemetics must be administered prior to anesthesia itself [45]. Postoperative ileus could occur due to prolonged opiate use during anesthesia, decreased potassium levels, trauma or due to iliac bone harvesting as a complication or resultant severe pain.

## 3.10 Pregnancy

Pregnancy is often associated with changes in cardiovascular, endocrine, hematological, respiratory, gastrointestinal, and genitourinary system. These alterations may occasionally be subtle and can lead to disastrous complications if not identified [46].

### 3.10.1 Physiologic Changes

There will be increase in the heart rate leading to an increase in cardiac output. Cardiac output increases mostly in the first trimester and remains fairly unchanged with minimal increase in the final trimester.

During the second and final trimesters, a decrease in blood pressure and cardiac output may occur while the patient is in a supine position. This is caused by the gravid uterus compressing the inferior vena cava leading to a decreased venous return to the heart leading to hypotension, bradycardia, and syncope. This phenomenon is called *supine hypotension syndrome* [47].

The concentration of all coagulation factors, other than factors XI and XIII, is increased. As Thrombin-mediated fibrin generation increases during pregnancy, this combines with an increase in the aforementioned clotting factors and hematocrit, leading to the hypercoagulable state of pregnancy. This leads to a higher risk of deep vein thrombosis (DVT) and pulmonary embolism (PE).

In the abdomen, the enlarging uterus displaces the stomach onto the spleen and liver leading to high intragastric pressure. This and the delayed gastric emptying leads to regurgitation and gastric reflux. Hyperventilation that begins in the first trimester might increase throughout pregnancy. This has obvious implications on drug dosage, route and timing of administration.

In the first trimester, glomerular filtration rate increases 30–50%, which results in an increase in clearance of creatinine, uric acid, and urea. This leads to a decrease in levels of the same. While prescribing drugs, doses may need to be increased to account for this rapid clearance [48].

### 3.10.2 Treatment Protocol

#### 3.10.2.1 Minor Surgery

While minor oral surgery is not a contraindication in the pregnant patient, it is advised that the oral surgeon should consult with the patient's obstetrician to address specific concerns should dental emergencies arise during the first trimester.

Unless emergency treatment is required, it is advisable to defer treatment during the first trimester because of the potential vulnerability of the fetus. The second trimester is the safest time to perform the routine dental treatment. No elective treatment is advisable late in the third trimester.

#### 3.10.2.2 Dental Radiology

Two important factors to be considered are the dose of radiation to be given and the time of gestation. Animal and human data clearly support the conclusion that no increase in congenital anomalies due to exposures totaling less than 0.05–0.1 Gy during pregnancy. The amount of radiation used in dental radiographs is well below the threshold dose [47]. With modern features such as high-speed film, filtration, collimation, and use of lead aprons, dental radiography is deemed quite safe.

#### 3.10.2.3 Major Surgery

Elective surgery should be postponed until after delivery. If possible, nonurgent surgery should be performed in the second trimester when preterm contractions and spontaneous abortion are least likely. Fetal safety requires that potentially dangerous drugs are avoided and adequate uteroplacental perfusion is ensured. No anesthetic drugs have been proven to be clearly hazardous to the human fetus. However, teratogenic effects of nitrous oxide have been demonstrated in animal models following prolonged administration in high concentration [49].

Anxiety in itself leads to decrease in uteroplacental perfusion secondary to increase in circulating catecholamines. Appropriate timing of surgery and anxiolysis is of paramount importance.

### 3.10.3 Drug Usage in Pregnancy

Most drugs cross the placental barrier by simple diffusion. Hence, the major concern of drug administration during pregnancy is the potential of teratogenic adverse effects. The period of maximum risk for teratogenicity is during organogenesis. This occurs from the end of the predifferentiation period until the end of the 10th week after the last menstrual period (Table 3.7).

**Table 3.7** Commonly used safe and unsafe drugs during pregnancy [46]

| Drug | Safe | Unsafe |
|---|---|---|
| Local anesthetics | Articaine<br>Lignocaine<br>Prilocaine | Bupivacaine |
| Analgesics | Paracetamol<br>Ibuprofen (first and second trimesters) | Aspirin<br>Diclofenac<br>Ibuprofen (third trimester)<br>Naproxen |
| Antibacterials | Amoxicillin<br>Azithromycin<br>Cephalosporins<br>Erythromycin | Aminoglycosides<br>Metronidazole<br>Sulfonamides<br>Tetracyclines |
| Antifungals | Fluconazole<br>Nystatin | Ketoconazole |
| Anxiolytics | None | Alprazolam<br>Diazepam |

## 3.11 Endocrine Disorders

### 3.11.1 Diabetes

Diabetes is an endocrine disease manifesting as hyperglycemia, leading to microvascular and cardiovascular complications. Type 1 diabetes mellitus is an autoimmune pancreatic beta cell destruction leading to inadequate production of insulin. In type 2 diabetes mellitus, there is a condition of insulin resistance in addition to defects in insulin secretion by the pancreatic beta cells, and increased endogenous glucose production, primarily by the liver [50].

The current recommendation for diagnosis of diabetes stands at >126 mg/dl of fasting plasma glucose levels or a 2-h plasma glucose level of 200 mg/dl [51]. The Endocrine Society guidelines indicate that patients with hyperglycemia and glycated haemoglobin (HbA1c) of 6.5% or higher can be identified as having diabetes [52].

Optimal glycemic control is advised in each patient to avoid hyperglycemia or hypoglycemia. The surgical patient with diabetes is at higher risk of perioperative morbidity and mortality and subsequently longer length of hospital stays. This is mainly due to increased chances of surgical site infections and systemic infections, other complications like acute kidney injury, acute coronary syndromes, acute cerebrovascular accidents, hospital-acquired diabetic ketoacidosis, etc [53].

The stress of surgery and anesthesia derails the glycemic control of the patient due to the metabolic response to surgery. Nondiabetic patients evoke a catabolic response with a release of cortisol, glucagon, catecholamines, etc., promoting hepatic glycogenolysis and gluconeogenesis causing hyperglycemia. There is a catecholamine-induced inhibition of insulin production as well as insulin resistance. The type of anesthesia and the length of the procedure are also said to influence the amount of catabolism [54].

The preoperative preparation for a diabetic patient begins with a thorough history, including the type and dosing of medications, any history of cardiac events, or diabetic ketoacidosis. ECG is mandated as these patients have a higher occurrence of hypercholesterolemia, hypertension, macrovascular disease, autonomic neuropathy, and hence silent ischemia. If the ECG does suggest so, further investigation is indicated [55].

Renal function tests should include serum urea and creatinine. Hypertension should be ruled out or treated if present. Diabetic neuropathy should be evaluated as it may cause aspiration, silent myocardial ischemia, or even sudden death. It may manifest as postural hypotension, heartburn, or resting tachycardia [56].

HbA1c is usually advised in diabetic patients undergoing treatment as it reflects mean control over the previous 3 months. This allows one to estimate the quality of glycemic control before the consultation and adaptation of treatment to fixed objectives. It is also important to know the duration of the diabetes, dependence on insulin, and whether the glycemic control is achieved by oral hypoglycemics and lifestyle modification.

#### 3.11.1.1 Management of Patients Undergoing Procedures

The recommendations for target glycemic control vary. The Endocrine Society and the American Diabetes Association/AACE Practice Guidelines recommend that patients on insulin maintain a target preprandial glucose of less than 140 mg/dl and a random Blood Glucose (BG) of less than 180 mg/dl for patients treated [52]. The Joint British Diabetes Societies guideline, however, recommends that insulin therapy be commenced when random blood glucose levels exceed 180 mg/dl [53].

#### 3.11.1.2 Preoperative Glycemic Control in patients on Oral Hypoglycemic Agents

##### 3.11.1.2.1 Minor surgery

Patient should adhere to his daily oral diabetic medication and follow his usual diet [50].

##### 3.11.1.2.2 Major surgery

- Most oral hypoglycemics can be continued till the day before surgery. Sulfonylureas and insulin secretagogues should be stopped on the day of surgery to reduce the chances of hypoglycemia [52].
- If normal oral intake is expected to resume on the day of surgery, metformin may be given on the day of surgery [53].
- Metformin is discontinued if there is either prolonged state of fasting or use of i.v contrast dyes or reduced renal function
- (Dipeptyl Peptidase-4) DPP-4 inhibitors are not contraindicated throughout the perioperative period [54].

#### 3.11.1.3 Preoperative Glycemic Control in Type 2 Diabetics on Insulin

Patients on basal insulin: If they are on twice daily dosing then morning dose to be reduced to 80% of normal dose; whereas if those on single dose then evening dose to be reduced to 80% [57].

If the morning glucose levels are above 120 mg/dl, Neutral protamine Hagedorn (NPH) insulin and premixed formulations are reduced by 20% the evening before surgery and by 50% the morning of surgery. If not, morning insulin dose is withheld [58].

Naturally, these are guidelines and the diabetologist will tailor the doses to the individual requirement of the patient.

#### 3.11.1.4 Preoperative Glycemic Control in Type 1 Diabetics on Insulin

##### 3.11.1.4.1 Minor surgery:

- Well-controlled patients should halve their daily dose of insulin the morning of surgery and also eat their normal breakfast.
- Morning appointments are preferred. If preoperative glucose is between 100 and 200 mg/dl, surgery can be performed.
- If blood glucose is >200 mg/dl, an intravenous infusion of 10% dextrose in half-normal saline is initiated. 10-mEq potassium chloride should be added to each 500 ml of dextrose/saline infusion.
- Rapid-acting insulin is administered subcutaneously.
- Blood glucose should be monitored hourly if the surgery lasts beyond 1 h [50].

##### 3.11.1.4.2 Major surgery:

These patients are at risk of developing stress-induced hyperglycemia and ketoacidosis and hence need insulin coverage during perioperative period. These patients should receive 80% of basal insulin dose the evening before surgery and on the morning of surgery in order to prevent hypoglycemia [54].

##### 3.11.1.4.3 Intraoperative glycemic control:

The endocrine society recommends an intraoperative BG level within 180 mg/dl [52].

Levels above that are treated either with subcutaneous rapid-acting insulin analogs or with an IV infusion of regular insulin. In patients undergoing short surgeries (under 4-h operative time), ambulatory surgeries, expected hemodynamic stability and those expected to resume oral diet soon can be managed with subcutaneous rapid-acting insulin correction scales [3]. When it is used, the BG should be checked every 2 h [52].

An IV insulin infusion is preferred where there is anticipated hemodynamic disturbance, significant fluid shifts, expected changes in temperature, inotropic support, or lengthy operative times (greater than 4 h). In this situation, hourly insulin monitoring is needed.

#### 3.11.1.4.4 Postoperative glycemic control:

For noncritical and non-ICU patients, the subcutaneous sliding scale insulin is used with BG being checked every 2 h. If BG drops below 70 mg/dl, insulin is stopped and oral dextrose or iv dextrose is given. For patients in the ICU, continuous iv insulin infusion is given instead of the subcutaneous sliding scale for BG > 180 mg/dl. Oral antidiabetic agents are best avoided in hospitalized patients due to the limited data available on their safety and efficacy. DPP-4 has shown promising results for in-patient hyperglycemia control [54].

### 3.11.2 Hypo/Hyperthyroidism

The thyroid gland releases the hormone thyroxine (T4) and its active form T3. The thyroid hormones are released upon stimulation by the thyroid-stimulating hormone (TSH) released from the pituitary gland. This is, in turn, stimulated by thyrotropin release hormone (TRH). Secretion of T3 and T4 is regulated by the negative feedback loop modulating release of TSH [59].

Thyroid hormones play a critical role in maintaining metabolic homeostasis in the adult. Thyroid-related disorders are due to either overproduction of thyroid hormones (thyrotoxicosis) or hormone deficiency (hypothyroidism). These situations may arise due to infectious, autoimmune, proliferative, or tumorous pathologies [60].

Most patients with well-compensated thyroid disease do not need special consideration prior to surgery. Patients with a newly diagnosed thyroid disorder around the time of surgery will need to undergo risk assessment and optimization before surgery.

Routine thyroid screening is not done for asymptomatic patients unless there is a reason to suspect thyroid dysfunction. Thyroid disease present with a myriad of symptoms clinically. These include-unexplained weight changes, and fine tremor or changes in bowel habits, skin, hair, exophthalmos, goiter, abnormal reflexes. Palpitations, tachycardia, or bradycardia are common cardiovascular manifestations. In such situations as well as in patients with a known thyroid disorder, a TSH test should be included in the preoperative analysis [61].

#### 3.11.2.1 Hypothyroidism

Hypothyroidism may be primary (due to thyroid disease) or secondary due to hypothalamo-pituitary disorders. Commonly, it is due to thyroid loss from surgery, irradiation, autoimmune diseases, or drug induced [59]. The diagnosis is confirmed by blood tests revealing low T3 and T4 levels and high TSH in primary and decreased TSH in secondary hypothyroidism. These patients pose challenges during perioperative period due to their effects on various organ systems.

#### 3.11.2.1.1 Physiologic Challenges

Cardiac disturbances like increased peripheral vascular resistance, decreased cardiac output; Respiratory implications like increased incidence of pneumonia, impaired respiratory drive, respiratory muscle weakness. Decreased renal perfusion, decreased gastric motility, and slower drug metabolism need to be considered.

One of the most serious complications of surgery in hypothyroid patients is myxedema coma. It is associated with a mortality rate as high as 80%. It is characterized by altered mental status, which may manifest as coma or seizure, and hypothermia, bradycardia, hyponatremia, heart failure, and hypopnea. It is precipitated by surgery, infection, cold exposure, and administration of sedatives [61].

#### 3.11.2.1.2 Management

A condition of euthyroidism is usually targeted preoperatively and elective surgery is usually postponed. Once TSH values normalize, surgery can be performed. Use of sedatives, benzodiazepenes and Opiods should be avoided [59].

For urgent and emergent procedures, surgery may be performed in mild-to-moderate hypothyroidism with levothyroxine cover preoperatively. Surgery should be postponed in patients with severe hypothyroidism in case of nonemergent surgery. In an emergency, thyroid hormone levels should be normalized as rapidly as possible, using IV levothyroxine in a loading dose of 200–500 μg followed by 50–100 μg IV daily [62].

#### 3.11.2.2 Hyperthyroidism

It is commonly due to autoimmune disease (e.g., Graves' disease), multinodular goiter, or adenoma presenting as thyroid nodule. The diagnosis is confirmed by elevated serum T3 and T4. It usually causes exopthalmos, heat intolerance, anxiety, sweating, diarrhea, and weight loss [59]. It has a positive ionotropic and chronotropic effect on the heart coupled with decreased vascular resistance [61]. Hence, these patients manifest tachycardia, arrhythmias, or cardiac failure frequently.

Thyroid storm is a severe manifestation of uncontrolled hyperthyroidism and is characterized by tachycardia, confusion, fever, gastrointestinal complaints, and potentially leading to cardiovascular collapse. It is precipitated by pain, anxiety, trauma, or GA. Hence, elective surgery should always be postponed in patients with overt untreated hyperthyroidism. Hyperthyroidism is usually treated by β-blockers like atenolol or metoprolol as they decrease the sympathetic overactivity. When there is no time to render a patient euthyroid as in emergency cases, cardiac monitoring and adequate β-blockers with antithyroid medication should be given [61]. While epinephrine with lidocaine is not contraindicated, caution should be exercised. Benzodiapines should be avoided. Carbamizole causes agranulocytosis and this can manifest as oral ulcers.

### 3.11.3 Adrenal Gland Disorders

#### 3.11.3.1 Primary Adrenocortical Hypofunction

Addison's disease occurs due to autoantibody-mediated destruction of the adrenal cortex leading to failed cortisol and aldosterone secretion. It may also occur due to tuberculosis, histoplasmosis, sarcoidosis, etc [59]. Due to lack of adequate corticosteroid production, these patients are prone to hypotensive collapse, hypoglycemia, profound weakness, and dehydration (Adrenal crisis).

Adrenal crisis is rare in outpatient oral surgery. However, patients with Addison's disease who need surgery should be covered with supplemental steroids. Drugs like barbiturates, azole antifungals, etomidates, phenytoin, and rifampins should be avoided as they accelerate cortisol metabolism.

#### 3.11.3.2 Secondary Adrenocortical Insufficiency

Corticosteroids are prescribed as long-term treatment for various ailments such as inflammatory bowel disease, blood dyscrasias like idiopathic thrombocytopenia, rheumatologic disease, reactive airway disease, and immunosuppression for transplant recipients, etc. due to their immunosuppressive, anti-inflammatory, metabolic, and hemodynamic properties. This external source of long-term steroid can lead to secondary adrenal insufficiency that may manifest in the perioperative period [63].

In a healthy individual, corticotrophin-releasing hormone (CRH) has a diurnal pattern of release from the hypothalamus. This in turn acts on the anterior pituitary to release the Adrenocorticotrophic hormone (ACTH). ACTH acts on the adrenal cortex to release cortisol (hydrocortisone), corticosterone, and mineralocorticoids. Circulating corticosteroids have a subsequent negative feedback effect on CRH and ACTH release. This constitutes the hypothalamic-pituitary adrenocortical (HPA) axis [59].

Normally, an unstressed adrenal gland secretes approximately 8–10 mg of cortisol per day (Table 3.8). Stress, such as illness or surgery, is the stimulus for raised production of cortisol. During surgical stress, the rate varies between individuals and also upon the type of surgery. It is usually up to 50 mg/day for minor procedures and up to 75–150 mg/day for more complex procedures, rarely exceeding 200 mg/day. However, patients on exogenous corticosteroids aren't able to secrete adequate amounts of corticosteroids in response to stress due to HPA axis suppression and a resulting low level of ACTH and CRH leading to atrophy of the zona fasciculate of adrenal cortex [63].This may predispose them to develop adrenal crisis, with rapidly developing hypotension, hypoglycemia, collapse, and even death [59].

Even though there is no consensus on the exact dosage of corticosteroids that leads to hypofunction of the adrenal cortex, doses greater than physiologic doses of cortisol lead to suppression [59]. HPAA suppression does not extend beyond 1 year after exogenous steroid therapy is stopped [64]. Hence, those at risk are:

- Patients currently taking >5 mg of systemic prednisolone
- Corticosteroids been taken in the past 30 days
- Corticosteroids taken for more than a month during the past 1 year.

These patients require steroid cover/supplementation when undertaken for surgeries. Most dentoalveolar and maxillofacial surgeries result in stress and hence require steroid supplements, but most other dental procedures do not require any additional steroid supplements [59].

Following table shows the normal corticosteroid response to the particular level of stress and the appropriate steroid cover needed in cases of adrenal suppression (Table 3.9):

During the procedure, blood pressure and blood sugar levels should be monitored. NSAIDs should be avoided to avoid increasing risk of peptic ulceration. Prophylactic antibiotics should be given in such patients to avoid postoperative infections.

### 3.11.4 Renal Disorders

The kidneys are responsible for eliminating metabolic waste; fluid and electrolyte homeostasis; and to maintain acid and base balance. The kidneys also affect the cardiovascular and hematologic systems.

**Table 3.8** Approximate potencies of systemic corticosteroids relative to cortisol [59]

| Steroid | Glucocorticoid activity | Mineralocorticoid activity | Equivalent dose (IV/PO) |
|---|---|---|---|
| Cortisol (hydrocortisone) | 1 | 1 | 20 |
| Cortisone | 0.8 | 0.8 | 25 |
| Prednisone | 4 | 0.8 | 5 |
| Prednisolone | 4 | 0.8 | 5 |
| Methylprednisolone | 5 | 0.5 | 4 |
| Dexamethasone | 30–40 | 0 | 0.5–0.75 |

**Table 3.9** Normal corticosteroid response to the particular level of stress and the appropriate steroid cover needed in cases of adrenal suppression [63]

| Surgery type | Endogenous cortisol secretion rate | Examples | Recommended steroid dosing |
|---|---|---|---|
| Superficial | 8–10 mg/day (baseline) | Dental surgery<br>Biopsy | Usual daily dose |
| Minor | 50 mg/day | Multiple extractions LA, Dental implant surgery<br>Inguinal hernia repair<br>Colonoscopy<br>Uterine curettage<br>Hand surgery | Usual daily dose<br>plus<br>Hydrocortisone: 50 mg IV before incision<br>Hydrocortisone: 25 mg IV every 8 h × 24 h<br>Then usual daily dose |
| Moderate | 75–150 mg/day | Minor maxillofacial trauma,<br>Orthognathic surgery<br>Lower-extremity revascularization<br>Total joint replacement<br>Cholecystectomy<br>Colon resection<br>Abdominal hysterectomy | Usual daily dose<br>plus<br>Hydrocortisone: 50 mg IV before incision<br>Hydrocortisone: 25 mg IV every 8 h × 24 h<br>Then usual daily dose |
| Major esophagectomy | 75–150 mg/day | Total proctocolectomy<br>Major cardiac/vascular<br>Hepaticojejunostomy<br>Delivery<br>Trauma | Usual daily dose<br>plus<br>Hydrocortisone: 100 mg IV before incision<br>Followed by continuous IV infusion of 200 mg of hydrocortisone<br>more than 24 h<br>or<br>Hydrocortisone: 50 mg IV every 8 h × 24<br>Taper dose by half per day until usual daily dose reached<br>plus<br>Continuous IV fluids with 5% dextrose and 0.2–0.45% NaCl<br>(based on degree of hypoglycemia) |

The best parameter to assess the function of the kidneys is the glomerular filtration rate (GFR). It is measured by calculating the creatinine clearance based on serum creatinine (SC). The normal value of GFR for an adult male is 130 ml/1.73 $m^2$ and is 120 ml/1.73 $m^2$ for an adult female. Chronic kidney disease occurs when the GFR is reduced by at least 50 ml/min [65].

Patients with chronic kidney disease who are either on dialysis, dialysis naive, or renal transplant recipients or post-transplant patients require modification of treatment plan from a surgical point of view. These patients always have a risk of developing acute renal failure in the postoperative period either due to pre-existing renal dysfunction or solely due to the effects of surgery.

#### 3.11.4.1 Acute Renal Failure (ARF)

ARF is the rapid loss of renal function over the course of days to weeks, resulting in the patient's inability to clear nitrogenous waste, including creatinine and urea, from the body [66]. The term Acute Kidney Injury (AKI) has replaced acute renal failure in current literature. Perioperative AKI is a leading cause of morbidity and mortality due to increased risk of sepsis, anemia, coagulopathy, and mechanical ventilation.

There are three types of ARF based on etiology: prerenal, renal, and postrenal causes. The most common cause of AKI in perioperative period is the prerenal cause and the ischemic acute tubular necrosis (renal AKI) due to hypoxic damage to medullary region secondary to hypovolemia, hypotension, and dehydration [67]. Prerenal AKI and ischemic ATN are a part of a spectrum of manifestations of renal hypoperfusion. Hypotension or hypovolemia may be due to preoperative factors like hemorrhage, diarrhea, fasting, use of diuretics, due to intraoperative factors like ongoing blood loss, activation of sympathetic reflexes, and due to postoperative factors like intravascular volume depletion, myocardial infarction, etc [68]. Hypotension and hypovolemia result in activation of the sympathetic nervous system and the renin–angiotensin–aldosterone axis, which compromises GFR by inducing afferent arteriolar renal vasoconstriction. Other common causes of AKI are the use of NSAIDs, ACE inhibitors, nephrotoxic drugs like aminoglycosides, radiocontrast materials, myoglobin, hemoglobin, and amphotericin B. Pre-existing diseases like diabetes, hypertension, and obstructions of the urinary system also lead to perioperative AKI [68].

The strategy around perioperative AKI is ideally prevention. Preoperatively potential risk factors such as volume depletion, hypotension, sepsis, nephrotoxin exposure, and pre-existing chronic kidney disease should be identified and elective surgery should be postponed till optimization is complete. Anemia should be corrected before surgery. The choice of fluid in intraoperative resuscitation is usually a balanced crystalloid solution like Ringer's lactate and not a chloride-rich crystalloid. Hydroxyethyl starch is best avoided. Mean arterial pressure should be maintained and hemodynamic stability is of utmost importance. Diuretics should be only given in cases of volume overload and not for increasing GFR. Norepinephrine is preferred over dopamine as it maintains renal perfusion pressure, but the role is still not very clear [67].

#### 3.11.4.2 Chronic Renal Failure (CRF)

CRF is permanent renal insufficiency that develops over months or years caused by the structural and intrinsic damage of the glomerulus or tubulointerstitial system. This usually occurs when GFR is reduced by 50 ml/min. If necessary treatment is not started, most cases of CRF would lead to End Stage Renal Disease (ESRD). ESRD is maintained by regular dialysis or by transplant, in the absence of which, death may occur [68].

Preoperative assessment:

Detailed history and physical examination;
Cardiac work up as dictated by clinical symptoms. ECG and Echocardiogram
Complete blood count
Metabolic panel, serum magnesium, and phosphorus levels
Coagulation profile.

Coronary artery disease and congestive heart failure are commonly found in patients with ESRD and those on dialysis. Hence, cardiac workup and monitoring is required in the perioperative period. Maintaining euvolemia perioperatively in ESRD patients is mandatory. For patients not undergoing dialysis, euvolemia can be achieved with appropriate hydration or diuresis. Dialysis is usually performed a day before surgery to prevent fluid overload and to reduce uremic complications (bleeding). Postoperative dialysis helps to achieve euvolemia if large amounts of fluids were given during surgery. Heparin is withheld if dialysis is performed on the day of surgery.

Anemia complicates CKD due to the decreased production of erythropoietin. Transfusion should be considered in the perioperative period when hemoglobin levels fall below 8–10 g/dl due to surgical blood loss in patients with ESRD. If anemia has been detected, erythropoietin should be initiated several weeks before the elective surgery with iron supplementation to raise hemoglobin to the desired level. Patients who have ESRD may be susceptible to more intraoperative and postoperative bleeding due to platelet dysfunction caused by uremia. Hence, NSAIDs and dipyridamole should not be given within 72 h before surgery to patients who have ESRD due to their effects on platelet function. Hypertension and glycemic control should be tightly monitored in such patients as well.

These patients have inefficient mechanisms of drug clearance that inherently predispose them to adverse drug responses. Hence, NSAIDs, aminoglycosides, benzodiazipines, morphine, and radiocontrast media are avoided. Drugs like propofol, fentanyl, and inhalational anesthetics are usually the preferred drugs of choice.

## 3.12 Patients with Non-head and Neck Malignancies

### 3.12.1 Introduction

The most common cancers in India in women are Breast, Oral, Cervical, ovary, and esophagus. Men tend to be afflicted with head and neck cancers, lung, esophagus, stomach, and colorectal cancer [69]. The cancers that most commonly metastatize to the jaws and oral soft tissues are breast, lung, prostrate, thyroid, kidney, stomach, and colon [70]. Another group of malignancies that receive chemoradiotherapy are the lymphoproliferative and hematologic malignancies [70].

*Chemotherapy* is often employed either with an intent of palliation or for cure. It may be administered as adjuvant therapy or as neoadjuvant therapy. Cytotoxic chemotherapeutic agents have hematologic effects (myelosuppression) as well as nonhematologic effects. The effects of myelosuppression, i.e., leukopenia, thrombocytopenia, and anemia start after 5–7 days with the nadir occurring at 10–14 days. It is usually followed by bone marrow recovery [71]. Hence, the oral surgical treatment should be planned in a manner that it doesn't coincide with the nadir of the myelosuppression where the neutropenia can be as low as 500.

*Radiotherapy* is a part of treatment for a variety of Head and neck cancers either as primary treatment modality or as adjuvant therapy to the primary tumor or to the associated lymphatic structures. Unlike the effects of chemotherapy, effects of radiotherapy are more long lasting. These include mucositis, xerostomia, trismus, radiation-induced fibrosis, and dysguesia.

### 3.12.2 Treatment Protocol

#### 3.12.2.1 Chemotherapy

It is best to undertake a dental screening before the start of the chemotherapy so that the hopeless teeth can be extracted, be restored, periodontal therapy, alveoloplasty be performed, and primary closure be done. After extraction, it takes approximately 10 days to 6 weeks for healing to be enough for chemotherapy to start [72]. Ill-fitting and loose dentures should be discontinued and replaced ideally with implants especially in patients scheduled to take systemic bisphosphonates or RANK-L therapy as it might lead to osteonecrosis of the jaws [73]. Fluoride treatment can also be done.

However, patients suffering from leukemia, lymphomas have a state of myelosuppression even before the start of the

**Table 3.10** Modification of invasive dental treatment according to hematologic indices [75]

| Platelet count | Treatment modification | Neutrophil count | Treatment modification |
|---|---|---|---|
| >75,000 cells/mm$^3$ | No modification | >1000 cell/mm$^3$ | No need for antibiotic prophylaxis. |
| 40,000–75,000 cell/mm$^3$ | Platelet transfusion may be considered in the preoperative and postoperative (24 h). | <1000 cell/mm$^3$ | Postpone the dental treatment. In cases of emergency, discuss antibiotic coverage and endocarditis prophylaxis before treatment with the medical team. Hospitalization may be required |
| <40,000 cell/mm$^3$ | Postpone the dental treatment. In the case of dental emergency, contact the patient's physician before dental treatment to discuss supportive measures, such as platelet transfusion, control of bleeding, and need for hospitalization. Other coagulation tests may be necessary in some cases. | | |

chemotherapy. Only acute situations need to be dealt with. Elective treatments can wait till the time the patient is in optimal clinical and hematological parameters, which is usually until after chemotherapy is over. Hence, extractions of grossly carious and severely periodontally compromised teeth, ill-fitting denture, etc. should be addressed. For extractions to be done, or other invasive dental procedures, hematologic indices should be evaluated and antibiotic prophylaxis should be considered [74] (Table 3.10).

Once the chemotherapy starts, a gap of 1 week before the next cycle is essential before any dental intervention. For surgical procedures that cannot wait, like facial trauma or infection, the complete blood counts should be assessed and consultation should be sought with the medical oncologist to determine the nadir in blood counts, the timing of the chemotherapy cycle, and duration [72]. For platelet levels below 40,000/mm$^3$, platelet transfusions are usually needed [76].

Opportunistic infections may complicate mucositis and may be of viral, fungal, or bacterial origins. Treatment should be guided by culture and sensitivity. Febrile neutropenia needs to be treated usually by intravenous antibiotics like amoxicillin and clavulanic acid with a fluoroquinolone or clindamycin with fluoroquinolone. Hematopoeitic growth factors like granulocyte colony-stimulating factors or granulocyte-macrophage colony-stimulating factors are effective drugs for prophylaxis and treatment of febrile neutropenia. Mucositis occurs in almost all patients and causes great difficulty in feeding, hydrating, and causes pain. It is preferable to manage it with saline mouth rinses rather than with chlorhexidine mouthwashes. Some chemotherapeutic agents are also neurotoxic and cause a deep mandibular pain as well as altered taste sensation and dysguesia. Most of these symptoms subside after cessation of treatment [72].

#### 3.12.2.2 Radiotherapy

The same prophylactic measures of extraction, restoration, alveoloplasty, etc. have to be taken before radiotherapy as for chemotherapy. Additionally, jaw-opening exercises should be initiated and coronoidectomy should be considered as a part of the ablative procedure [72].

### 3.12.3 Prevention and Treatment of Osteonecrosis After Chemotherapy and Radiation

Osteonecrosis of the jaws occurring in an irradiated bone is called osteoradionecrosis (ORN). Those occurring in a patient on antiresorptive therapy like bisphosphonates or monoclonal antibodies to RANK-L is termed Antiresorptive osteonecrosis of jaws (AONJ) [72]. The incidence of ORN in areas of jaws that have received greater than 60 Gy of radiation is 5–15%. Incidence of AONJ in patients who have received denosumab is 1.3% and is 1.8% in patients treated with nitrogen-containing bisphosphonates [77, 78].

**Acknowledgments** Dr Prithvi Bachalli, Consultant Oral and Maxillofacial Surgeon

Rangadore Memorial Hospital, Bangalore

Dr. Prashanth Bhat, Consultant Oral and Maxillofacial Surgeon

Rangadore Memorial Hospital, Bangalore

Dr Shobha Hegde, Registrar Oral and Maxillofacial Surgeon

Rangadore Memorial Hospital, Bangalore

## References

1. 'Indians have gained 10 years of life expectancy since 1990'. The Business Line [Document on internet]. Updated on 09 Jan 2018. https://www.thehindubusinessline.com/news/science/indians-have-gained-10-years-of-life-expectancy-since-1990/article9958774.ece. Accessed 14 Nov 2017.
2. Central Bureau of Health intelligence. National Health profile 2018 [Document on internet]. New Delhi: India Offset Press. https://cdn.downtoearth.org.in/pdf/NHP-2018.pdf. Accessed 27 Apr 2018.
3. Arokiasamy P. India's escalating burden of non-communicable diseases. The Lancet; Global Health. 2018;6(12):1262–3.
4. Indian council of medical research, Public health foundation of India, and Institute for health metrics and evaluation. India: Health

of the Nation's states-The India state-level disease burden initiative. New Delhi: ICMR, PHFI and IHME; 2017. https://www.healthdata.org/sites/default/files/files/policy_report/2017/India_Health_of_the_Nation%27s_States_Report_2017.pdf
5. Government of India: Ministry of Housing and Urban Affairs. Urban Growth [document on the internet]. New Delhi; 2019. Last updated 9 May 2019. http://mohua.gov.in/cms/urban-growth.php#skip
6. India is the most depressed country in the world: Mental Health Day 2018. India Today Web Desk, 2018 [Document on the internet]. New Delhi; 2018. Updated: 10 Oct 2018. https://www.indiatoday.in/education-today/gk-current-affairs/story/india-is-the-most-depressed-country-in-the-world-mental-health-day-2018-1360096-2018-10-10. Accessed 10 Oct 2018.
7. Misra S. Systemic hypertension and noncardiac surgery. Indian J Anaesth. 2017;61:697–704.
8. Shahbabu B, Dasgupta A, Sarkar K, Sahoo SK. Which is more accurate in measuring the blood pressure? A digital or an aneroid sphygmomanometer. J Clin Diagn Res. 2016;10(3)
9. Hogan J, Radhakrishnan J. The assessment and importance of hypertension in the dental setting. J Dent Clin N Am. 2012 Oct;56(4):731–45.
10. Foëx P, Sear JW. The surgical hypertensive patient. Continuing Education in Anaesthesia Critical Care & Pain. 2004 Oct;4(5):139–14.
11. Southerland JH, Gill DG, Gangula PR, Halpern LR, Cardona CY, Mouton CP. Dental management in patients with hypertension: challenges and solutions. Clin Cosmet Investig Dent. 2016;8:111–20.
12. Niwa H, Sato Y, Matsuura H. Safety of dental treatment in patients with previously diagnosed acute myocardial infarction or unstable angina pectoris. Oral Surg Oral Med Oral Pathol Oral Radiol Endod. 2000;89(1):35–41.
13. Ferrari E, Benhamou M, Cerboni P, Marcel B. Coronary syndromes following aspirin withdrawal. J Am Coll Cardiol. 2005;45(3):456–9.
14. Zain MA, Siddiqui WJ. Coronary stents. [Updated 24 Jan 2019]. In: StatPearls [Internet]. Treasure Island (FL): StatPearls Publishing; 2019. https://www.ncbi.nlm.nih.gov/books/NBK507804
15. Oprea AD, Popescu WM. Perioperative management of antiplatelet therapy. Br J Anaes. 2013;111(Suppl 1):i3–i17.
16. Yeung LYY, Sarani B, Weinberg JA, McBeth PB, May AK. Surgeon's guide to anticoagulant and antiplatelet medications. Part Two: Antiplatelet agents and perioperative management of long-term anticoagulation. Trauma Surg Acute Care Open. 2016;1:1–7.
17. León AMD, López BC, Esteve CG. Dental management of patients receiving anticoagulant and/or antiplatelet treatment. J Clin Exp Dent. 2014 Apr;6(2):e155–61.
18. Abdullah WA, Khalil H. Dental extraction in patients on warfarin treatment. Clin Cosmet Investig Dent. 2014;6:65–9.
19. Shah SN. Oral anticoagulation in special population and conditions. J Assoc Phy Ind. 2014;62. http://www.japi.org/june_2014_special_issue/07_oral_anticoagulation_in.htm
20. Lam DK, Jan A, Sándor GK, Clokie CM. Prevention of infective endocarditis: Revised guidelines from the American Heart Association and the implications for dentists. J Can Dent Assoc. 2008;74(5):449–53.
21. Shah AH, Khalil HS, Kola MZ. Dental management of a patient fitted with subcutaneous Implantable Cardioverter Defibrillator device and concomitant warfarin treatment. Saudi Dent J. 2015;27(3):165–70.
22. Turner MD, Glickman RS. Epilepsy in the oral and maxillofacial patient: current therapy. J Oral Maxillofac Surg. 2005;63:996–1005.
23. Jacobsen PL, Eden O. Epilepsy and the dental management of the epileptic patient. J Contemp Dent Pract. 2008;9(1):1–13.
24. Scheffer IE, Berkovic S, Capovilla G, Connolly MB, French J, Guilhoto L, et al. ILAE classification of the epilepsies: position paper of the ILAE Commission for Classification and Terminology. Epilepsia. 2017;58(4):512–21.
25. Scully C. Neurology. In: Scully's medical problems in dentistry. 7th ed. Haryana: Churchill Livingstone, Elsevier; 2014. p. 345–93.
26. Mehmet Y, Senem O, Sülün T, Hümeyra K. Management of epileptic patients in dentistry. Surg Sci. 2012;3:47–52.
27. Bodnar DC, Varlan CM, Varlan V, Vaideanu T, Popa MB. Dental management in Stroke patients. TMJ. 2008;58(3–4):228–35.
28. Arboix A, Pérez Sempere A, Alvarez SJ. Ictus: etiological types and diagnostic criteria. In: Díez Tejedor E, editor. Guide for the diagnosis and treatment of stroke. Barcelona: Prous Science; 2006. p. 1–23.
29. British Society of Gerodontology. Guidelines for the oral healthcare of stroke survivors. June 2010. p. 4–10.
30. MBA A, Abbas G, Latifeh Y, Hamadah O. The oral manifestations of psychiatric disorders. Oral Health Dent Manag. 2018;17(4):1–6.
31. Al-Atram Majmaah AA. The ability of dentists to identify psychiatric symptoms in their patients. J Health Sci. 2017;5(2)
32. Tomar B, Bhati NK, Kumar P, Bhatia MS, Shah RJ. The psychiatric and dental inter-relationship. Delhi Psychiatry Journal. 2011;14(1)
33. Sousa AD. Psychological issues in oral and maxillofacial reconstructive surgery. Br J Oral Maxillofac Surg. 2008;46(8):661–4.
34. Nassab ISAHG, Samieirad S, Zadeh MV, Aghahi RK, Hashemipour MA. Depression and anxiety disorders in a sample of facial trauma: a study. Med Oral Patol Oral Cir Bucal. 2016 Jul 1;21(4):e477–82.
35. Pamplona MC, Muñoz MM, Pérez MGS. Dental considerations in patients with liver disease. J Clin Exp Dent. 2011;3(2):127–34.
36. Grau-García-Moreno DM. Dental management of patients with liver disease. Med Oral. 2003;8:231.
37. Golla K, Epstein JB, Cabay RJ. Liver disease: current perspectives on medical and dental management. Oral Surg Oral Med Oral Pathol Oral Radiol Endod. 2004;98:516–21.
38. Dienstag JL, Isselbacher KJ. Acute viral hepatitis [Internet]. Columbus, OH: The McGraw-Hill. http://harrisons.accessmedicine.com.proxy.cc.uic.edu. Accessed 12 Sep 2004.
39. Al-Khalidi JA, Czaja AJ. Current concepts in the diagnosis, pathogenesis, and treatment of autoimmune hepatitis. Mayo Clin Proc. 2001;76:1237–52.
40. Iredale JP. Cirrhosis: new research provides a basis for rational and targeted treatments. Br Med J. 2003;327:143–7.
41. Haddad J, Deny P, Munz-Gotheil C, Ambrosini JC, Trinchet JC, et al. Lymphocyte sialadenitis of Sjogren's syndrome associated with chronic Hepatitis C virus liver disease. Lancet. 1992;339:1425–6.
42. Greenwood M, Meecham JG. General medicine and surgery for dental practitioners. Part 5: Liver disease. Br Dent J. 2003;195:71–3.
43. John Firriolo F. Dental management of patients with end stage liver disease. Dent Clin N Am. 2006;50:563–90.
44. Edwards CR, Boucher IA. Davidson's principles and practice of medicine. 17th ed. London: Churchill Livingston; 1996. p. 405–82.
45. Gan TJ. Postoperative nausea and vomiting-can it be eliminated? JAMA. 2002;287:1233–6.
46. Scully C. Age and gender issues. In: Scully's medical problems in dentistry. 7th ed. Haryana: Churchill Livingstone, Elsevier; 2014. p. 642–6.
47. Cengiz SB. The pregnant patent: consideration for dental management and drug use. Quintessence Int. 2007;38:777e733-742.

48. Turner M, Aziz SR. Management of the pregnant oral and maxillofacial surgery patient. J Oral Maxillofoc Surg. 2002;60:1479–88.
49. Upadya M, Saneesh PJ. Anaesthesia for non-obstetric surgery during pregnancy. Indian J Anaesth. 2016 Apr;60(4):234–41.
50. Bergman SA. Perioperative management of the diabetic patient. Oral Surg Oral Med Oral Pathol Oral Radiol Endod. 2007;103:731–7.
51. Definition and diagnosis of diabetes mellitus and intermediate hyperglycemia: Report of a WHO/IDF consultation (Document on the internet). WHO Document Production Services, Geneva. 2006. https://www.who.int/diabetes/publications/Definition%20and%20diagnosis%20of%20diabetes_new.pdf
52. Umpierrez GE, Hellman R, Korytkowski MT, Kosiborod M, Maynard GA, Montori VM, Seley JJ, Van den Berghe G. Endocrine Society: Management of hyperglycemia in hospitalized patients in non-critical care setting: an endocrine society clinical practice guideline. J Clin Endocrinol Metab. 2012;97:16–38.
53. Dhatariya K, Levy N, Kilvert A, et al. NHS Diabetes guideline for the perioperative management of the adult patient with diabetes. Diabetic Med. 2012;29:420–33.
54. Duggan EW, Carlson K, Umpierrez GE. Perioperative hyperglycaemia management: an Update. Anesthesiology. 2017;126:547–60.
55. Plodkowski RA, Edelman SV. Pre-surgical evaluation of diabetic patients. Clin Diabetes. 2001;19:92–5.
56. Yoo HK, Serafin BL. Perioperative management of the diabetic patient. Oral Maxillofacial Surg Clin N Am. 2006;18:255–60.
57. Rosenblatt SI, Dukatz T, Jahn R, Ramsdell C, Sakharova A, Henry M, et al. Insulin glargine dosing before next-day surgery: comparing three strategies. J Clin Anesth. 2012;24:610–7.
58. Likavec A, Moitra V, Greenberg J, Drum M, Sweitzer BJ. Comparison of preoperative blood glucose levels in patients receiving different insulin regimens. Anesthesiology. 2006;105:A567.
59. Scully C. Endocrinology. In: Scully's medical problems in dentistry. 7th ed. Haryana: Churchill Livingstone, Elsevier; 2014. p. 171–99.
60. Fauci AS, Kasper DL, Longo DL, Braunwald E, Hauser SL, Jameson JL, Loscalzo J. Harrison's internal medicine. 17th ed. https://doi.org/10.1111/j.1445-5994.2008.01837.
61. Palace MR. Perioperative management of thyroid dysfunction. Health Serv Insights. 2017; https://doi.org/10.1177/1178632916689677.
62. Bennet Guerrero E, Kramer DC, Schwinn DA. Effect of chronic and acute thyroid hormone reduction on perioperative outcome. Anesth Analg. 1997;85:30–6.
63. Liu MM, Reidy AB, Saatee S, et al. Perioperative steroid management: approaches based on current evidence. Anesthesiology. 2017;127:166–72.
64. Axelrod L. Perioperative management of patients treated with glucocorticoids. Endocrinol Metab Clin N Am. 2003;32:367–83.
65. Horio M, Orita Y, Fukunaga M. Assessment of renal function. In: Johnson RJ, Feehally J, editors. Comprehensive clinical nephrology. Philadelphia: Mosby; 2000. p. 3.1–6.
66. Anderson RJ, Schrier RW. Clinical spectrum of oliguric and nonoliguric acute renal failure. Contemporary issues in nephrology, Vol. 6. New York: Churchill Livingstone; 1980. p. 1–16.
67. Goren O, Matot I. Perioperative acute kidney injury. Br J Anaesth. 2015;115(Suppl 2):ii3–14.
68. Carrasco LR, Chou JC. Perioperative management of patients with renal disease. Oral Maxillofacial Surg Clin N Am. 2006;18:203–12.
69. India: Globocan 2018. International Agency for research on cancer. 2019. http://gco.iarc.fr/today/data/factsheets/populations/356-india-fact-sheets.pdf
70. Scully C. Malignant disease. In: Scully's medical problems in dentistry. 7th ed. Haryana: Churchill Livingstone, Elsevier; 2014. p. 576–93.
71. Motzer RJ, Geller NL, Bosl GJ. The effect of a 7-day delay in chemotherapy cycles on complete response and event-free survival in good-risk disseminated germ cell tumor patients. Cancer. 1990;66(5):857–61.
72. Demian NM, Shun JW, Kessel IL, Eid A. Oral surgery in patients undergoing chemoradiation therapy. Oral Maxillofacial Surg Clin N Am. 2014;26:193–207.
73. Yamashita J, Mc Cauley LK. Antiresorptives and osteonecrosis of the jaw. J Evid Based Dent Pract. 2012;12(Suppl 3):233–47.
74. Zimmermann C, Meurer MI, Grando LJ, et al. Dental treatment in patients with leukemia. J Oral Oncol. 2015;2015:Article ID 571739, 14 pages. https://doi.org/10.1155/2015/571739.
75. American Academy of Pediatric Dentistry. Guideline on dental management of pediatric patients receiving chemotherapy, hematopoietic cell transplantation, and/or radiation. J Pediat Dentistry. 2013;35(5):E185–93. http://www.ncbi.nlm.nih.gov/pubmed/24290549.
76. Lopez BC, Esteve CG, Perez MG. Dental treatment considerations in the chemotherapy patient. J Clin Exp Dent. 2011;3(1):e31–2.
77. Jacobson AS, Buchbinder D, Hu K, et al. Paradigm shifts in the management of osteoradionecrosis of the mandible. Oral Oncol. 2010;46(11):795–801.
78. Saad F, Brown J, Van Poznack C, et al. Incidence, risk factors and outcomes of osteonecrosis of the jaws: integrated analysis from three blinded active controlled phase III trials in cancer patients with bone metastasis. Ann Oncol. 2012;23(5):1341–7.

4

# Handling Medical Emergencies

Nallamilli V. S. Sekhar Reddy

## 4.1 Introduction

Oral and Maxillofacial Surgery has evolved over the last few decades. Although it is now practiced as a full-fledged hospital-based specialty, a significant amount of work is still carried out under local anesthesia; predisposing toward a medical emergency precipitated particularly by stress. Oral and Maxillofacial surgeons thus deal with the medical emergencies in an office or hospital setting on a regular basis.

Emergency team response in most countries is prompt. The published guidelines from these countries reflect this in the advice for the general practitioner; doing the essential minimum toward the sustenance of life in case of a medical emergency and to prioritize escalation of call for help to the emergency team. However, in some parts of the world, the response time of the emergency team is expected to be comparatively longer, due to various policy issues. The chapter considers these special circumstances, to suggest some additional measures toward the management of the emergency, while waiting for the arrival of the emergency team.

Also, the general advice in the management of a medical emergency during an outpatient procedure in a clinic is aimed at general practitioners, who may not necessarily be exposed to training in clinical skills like the placement of an intravenous cannula. Oral and Maxillofacial surgeons are expected to be well versed with this life-saving simple clinical skill and the protocols discussed here take this into consideration.

The management of emergency should follow the universally accepted ABCDE approach [1], which helps the clinician to follow a systematic approach in an emergency situation where the most life-threatening condition is assessed and is given the top priority. Lack of airway kills the patient first, then the lack of ability to breathe followed by the absence of circulation. ABCDE approach incorporates:

N. V. S. Sekhar Reddy (✉)
Panineeya Institute of Dental Sciences and Research Centre, Hyderabad, Telangana, India

A: Airway
B: Breathing
C: Circulation
D: Disability (refers to neurological function)
E: Exposure

Medical Emergencies that are life threatening and need immediate remedial measures on an emergency basis are discussed here:

1. Acute Asthmatic Attack
2. Adrenal Crisis
3. Airway Obstruction
4. Anaphylaxis
5. Chest Pain
6. Cardiac Arrest
7. Hypoglycemia
8. Tonic-Clonic Seizure
9. Syncope.

## 4.2 Acute Asthmatic Attack

Stress, Anxiety, and Infection can precipitate an asthmatic attack in individuals who are prone. Unfortunately, all three of them can be part of OMFS practice.

**Box 4.1**
Note: Asthma that is part of a generalized anaphylactic reaction needs Adrenaline via intramuscular route.

**Signs and Symptoms:**

- Difficulty in breathing
- Cough
- Wheezing
- Use of accessory muscles of respiration
- Tightness of chest

- Rapid breathing and Tachycardia
- Pale and anxious-looking face

**Management:**

- Keep the patient in a sitting position.
- Give two puffs of Salbutamol (100 µg/puff) inhaler [2, 3].
- If no rapid response, give further puffs through a spacer device.
- Consider oxygen supplementation.
- If no improvement, consider urgent transfer to a medical center.

### 4.2.1 Life-Threatening Acute Asthma

Asthmatic attack can sometimes be severe and may fail to respond to standard bronchodilator therapy. This can be fatal if no proper treatment is given. When an asthmatic attack failed to respond to the treatment and getting worse, the patient will need urgent transfer to appropriate medical center.

**Signs and symptoms of severe life-threatening asthma:**

- Silent chest, poor respiratory effort, cyanosis
- $SPO_2 < 92\%$
- Exhaustion
- Altered consciousness
- Weak or irregular pulse

**Treatment:**

- Urgent transfer to hospital is needed.
- Oxygen supplementation.
- Salbutamol 100 µg/puff; give four puffs through spacer device, followed by two puffs every 2 min according to response, up to a maximum of ten puffs or if there is nebulizer available, give salbutamol 5 mg [4].
- Hydrocortisone: 100 mg IV, or Prednisolone: 40–50 mg Orally [4].
- For children 5 years and above, use Oral Prednisolone 30–40 mg.
- For children less than 5 years, give salbutamol inhalation up to a maximum of ten puffs while awaiting transfer to an appropriate medical facility [2].

## 4.3 Acute Adrenal Insufficiency/Adrenal Crisis/Steroid Crisis/Addisonian Crisis

Sudden and severe hypotension in patients who cannot mount a normal stress-induced cortisol response. The stress can be physiological or psychological. Adrenal crisis can be seen in patients who were taking glucocorticoids regularly or who have taken glucocorticoids for a considerable period of time in the past, patients with Addison's disease, hypopituitarism, or in other conditions associated with decreased adrenocorticotropic hormone (ACTH) production.

> **Box 4.2**
> *Oxygen—Supports Combustion*
> *Keep cylinders away from open flames and heat sources*
> *Oxygen cylinder should be stored in a well-ventilated area*
> *Do not oil, grease, or lubricate cylinder controls.*

**Signs and Symptoms:**

- Severe hypotension, which can manifest as weakness, confusion, dizziness, drowsiness, loss of consciousness.
- Nausea, vomiting.
- Seizure may occur following deep faint.

**Treatment:**

- Lay patient flat.
- Give high flow oxygen.
- Arrange for urgent transfer to a medical center.
- Establish Intravenous access.
- Administer Hydrocortisone sodium succinate by IV. Dosage given below [5, 6]:
  - Children from age 2 to 11 years, 2–4 mg/kg body weight.
  - Above 11 years: give adult dose.
  - Adult dose: 100 mg by IV.
  - If unable to secure IV access, give the same dose by IM route.
- Start IV infusion of 0.9% Normal Saline.

## 4.4 Airway Obstruction

As the mouth is the primary area of our specialty, clinicians may have to deal with acute airway obstruction. As with everything else, prevention is the most important thing.

**Signs and Symptoms:**

- Distressed patient.
- Abnormal noises like gurgling, crowing, snoring.
- Forced inspiratory efforts.
- No sounds at all in complete airway obstruction
- Various degrees of cyanosis leading to loss of consciousness.

**Treatment** [7]:

- Encourage the patient to cough.
- If an object could be visualized, retrieve it with an appropriate instrument.
- If obstruction is caused by fluids, use high-volume suction.
- Back slaps: up to five back blows between the scapulae while the patient is supported leaning forward.
- Abdominal thrusts: (Heimlich maneuver) up to five abdominal thrusts by standing behind the patient.

- If obstruction fails to relieve, continue with five back blows alternating with abdominal thrusts.
- If these measures fail, the patient will lose consciousness. Lay the patient down on floor and start with CPR.
  - Start with chest compressions even if there is pulse, as chest compressions can help relieving the obstruction.
- If there is partial obstruction, which could not be relieved by the foregoing means, arrange for emergency transfer to appropriate medical care.
  - Patient may need oxygen supplementation.
- In patients with a completely obstructed airway, where the obstruction could not be relieved with these measures, where there are no facilities or skill to use a laryngoscope, emergency invasive procedures like jet insufflation or cricothyroidotomy may be needed as life-saving measures.
- Jet Insufflation involves placing a wide bore cannula (12–14 gauge) through cricothyroid membrane and connect this to a high flow oxygen source.
- It is advised to read further about Jet insufflation and Cricothyroidotomy as the full detailed description is beyond the scope of this textbook.

**Box 4.3**

Aspiration of small objects like burs, endodontic files, and reamers may not cause immediate life-threatening airway obstruction, but retrieval of these rather small and prickly instruments from lungs is a very difficult task needing bronchoscopy and can result in serious lung infections and damage. Prevention takes priority.

## 4.5 Anaphylaxis

Sudden onset, severe form of life-threatening allergic reaction, which can be seen following exposure to an allergen. Remember topical anesthetic gels, chlorhexidine mouth wash, and even contact with latex gloves can trigger anaphylaxis in individuals who are sensitive [8].

Prompt recognition and immediate response are key to success.

**Signs and Symptoms:**

- Face—red and hot.
- Generalized skin rash with itching.
- Various degrees of breathing difficulties manifested as stridor, wheezing, or hoarseness.
- Pulse may initially be rapid but can gradually become weak or impalpable.
- Hypotension can progress to cardiac arrest.

**Treatment:**

- Make sure airway is clear.
- Administer Adrenaline [9].
- Position the patient in supine position unless the patient prefers to sit up due to breathing difficulties.
- Make arrangements for emergency transfer to appropriate medical center.
- While waiting for transfer [10],
  - Oxygen supplementation at 15 L/min.
  - Keep assessing the airway and provide necessary support.
  - Chlorpheniramine maleate IM or IV.
  - Hydrocortisone sodium succinate IM or IV.
  - Establish Intravenous access.
  - Ringer's lactate solution or 0.9% Normal saline to support circulation.
  - Reassess the need for further adrenaline.
- Start CPR in case of cardiac arrest.

**Box 4.4**

Adrenaline is to be administered if there is severe respiratory distress or when there are signs of shock.

**Box 4.5**

Adrenaline—Life-saving drug for Anaphylaxis
Repeat after 5 min if not getting better
Supply: 1 mL ampoule containing 1 mg adrenaline in 1:1000 concentration
Site: I.M Anterolateral thigh
Dosage:
Adult: 500 μg IM 0.5 mL
Child More than 12 years: 500 μg IM 0.5 mL
Child 6–12 years: 300 μg IM 0.3 mL
Less than 6 years: 150 μg IM 0.15 mL

**Box 4.6**

**Second-line drugs:**
Hydrocortisone sodium succinate: 100 mg
Route: IM or Slow IV
12 years and adults: 200 mg IM/IV
6–12 years: 100 mg IM/IV
6 months to 6 years: 50 mg IM/IV
Chlorpheniramine Maleate
Supply: Chlorpheniramine Maleate 10 mg/1 mL Ampoule
Route: IM or IV
12 years and adults: 10 mg IM/IV
6–12 years: 5 mg IM/IV
6 months to 6 years: 2.5 mg IM/IV

## 4.6 Chest Pain

Experiencing chest pain in an outpatient office can be a frightening experience for both the patient and to the attending clinician. Thorough understanding of the pathophysiology of these acute cardiac events is very important for the clinician to stay composed and initiate appropriate measures to prevent mortality. Myocardial infarction may not always have the typical features of chest pain and especially diabetic patients may not have pain. Hence, a high index of suspicion is what is required.

Causes of chest pain:

- Angina
- Myocardial Infarction
- Hyperventilation

Hyperventilation is associated with anxiety and often a young person who is quite frightened of the intended treatment, the breathing gets very heavy resulting in decreased carbon dioxide levels in the blood.

### 4.6.1 Angina

Transient decrease of oxygen supply to cardiac muscle precipitates pain.

Precipitating factors:

Anxiety, stress, exertion, strong emotions, heavy meal, and extreme weather conditions.

**Signs and Symptoms:**

If you are looking for typical symptoms of chest pain, you may miss some cases. List of all possible presentations being:

- Pain, heaviness, or tightness in the chest.
- Pain in the neck, throat, arms, stomach, and back.
- Pain can be associated with light-headedness, nausea, shortness of breath, and sweating.

**Management:**

- Stop the procedure and reassure the patient.
- Clear the mouth from any foreign bodies.
- Let the patient attain a comfortable position (may not like to lie flat).
- Administer Glyceryl trinitrate sublingual spray or Glyceryl trinitrate sublingual tablets [11].
- Oxygen supplementation.
- Check for any irregularities of pulse.

Simple angina should resolve very quickly with rest alone or with sublingual glyceryl trinitrate spray or tablets. In simple angina, the cardiac output is not impaired, and pulse should be regular. In a patient with chest pain, having an irregular pulse, suspect MI.

### 4.6.2 Myocardial Infarction (Heart Attack)

Progressive/Sudden ischemia of the cardiac muscle leads to necrosis of cardiac muscle. This can cause cardiac arrest.

**Signs and Symptoms:**

- Same as angina but can be more severe in intensity and lasts long.
- Pain in the center of the chest.
- Pain radiates to neck, arms, jaw, back, or stomach.
- Pain associated with sweating, vomiting, shortness of breath, lightheadedness, or dizziness.
- Chest discomfort associated with a feeling of weakness and unwell.
- Chest pain associated with an irregular pulse.
- Chest pain fails to relieve with two doses of Nitroglycerin sublingual Spray.
- Chest pain getting progressively worse.
- Patient with previous experience of angina, now experiencing an unusual type of chest discomfort.
- Weak pulse.
- Falling Blood pressure.
- Skin—pale and clammy.

**Management:**

- The moment MI is suspected, arrange for an emergency transfer of the patient to an appropriate medical facility.
- Let the patient attain the most comfortable position. The patient may like to sit up to avoid venous congestion on the heart and lungs.
- Administer soluble Aspirin, 300 mg [12]. Chew and swallow for rapid action.
- By this time, the patient should have received at least two doses of sublingual Glyceryl trinitrate spray or tablets [12], this may need a repeating.
- While waiting for transfer, the following measures can be done, but do not delay transfer, early expert care improves outcome.
  - Establish IV access.
  - Give antiemetic Metoclopramide hydrochloride by IV [13].

    Adult > 60 kg, dose 10 mg

    Small-sized Adult <60 kg, dose 5 mg
  - Administer analgesia - Paracetamol by slow IV (Morphine, diamorphine 7 fentanyl, are not easily available in India) [13].

Adult >50 kg, dose 1000 mg in 100 mL
Small-sized Adult <50 kg, dose 750 mg in 75 mL
When no IV access, alternatively, give Oral Paracetamol 650 mg

- Do not routinely administer oxygen. Supplemental oxygen only when hypoxic.
- Patients where consciousness level deteriorates.
  - Watch for signs of cardiac arrest.
  - Start CPR, if cardiac arrest occurs.

**Box 4.7**
Drugs for MI:
Glyceryl Trinitrate Aerosol Spray: 400 µg/metered dose
Glyceryl Trinitrate: 300-µg tablets
Soluble Aspirin: 300-mg tablets
Metoclopromide: 10-mg solution for IV
Paracetamol: 1000-mg/100-mL solution for IV
Paracetamol: 500-mg tablets
Paracetamol 650 mg tablets

## 4.7 Cardiac Arrest

Cardiac arrest is a sudden loss of heart function resulting in hypoxic damage to body organs. Lack of oxygen to the brain causes loss of consciousness, victim falls to the ground and stops breathing. Cardiac arrest can occur suddenly with or without any symptoms.

Following cardiac arrest neurons start to die within 4–6 min without oxygen. Chances of survival can be increased by early defibrillation (where indicated) and good-quality Cardiopulmonary Resuscitation, that's instituted quickly and performed with minimal interruptions. Automated External Defibrillators (AED) are increasingly available and these can analyze the rhythm, whether it's shockable or not and can suggest you through the process of CPR by voice commands. In centers where AEDs are not available, CPR is continued until appropriate help arrives. Often, in busy countries like India, this can take quite a considerable amount of time, so hospitals and healthcare establishments should be encouraged to buy AEDs.

Recognition of cardiac arrest:

- Unconscious
- Unresponsive
- Not breathing normally (agonal breathing/gasping) or absent breathing
  - Some people may have a seizure when cardiac arrest occurs as a result of severe cerebral hypoxia.

**Box 4.8**
Chest pain in a patient with previous history of stable angina: Urgent transfer to appropriate medical facility is to be done, if the patient feels the pain is unusual or if the pain doesn't resolve with rest and Sublingual Glyceryl Trinitrate.

**Box 4.9**
Do not waste time, for example, trying to find a vein while the ambulance is waiting! Antiplatelet medication (aspirin) within few minutes of suspecting MI and early thrombolysis by the Physicians can significantly reduce the mortality associated.

**Management:**

- Call for help and ask to bring defibrillator and emergency drug kit.
- Second person can call for ambulance.
- Start CPR [14]
  - CPR can be executed in the dental chair.
- Start with chest compressions.
  - Second person checks airway, gets ready for ventilations, preferably using a bag valve mask.
- Give 30 chest compressions.
- Give two ventilations.
- Carry on CPR at 30:2 until expert help or AED arrives.
- Stop CPR when patient shows signs of life.

CPR with AED:

- Continue with CPR while the pads of AED are being attached.
- Stop CPR and do not touch victim while the AED starts analyzing the rhythm [15].
  - Nonshockable rhythm observed by AED—continue CPR until signs of life or AED starts analyzing rhythm again [16].
  - Shock advised by AED—Make sure no one touches the patient directly or indirectly—Deliver the shock.
- Continue CPR at 30:2 while the pads remain attached.
- After 2 min, AED will start reanalyzing the rhythm and the cycle to be continued until the patient shows signs of life.

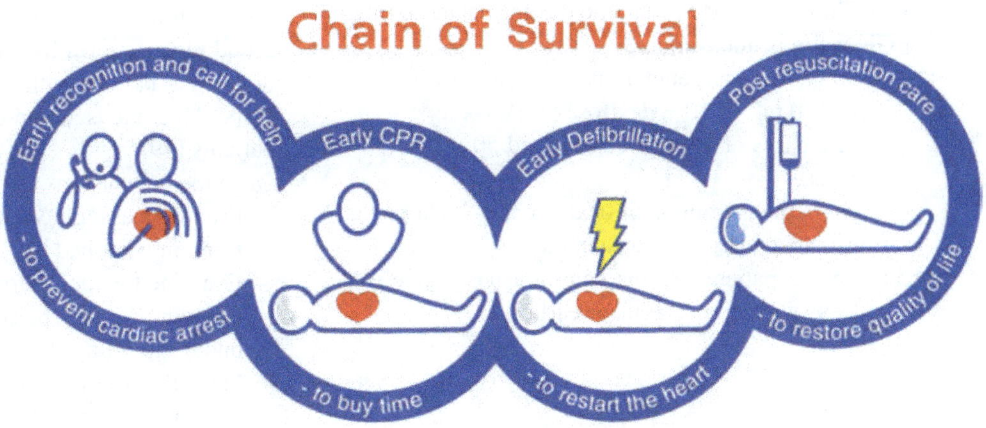


**Fig. 4.1** Chain of survival

- Once the patient regains consciousness, put the patient in recovery position and maintain saturations above 94%, supplemental oxygen may be needed.
- The patient should receive appropriate post-resuscitation care and keep monitoring as chances of a second cardiac arrest is high in the immediate post-resuscitation period.

To improve overall outcome in cardiac arrest patients, it is necessary to follow these four important aspects of care:

1. *Early recognition and call for help*—do not waste time trying to ascertain if pulse is there or not. A patient who is unresponsive and not breathing should be considered in cardiac arrest unless until proven otherwise.
2. *Early CPR*—the victim soon after cardiac arrest will have some oxygen in the blood and starting with chest compressions early will be extremely beneficial to the cells starved of oxygen.
3. *Early Defibrillation*: The chances of reversing a shockable rhythm diminish with the passage of time.
4. *Post resuscitation care:* All patients who have been successfully reversed from cardiac arrest should be transferred to an appropriate center with cardiac care facilities.

The four points are incorporated into this internationally recognized "chain of survival," which is given here (adapted from the Resuscitation Council UK; website: https://www.resus.org.uk/EasysiteWeb/getresource.axd?AssetID=3907&type=Full&servicetype=Attachment) (Fig. 4.1):

**Box 4.10**

All healthcare workers should undergo proper training in CPR. Healthcare organizations throughout the world are now insisting on a CPR certificate. Such a training has to be done on a periodic basis so that the skills are retained. The reader is strongly advised to undergo training periodically and a valid certificate will prevent you from future litigation if an unfortunate event occurs to one of your patients.

## 4.8 Hypoglycemia

Glucose is essential for the effective functioning of neurons. When the glucose levels in blood drop to a very low level, brain function will get affected and if the glucose levels are not restored quickly, permanent neurologic damage can occur within 4–6 min. Hypoglycemia can occur in diabetic patients taking Insulin, who skipped meal, and is also the leading cause of loss of consciousness in children. Hypoglycemia occurs when blood glucose level falls below 70 mg/dL.

**Signs and Symptoms:**

- Anxious, confused, irritable, or aggressive behavior.
- Sweating
- Nausea and vomiting
- Hungry
- Visual disturbances
- Convulsions
- Loss of consciousness.

**Management** [17]:

Management depends on consciousness level and the ability of the patient to take food orally without the risk of aspiration.

- Conscious patient:
  - 10–20 g of glucose

    10 g of glucose in two teaspoons of granulated sugar
    Two teaspoons of Glucon-D powder contain 15 g of Glucose
  - Can be repeated in 10–15 min
  - Once the patient's condition improves, provide a carbohydrate snack or meal as appropriate to raise blood glucose level.
- Unconscious patient:
  - Check if airway is clear—ABCDE approach
  - Put patient in recovery position
  - Oxygen supplementation at 15 L/min

- Give Glucagon by IM route into the anterolateral thigh
- If Glucagon is not available

  Arrange for emergency transfer of patient

  Give 100 mL of 10% dextrose by IV route

  Severe cases of hypoglycemia need 50 mL of 50% Dextrose

  Higher concentrations of dextrose are thicker solutions, need a larger bore cannula.

  Once the patient regains consciousness, give oral glucose and carbohydrate as earlier.

**Box 4.11**

Glucagon either by IM or SC route

Dose: Adult—1 mg

Child under 8 years or less than 25 kg should be given 500 µg (0.5 mg)

Keep patient in lateral position to prevent risk of aspiration

## 4.9 Grand Mal Seizures

Enquire with patients about how frequently they get seizures and their compliance with medication. Patients with frequent seizure history or patients who are irregular with their medications are more likely to have a seizure while having dental procedures. Provide the treatment in a calm, stress-free environment, avoid any seizure-triggering factors.

**Signs and Symptoms:**

- Seizure activity may have a brief period of aura, where the patient can behave indifferently, spaced out, and detached.
- The patient will go rigid, lose consciousness, lose balance, and may cry-tonic (rigidity) phase.
- After a few seconds, sudden rhythmic jerking movements of the body lasting for up to 2 min.
- Mouth goes rigid. Frothy saliva can be noticed.
- Cyanosis around the mouth can be noticed as breathing stops.
- Possible urination.
- Following the seizure, patient can go into varying periods of confused state and may fall asleep.

**Treatment** [18]:

- Prevent injury to patient
  - Remove all the sharps away
  - Create safe space around a fitting patient
  - Provide cushions like a pillow or blanket
  - Pay particular attention to head
- Do not restrain
- Do not attempt to insert any object between teeth
- Supplemental oxygen at 15 L/min
- Have a suction readily available, with a yankauer suction tube clear oral cavity of any fluids after seizure stops [19].
- Ascertain hypoglycemia as a possible cause by checking blood glucose level by a finger prick test. This should be done in a patient with no previous history of epilepsy. Hypoglycemia is common in children and in diabetic patients [19].
- Once the convulsions are stopped:
  - Provide reassurance and empathy to the patient
  - Explain what had happened
  - Examine the mouth for any fluids and use suction
  - Examine for any bleeding, lacerations of tongue secondary to biting
  - Place the patient in a recovery position
  - Examine for any other injuries
  - Provide oxygen as required
  - Stay with the patient until the patient is fully recovered
  - Do not give anything orally until the patient is fully conscious, to avoid the risk of aspiration
  - Do not attempt to arouse a patient who is sleeping after a convulsive episode
- Prolonged Convulsions beyond 5 min or repeated seizure activity without proper recovery constitutes—status epilepticus [20], which can be fatal and needs to be managed as:
  - Make arrangements for urgent transfer to appropriate medical center
  - Administer midazolam intravenously [21]
  - Where IV access is not possible:

    Rectal route can be used effectively, especially in children.

    Buccal midazolam gel can be instilled into buccal vestibule with the help of a syringe with no needle.

    Midazolam sprays, which can be used via nasal route, are slowly being available in India.

    Buccal and nasal routes are increasingly being used and the reader is advised to look up for more up-to-date information as suitable formulations are not routinely available in India.

**Box 4.12**

Midazolam Dosage:

I.V route: Above 12 years, 5 mg slowly—patient may need encouragement to breathe after IV midazolam.

I.M route: Adult: 0.2 mg/kg, Not to exceed 10 mg in total.

Child: 0.1–0.2 mg/kg, not to exceed 10 mg in total

Nasal Spray: Child: 0.2 mg/kg body weight (Max: 5 mg/nares)

Rectal: Adult and children above 12 years: 10–20 mg, can be repeated once after 10–15 min if needed

Child 2–11 years: 5–10 mg, can be repeated once after 10–15 min

**Box 4.13**
Remember generalized tonic-clonic seizures can be seen in:

- Epilepsy
- Head injury
- Hypoglycemia
- Hypoxia
- Alcohol withdrawal
- Drugs
- Local anesthesia overdose or Intravascular injection
- Febrile convulsions

**Box 4.14**
Midazolam is a benzodiazepine that carries the risk of respiratory depression. Patients need close monitoring after drug administration and may need respiratory support.

**Box 4.15**
Typical grand mal seizure, in a known epileptic patient, where the seizure has subsided within a couple of minutes, patient can be discharged with the carer, provided all the vital signs are with in normal range. Urgent hospital transfer is indicated in all other epileptic seizures.

## 4.10 Syncope

Energy demands of the brain are met primarily by oxidation of glucose. A regular and constant supply of glucose and oxygen is essential for brain function. Supply of both glucose and oxygen depends on effective perfusion of the brain. When brain perfusion decreases beyond a critical level, the patient loses consciousness and the balance gets affected and the patient falls.

**Signs and Symptoms:**

- Feeling unwell
- Nausea, Lightheadedness
- Blurred vision
- Pallor
- Sweaty, especially forehead
- Sudden loss of consciousness and collapse
- Seizure, if the patient is not positioned in a horizontal position quickly.

**Management** [22]:

- Clear airway and reassure
- Change position to a flat or legs elevated
- Let fresh air by opening a window or a fan
- Do not let people to crowd around
- Place cold towel on forehead
- Supplemental Oxygen can be given, but usually, if it's simple faint consciousness should recover very quickly.
- Once recovered, encourage the patient to have a sugary drink.
- Examine for injuries secondary to fall.

## 4.11 Other Causes of Loss of Consciousness

Although syncope is the most common cause of loss of consciousness, the other causes should also be borne in mind, as some of them can be quite serious, such as:

- Postural Hypotension
- Hyperventilation
- Epilepsy
- Adrenaline crisis
- Hypoglycemia
- Stroke
- Cardiac Arrest

**Postural Hypotension:**

- Loss of consciousness following a sudden change of posture from supine or sitting to standing upright.
- Usually in patients who are taking antihypertensives or elderly.
- Place them in a supine position and bring them to the upright position slowly.

**Hyperventilation:**

Excessive breathing in an anxiety state or excessive crying resulting in drop of blood $CO_2$ level.

- Feeling lightheaded, dizzy
- Chest discomfort to chest pain
- Muscle spasms, especially in hands and feet
- Tingling or numbness in the arms and in the perioral region
- Control the crying/breathing through suggestion
- Use a paper bag to rebreath exhaled air to build up $CO_2$ levels

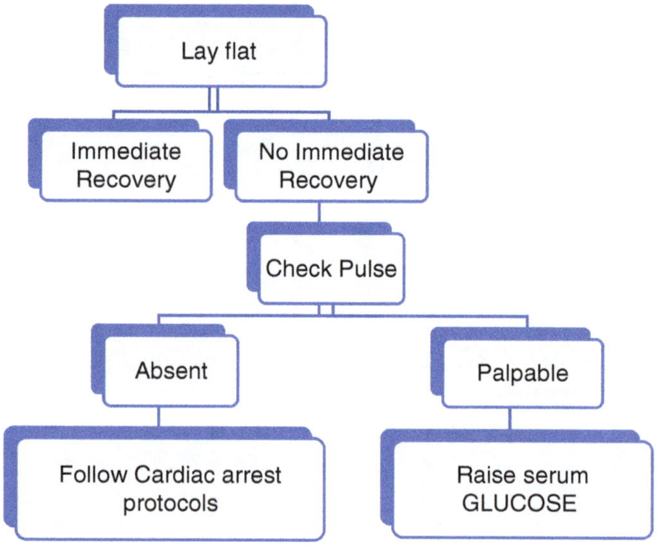


**Flowchart 4.1** Management algorithm for a collapsed patient where the cause of collapse is not known

## 4.12 Conclusion

Preparedness for emergency is the key and when you are prepared, emergencies are easier to manage. The maxillofacial surgeon should be able to recognize these conditions and initiate appropriate management before professional emergency help is available. More often, maxillofacial surgeon is the lone clinician and is the sole responder in an emergency. It is prudent for the surgeon to know what to do and what not to do to get the best out of the worst scenario or situation.

It is imperative that the maxillofacial surgeons thoroughly understand the pathophysiology and extend their skills to recognize and manage expeditiously and effectively the emergencies that may arise. It is advisable that the contemporary clinicians update their knowledge and skills periodically with proper training courses.

Protocols given here are based on the currently available evidence, keeping in view of the local healthcare systems and access. As protocols are only suggestive, the clinician is strongly advised to use his or her own discretion when dealing with medical emergencies (Table 4.1 Flowchart 4.1).

**Table 4.1** Causes of loss of consciousness and its age distribution

| Causes of unconsciousness | | |
|---|---|---|
| Child | Teen-mid 30 | Above 40 |
| Hypoglycemia | Syncope | Cardiovascular causes |
| Epilepsy | Hypoglycemia | |
| Congenital heart disease | Epilepsy | |

## References

1. Thim T, Krarup NHV, et al. Initial asseement and treatment with the Airway, Breathing, Circulation, Disability, Exposure (ABCDE) approach. Int J Gen Med. 2012;5:117–21.
2. Saglani S, Fleming L, Sonnappa S, et al. Advances in the aetiology, management, and prevention of acute asthmatic attack in children. Lancet Child Adolesc Health. 2019;3(5):354–64.
3. Fergeson JE, Patel SS, Lockey RF. Acute asthma, prognosis, and treatment. J Allergy Clin Immunol. 2017;139(2):438–47.
4. Marsh B, Drake MG. Outpatient management of acute exacerbations of obstructive lung diseases. Med Clin N Am. 2017;101(3):537–51.
5. Hahner S. Acute adrenal crisis and mortality in adrenal insufficiency. Ann Endocrinol. 2018;79(3):164–6.
6. Paur THK, Stikkelbroeck NMMI, et al. Adrenal crisis: still a deadly event in the 21st century. Am J Med. 2016;129(3):339.
7. Schwartz A. Airway mangement for the oral surgery patient. Oral Maxillofac Surg Clin N Am. 2018;30(2):207–26.
8. Chapman J, Lalkhen AG. Anaphylaxis. Anaesth Intensive Care Med. 2017;18(1):16–21.
9. Young NH, Nimmo GR. Anaphylaxis. Medicine. 2017;45(3):157–62.
10. Moore LE, Kemp AM, Kemp SF. Recognition, treatment, and prevention of Anaphylaxis. Immunol Allergy Clin N Am. 2015;35(2):363–74.
11. Waller JR, Waller DG. Drugs for systemic hypertension and angina. Medicine. 2018;46(9):566–72.
12. Dym H, Barzani G, et al. Emergency drugs for the dental office. Dent Clin N Am. 2016;60(2):287–94.

13. Herman WW, Ferguson HW. Dental care for patients with heart failure: an update. J Am Dent Assoc. 2010;141(7):845–53.
14. Yates EJ, Schmidbauer S, et al. Out of hospital cardiac arrest termination of resuscitation with ongoing CPR: an observational study. Resuscitation. 2018;130:21–7.
15. Fernando SM, Vaillancourt C, et al. Analysis of bystander CPR quality out of hospital cardiac arrest using data derived from AED. Resuscitation. 2018;18:138–43.
16. Pollack RA, Brown SP, et al. Bystander automated external defibrillator application in non-shockable out of patient cardiac arrest. Resuscitation. 2019;137:168–74.
17. Bansal N, Dhaliwal R, et al. Management of diabetes in elderly. Med Clin N Am. 2015;99(2):351–77.
18. Johnson EI. Seizures & epilepsy. Med Clin N Am. 2019;103(2):309–24.
19. Thijs RD, Surges R, et al. Epilepsy in adults. Lancet. 2019;393(10172):689–701.
20. Paris M, Reddy U. Update on the management of status epilepticus. Anaesth Intensive Care Med. 2018;19(3):83–6.
21. Papavasiliou AS, Kotsalis C, et al. Intravenous midazolam in convulsive status epilepticus in children with pharmacoresistant epilepsy. Epilepsy Behav. 2009;14(4):661–4.
22. Numeroso F, Mossini G, et al. Emergency department management of patients with syncope according to the 2018 ESC guidelines. Int J Cardiol. 2019;283:119–21.

# Part III

# Usage of Anesthesia

5

# OMS and Local Anesthesia

Reena Rachel John

## 5.1 Introduction

Pain, the dreaded symptom, is an unpleasant sensation that draws the attention of the individual as a whole. Its management has greatly evolved in the field of dentistry, starting from the leaves of a coca tree to articaine, Comfort Control Syringe (CCS) system, Transcutaneous Electrical Nerve Stimulation (TENS), Computer-Controlled Local Anesthetic Delivery System as well as oral and intravenous sedatives. Apart from all these, local anesthesia (LA) is the favored mode of pain control in the profession. The painless surgery under LA is must; otherwise, endogenous catecholamines are released if there is excessive pain during dental treatment, which can alter the hemodynamic status such as an increase in blood pressure and heart rate and even dysrhythmias [1].

### 5.1.1 Historical Background

The first local anesthetic isolated from the leaves of a coca tree in 1860 by Neiman was cocaine, and it was Karl Koller in 1884 who showed the anesthetic effect of Cocaine. In 1905, Einhorn popularized Procaine as an effective local anesthetic. It was derived from benzoic acid and diethyl amino ethanol. In 1948, the anesthetic property of lignocaine was discovered by Lofgren, and T. Gordh applied it in dental surgery [2].

### 5.1.2 Definition

Local anesthesia is defined as a reversible loss of sensation in the circumscribed area of the body caused by depression of excitation in the nerve endings or inhibition of the conduction process in peripheral nerves [2].

R. R. John (✉)
Department of Oral and Maxillofacial Surgery,
Vinayaka Mission's Sankarachariar Dental College and Hospital,
VMRF DU, Salem, India

### 5.1.3 Ideal Characteristic of Local Anesthesia

An ideal local anesthetic must have the following characteristics:

- It should be nonirritating and nonallergic.
- It should not cause structural changes to nerve and have low systemic toxicity.
- Its onset of action should be short and should be stable in solution.
- It should be effective as both injectable and topical application.
- Its action should be long enough to allow the procedure to be completed.

## 5.2 Classification (Tables 5.1 and 5.2)

**Table 5.1** Classification of local anesthetic agents: based on chemical structure

| Chemical structure | Example |
|---|---|
| Esters of benzoic acid | Cocaine, Benzocaine, Butacaine, Piperocaine, Tetracaine |
| Esters of para amino benzoic acid | Procaine, Chloroprocaine, Propoxycaine |
| Amides | Articaine, Bupivicaine, Lidocaine, Dibucaine, Mepivacaine, Prilocaine |
| Quinolone derivatives | Centbucridine |

**Table 5.2** Classification of local anesthetic agents: based on duration of action

| Duration of action | Example |
|---|---|
| Ultra short acting<br>Pulpal anesthesia: less than 10 min<br>Soft-tissue anesthesia: 30–45 min | Chloroprocaine, Procaine |
| Short acting<br>Pulpal anesthesia: 5–10 min<br>Soft-tissue anesthesia: 60–120 min | Lidocaine, Prilocaine |
| Medium acting<br>Pulpal anesthesia: 45–90 min<br>Soft-tissue anesthesia: 120–240 min | Mepivacine, Articaine |
| Long acting<br>Pulpal anesthesia: 90–180 min<br>Soft-tissue anesthesia: 240–540 min | Bupivicaine, Etidocaine |

## 5.3 Local Anesthetic Agents

The LA agents have been divided into Esters and Amides groups. The commonly used Amides are Lidocaine, Articaine, and Bupivacain [2].

### 5.3.1 Lidocaine (Lignocaine)

Lofgren in 1943 introduced the prototype amide local anesthetic [2], i.e., Lidocaine.

The other similar names are xylocaine, octocaine, dentocaine. Chemically, it is Diethyl 2, 6 dimethyl acetanilide. The maximum recommended dosage for Lignocaine with vasoconstrictor is 7 mg/kg not exceeding 500 mg and without vasoconstrictor is 4.4 mg/kg not exceeding 300 mg. Its onset of action is 2–3 min and duration of action with vasoconstrictor is 45–75 min, without vasoconstrictor is less than 30 min. Its contraindications include Ehlers Danlos syndrome and Attention-deficit hyperactive syndrome. Lignocaine is available in the form of jelly, spray, patches, and ointments. The toxicity arises from inadvertent intravascular administration or from overdose.

Recently, Howlader et al. [3] suggested open reduction and internal fixation (ORIF) of isolated subcondylar fractures under local anesthesia by using 2% lidocaine with 1:200,000 epinephrine for mandibular nerve block and superior cervical plexus blocks (SCPB).

To anesthetize the cutaneous branches of SCP (lesser occipital, greater auricular, transverse cervical, and supraclavicular nerve), the solution is deposited at the midpoint of the posterior border of sternocleidomastoid muscle border, as well as inferior and superior to that point subcutaneously creating a field block.

The anesthetic agent selection should be based on three main clinical considerations: anesthetic potency and latency, onset, and duration. The composition of the local anesthetic solution is shown in Table 5.3.

**Table 5.3** Composition of local anaesthetic solution (Lignocaine with Adrenaline)

| Ingredients | Functions |
|---|---|
| Lignocaine HCl 2% (21.3 mg) | Anesthetic agent |
| Adrenaline 1:80,000 (0.0125 mg) | Vasoconstrictor, decreased absorption of LA in blood |
| Sodium Metabisulfite (0.5 mg) | Preservative |
| Methyl Paraben (1.0 mg) | Preservative to increase shelf life |
| Sodium Chloride (0.6 mg) | Isotonicity of solution to the tissues |
| Sodium Hydroxide | To maintain and adjust pH |
| Thymol | Fungicidal |
| Distilled water | Dilution |
| Nitrogen Bubble | 1–2 mm in diameter, present to prevent oxygen from being trapped in cartridge and potentially destroying vasopressor or vasoconstrictor. |

### 5.3.2 Bupivacaine

Its chemical name is 1 butyl-2,6piperoloxylidine hydrochloride.

It is four times more potent than prilocaine, lidocaine, and mepivacaine. It is less toxic than lidocaine and mepivacaine and it is metabolized in the liver by amidases and excretion via kidney 16% unchanged. Its onset of action is similar to lidocaine, mepivacaine, and prilocaine. Effective dental concentration is 0.5% and anesthetic half-life is 2.5 h.

Maximum recommended dose is 1.3 mg/kg body wt to a maximum of 90 mg. Because of its long duration of action, it is advisable for use in lengthy surgical procedure and the management of postoperative pain. Hence, the patient's requirement for postoperative opioid analgesics is lessened when bupivacaine is used. Bupivacaine is not recommended in young patients as the risk of self-mutilation is increased.

The duration of soft-tissue anesthesia has been consistently shown to be longer than with lidocaine [4] and thereby reducing postoperative pain experience [5].

### 5.3.3 Articaine

Its chemical structure is 3-N Propylaminoproprionylamino 2-Carbomethoxy 4-Methylthiophene hydrochloride.

The potency of Articaine is 1.5 times more than lignocaine and 1.9 times than procaine. Its onset of action when used with vasoconstrictor is 1–2 min. Half-life is approximately 21 min and it is metabolized to pharmacologically inactive metabolite called articaine acid glucoronide. Since it is rapidly biotransformed to its inactive metabolite, it is a safe local anesthetic agent. It is excreted via kidney

**Table 5.4** Maximum recommended dose of common Local Anesthetic used

| Local Anesthetic | mg/kg | mg/lb | MRD (mg) |
|---|---|---|---|
| *Articaine* | | | |
| With vasoconstrictor | 7.0 | 3.2 | 500 |
| *Bupivacaine* | | | |
| With vasoconstrictor | 1.3 | 0.6 | 90 |
| *Lidocaine* | | | |
| No vasoconstrictor | 4.4 | 2.0 | 300 |
| With vasoconstrictor | 6.6 | 3.0 | 500 |

unchanged (5–10%) and as metabolite (90%). The maximum recommended dosage for articaine is 0.8 mg/kg body weight.

Contraindications for the use of articaine are Idiopathic or congenital methemoglobinuria, hemoglobinopathies, hypoxia, and in patients with cardio-respiratory failures. Prolonged paraesthesia has been reported as a complication following inferior alveolar nerve block (IANB) [6].

Articaine with epinephrine is the best choice to improve anesthesia in both inflamed and in uninflamed tissues with good results, and more effective anesthesia for longer duration can be achieved [7]. Table 5.4 shows maximum recommended dose of commonly used LA.

## 5.4 Vasoconstrictors

Importance of vasoconstrictors in local anesthetic solution include

1. To decrease the tissue perfusion and therefore to decrease the blood flow at the site of drug administration, which further decreases the absorption of local anesthetics into the circulatory system. Therefore, the blood levels of the anesthetic agents remain low, thereby decreasing the risk of toxicity [2].
2. It also increases the time taken by the local anesthetic to be absorbed from the site of administration and therefore increases the duration of action of the local anesthetic.

Most commonly used vasoconstrictors are epinephrine, norepinephrine, levonordefrin hydrochloride, phenylephrine hydrochloride.

### 5.4.1 Dilution of Vasoconstrictor

The explanation of 1:1000 vasoconstrictor concentration is that 1 g/1000 mg of solute is present in 1000 ml of the solution, which means 1 mg of solute in 1 ml of solution. In the local anesthetic solution, the concentration of vasoconstrictor is less. The concentrations used are 1:80,000 or 1:100,000 or 1:200,000. The concentration of 1:100,000 of the vasoconstrictor would contain 1000 mg in 100,000 ml of the solution. Therefore, 1 ml of 1:100,000 concentration would contain 0.01 mg in 1 ml.

**Table 5.5** Quantity of vasoconstrictor with varying dilutions

| Concentration (dilution) | Milligrams per milliliter (mg/ml) | Micrograms per milliliter (μg/ml) | Microgram per cartridge (1.8 ml) |
|---|---|---|---|
| 1:1000 | 1.0 | 1000 | |
| 1:2500 | 0.4 | 400 | |
| 1:10,000 | 0.1 | 100 | |
| 1:20,000 | 0.05 | 50 | 90 |
| 1:30,000 | 0.033 | 33.3 | 73 |
| 1:50,000 | 0.02 | 20 | 36 |
| 1:80,000 | 0.0125 | 12.5 | 27.5 |
| 1:100,000 | 0.01 | 10 | 18 |
| 1:200,000 | 0.05 | 5 | 9 |

The absorption of vasoconstrictors is dose dependent and may last from minutes to half an hour. The patients with cardiovascular compromise are at increased risk with endogenously released epinephrine in response to stress rather than the epinephrine, which is injected with the local anesthetic (Table 5.5).

## 5.5 Causes of Failure of LA

1. Anatomic variation
2. Bifid or double nerve supply
3. Secondary supply by a soft-tissue nerve
4. Inadequate dose
5. Injection into the blood vessel
6. Degradation of vasoconstrictor
7. Patient having sepsis

## 5.6 LA Toxicity and Antidote for Toxicity

Symptoms, which reflect toxicity from the administration of local anesthetic solution, may range from mild cutaneous reactions to severe life-threatening anaphylactic reactions. There are a variety of methods and drugs to treat these reactions symptomatically. However, the reversal of toxicity, including damage to vital organs such as the heart and brain, is still less understood. A clinically efficient antidote for a complete reversal of toxicity is still beyond our grasp currently.

### 5.6.1 Reversal of Cardiomyotoxicity

Intravenous lipid emulsion (IVLE) is being reported as a rescue measure for LA toxicity. This has been studied and proven in both animal models and in limited human trials with successful resuscitation outcomes. The lipid emulsion acts on the plasma and tissue and extracts the lipophilic anesthetic molecules, thereby reversing their inhibitory myocardial effects. Bolus doses of 1.2–2 ml/kg followed by continuous infusion of 0.25–0.5 ml/kg/min are currently advocated for adequate efficacy. This drug needs to be used judiciously as optimal dosages have not been established and the risks of overdosage are not clearly understood.

## 5.7 Reversal of Soft-Tissue Anesthesia

The duration of soft-tissue anesthesia often exceeds that of pulpal or bony anesthesia. This is an important reason for the occurrence of undesirable events like accidental lip or tongue biting, difficulties in speaking, eating, or drinking liquids, etc. Various drugs have been studied to decrease the postoperative duration of anesthesia. Of the various drugs tried clinically, phentolamine is one drug, which has demonstrated appreciable clinical efficacy.

Phentolamine is a nonselective alpha-adrenergic antagonist that is reversible. Its main action is vasodilatation. It has been used effectively for controlling hypertensive emergencies, especially in pheochromocytomas. In dental practice, Phentolamine in the form of phentolamine mesylate injections has been used as a reversal agent against LA by reversing the action of vasoconstrictors in the LA solution and expedites the metabolism of the LA molecules. The recommended dose for phentolamine is the administration of 1.8 ml of the solution containing 0.4 mg of phentolamine mesylate immediately after treatment.

## 5.8 Plain Local Anesthetic (Without Epinephrine)

It is preferred for patients having comorbidities such as circulatory disorder to avoid complications and adverse systemic effects of vasoconstrictors [8]. Lip laceration is one of the common cases, which are attended to by a maxillofacial surgeon in the emergency department for suturing. Localized blanching caused by the use of local anesthetic with adrenalin at the lacerated wound causes difficulty in locating the exact demarcation between skin, white roll, and lip. Therefore, LA without epinephrine is preferred in such cases before suturing [9].

## 5.9 Topical Local Anesthetic Agent

The solution used for this purpose is 5% Lignocaine, 10% Lignocaine, combination of 2.5% lignocaine and 2.5% prilocaine [10]. They are indicated in patients [11, 12]

- For removal of maxillary and mandibular arch bars
- Gingival probing
- Deep Scaling
- Closure of facial lacerations in younger children
- Before LA injections in small patients

In suture and staple removal

## 5.10 Surface Anesthesia

The form of drug used to obtain this includes ointment, gel, viscous, cream, spray, etc. Topical application of these forms can produce anesthesia on the surface, particularly of the oral mucosa.

This is used often, before an actual injection for L.A, at the site of injection, in order to reduce the pain of the needle prick itself. It can also be used to obtund pain in situations where the oral mucosa is breached, as in an ulcer in the oral mucosa. The gel may also be used to anesthetize the surface mucosa, e.g., nasal, pharyngeal, etc., before a diagnostic endoscopy.

The concentration of a local anesthetic applied topically is typically greater than the same drug administered by injection. Drugs that are commonly employed in topical L.A formulations are Benzocaine and Lidocaine.

EMLA, which is a eutectic mixture of local anesthetic agents, lignocaine, & prilocaine in the ratio 1:1 by weight, has been found to be a very useful topical agent to be applied on the skin, before painful procedures like injection, venipuncture, etc. and is used extensively in children. This particular cream, which is oil-in-water emulsion, may also be used for surface anesthesia of the oral mucosa for purposes listed earlier.

## 5.11 Methods of Local Anesthetic Administration

There are major three different types of methods:

- Local infiltration
- Field block
- Nerve block

In local infiltration, deposition of the local anesthetic solution in the area of the surgery to anesthetize small terminal nerve endings. Field block involves the deposition of anesthetic solution near the large terminal nerve branches to prevent the passage of impulses from teeth to the central nervous system. In nerve block, local anesthesia is deposited away from the site of surgery, but close to the main nerve trunk.

Different techniques for mandibular nerve block anesthesia have been published, including the mental/incisive nerve block [13–15].

1. The standard (Halsted) technique
2. The standard indirect technique
3. Mental nerve (incisive nerve) block
   - standard approach for mandibular anteriors and soft tissue
   - anterior approach
   - extraoral approach
4. Clarke-Holmes technique (1959)

5. Vazirani technique (1960)
6. Akinosi technique (1977) closed-mouth technique
7. Wolfe technique (1992)
8. Sargenti technique (1966)
9. Gow-Gates technique (1973)
10. Ipsilateral open-mouth technique (2007)
11. Morishita (positive aspiration) technique (2007)
12. Extraoral submandibular approach
13. Lateral extraoral approach
14. Anterior extraoral approach. (1969)

Different maxillary nerve block techniques have been described.

1. Anterior-superior alveolar nerve and infraorbital nerve blocks,
   - intraoral approach (bicuspid approach)
   - Bisecting approach (central incisor)
   - extraoral approach
   - nasal approach (1969)
2. Posterior-superior alveolar nerve block (tuberosity block)
3. Middle-superior alveolar nerve block (buccal approach)
4. Middle and anterior-superior alveolar nerve block (palatal approach)
5. Sphenopalatine (incisive) nerve block
6. Greater palatine nerve and lesser palatine nerves block
7. Maxillary nerve blocks,
   - High tuberosity approach
   - Greater palatine canal approach
   - nasal approach
   - lateral extraoral approach
   - suprazygomatic extraoral approach extraoral approach
   - anterior-lateral extraoral approach.

### 5.11.1 Percentage of Blood Vessel Penetration During IANB

During IANB, the intravenous injection of local anesthetic is very common. Frangiskos F et al. [16], in their study, found positive aspiration (the tip of the needle is in the blood vessel) 20% times. The positive aspiration was more commonly seen in young patient's age ranging from 9 to 19 years. To avoid systemic complications while giving local anesthesia, aspiration is must in each and every case.

### 5.11.2 Controversy in the Use of Bilateral IANB and Lingual Nerve Block [17]

Has bilateral IAN and Lingual nerve block been given? Some surgeons recommend, while some do not, but there are no published data available regarding its contraindications. The common complications associated with its use are

- Collection of fluid in the oral cavity
- Injury to tongue
- Loss of control of tongue, which can lead to respiratory embarrassment
- Unpleasant effects of bilateral anesthesia [18].

Many authors advocated the use of sodium bicarbonate in addition to the lignocaine solution to reduce the duration of onset of anesthesia, and it is very effective in reducing pain during the injection. Sodium bicarbonate ions also nonspecifically reduce the safety margin for nerve conduction and it has a direct action on the binding of Local anesthetic to the sodium channel [19–21].

## 5.12 Techniques

### 5.12.1 Inferior Alveolar Nerve Block (*Also Known as* Mandibular Nerve Block) [Along with Lingual & Long Buccal Nerve Blocks]

This is the single most important nerve block, whose technique needs to be mastered. With this, we can anesthetize the whole of the mandibular soft and hard tissues, including the cheek, and many procedures in this region can be carried out.

Secondly unlike in the maxilla, infiltration techniques do not provide adequate anesthesia to the hard tissue in the mandible, particularly the teeth. This is due to the dense cortical bone in the mandible, in contrast to the porous maxillary bone, where a paraperiosteal deposition of the solution can allow the solution to diffuse through the bone to the periapical region easily and cause anesthesia of the teeth and their supporting structures.

### 5.12.2 Technique

This description is for injection on the right side of the patient and for a right-handed operator. The surgeon is on the right side of the patient, in front of the patient. The patient is asked to open the mouth wide.

With the left hand, the operator palpates the posterior buccal sulcus, runs the index finger posteriorly to feel the external oblique ridge and the anterior border of the coronoid process. As the finger proceeds upwards, palpate the coronoid process up and down to determine the deepest point on its anterior border. This is the coronoid notch. [This is a very important landmark because this determines the vertical height at which the needle should be inserted, the reason being the Mandibular foramen on the medial aspect of the ramus where we want the needle to reach is in direct line with the coronoid notch] Fig. 5.1.

Once the coronoid notch is palpated with the pulp of the index finger, the finger is rotated such that the nail faces medially. At the same time, the finger retracts the soft tissue

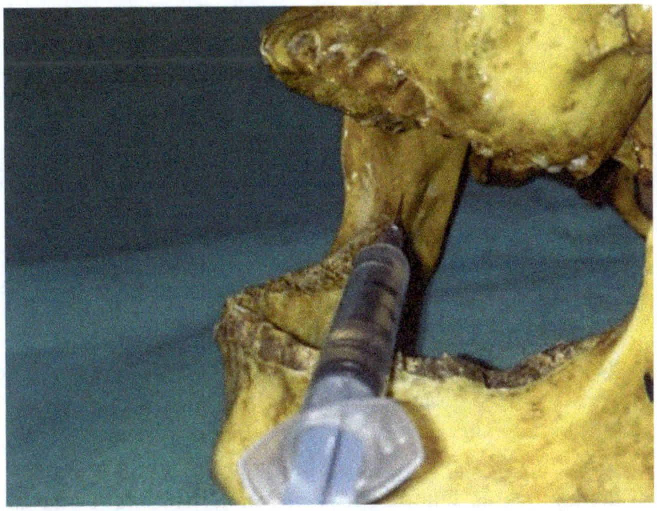



**Fig. 5.1** Dry mandible showing the position of needle and the coronoid notch

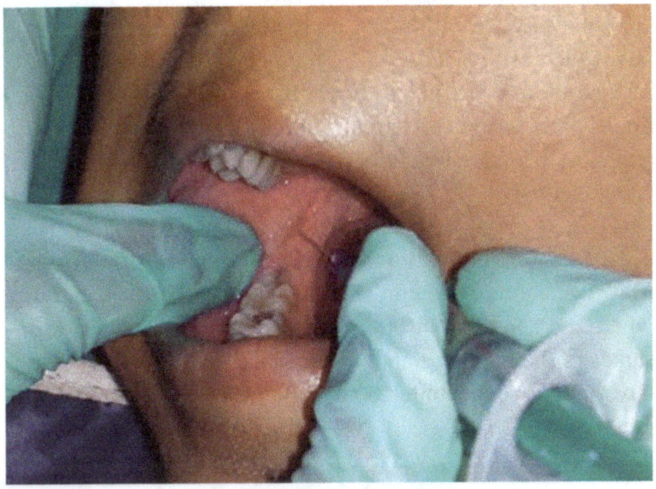



**Fig. 5.2** Picture showing needle insertion position from the soft tissue for IAN block

to reveal a depression called the pterygo mandibular depression, which is medial to the finger between the finger and the pterygo Mandibular raphe (Fig. 5.2).

Now the needle with solution in the syringe is taken in the right hand and is introduced into the mouth from the opposite side (i.e., left side) corner of the mouth/premolar area.

The syringe and needle are kept parallel to the Mandibular occlusal plane and are introduced into the pterygo temporal depression at the same height as the nail of the index finger (on the coronoid notch). The needle is advanced slowly in the soft tissue till the needle strikes the bone and resistance is felt. Now the needle is in the pterygo mandibular space bounded laterally by the medial surface of the ramus of the mandible and it is just above the lingula in the area of the opening of the mandibular foramen.

The syringe is aspirated and 1 ml of the solution is deposited. This will anesthetize the inferior alveolar nerve as it enters the mandible. Now, the needle with the syringe is swung on to the corner of the mouth on the same side, i.e., right, and is slowly withdrawn after about half the length is inserted and 0.5–0.8 ml of the solution is deposited here. This will take care of the lingual nerve, which is anteromedial to the inferior alveolar nerve.

Now the needle is withdrawn completely out of the soft tissue and is reinserted into the cheek, posterior to the last molar teeth at the level of the occlusal plane of the mandibular teeth for a short distance. After aspiration, the remaining 0.5 ml of the solution is deposited. This anesthetizes the long buccal nerve [for the left-sided block, the surgeon is slightly behind the patient on the right side with the left hand coming around].

This classical Mandibular Nerve block of inferior alveolar nerve with lingual & long buccal is done together if the mandibular molars and their adjoining soft tissues need to be anaesthetized. The reason being the pulp and the periodontium of these teeth are supplied by the inferior alveolar nerve. The lingual gingiva is supplied by the lingual nerve and the buccal gingiva by the long buccal nerve.

### 5.12.3 Areas Anesthetized by This Block

1. *Inferior Alveolar Nerve Block*
   (a) All mandibular teeth and the bone surrounding them.
   (b) The buccal gingiva in relation to the Mandibular anterior and premolar teeth.
   (c) Lower lip on the same half up to the midline.
2. *Lingual Nerve Block*
   (a) The lingual gingiva of the Mandibular teeth along with the lingual Mandibular mucosa.
   (b) The Anterior 2/3rd of the tongue on the same side.
3. *Long buccal nerve Block*
   (a) The cheek mucosa.
   (b) Buccal gingiva and mandibular mucosa in relation to the molar teeth.

### 5.12.4 Signs and Symptoms of Anesthesia

It usually takes about 3–5 min before adequate depth of anesthesia is obtained after any injection. In other words, although symptoms of anesthesia may be felt almost instantly after the injection, for the patient to feel no pain during the procedure a wait of at least 5 min is needed.

It has been conventional to confirm the anesthesia obtained with two parameters:

1. Subjective symptoms of anesthesia as experienced by the patient.
2. Objective signs elicited by the surgeon.

Subjective symptoms may or may not be present with certain nerve blocks, e.g., nasopalatine block. However with the classical inferior alveolar/mental nerve block, a *tingling and numbness* on one half of the lip (same side) will be felt. There will be an area of sharp demarcation between the numb side of the lip and the normal side at the midline. The tingling or numbness will start instantly to become heavy in about 3–5 min. Similar sensation of numbness will be felt on the same side of the tongue particularly the tip as a result of the lingual nerve block. There may be no symptoms of numbness felt by the patients in the other anaesthetized areas, e.g., the gingiva, teeth, or the cheek.

The objective sign as elicited by the surgeon is more reliable and may be the only means of ascertaining anesthesia in the absence of subjective symptoms. The objective sign of anesthesia is *lack of pain in the area anesthetized when stimulus is applied* with a blunt instrument, e.g., the end of a periosteal elevator. [It should be noted from the earlier discussion that the patient might feel the pressure of the instrument and an apprehensive patient might occasionally interpret this as pain.]

In checking for anesthesia of the inferior alveolar nerve, the blunt instrument must be applied on the buccal gingiva anterior to the mental foramen, because the lack of sensation in the posterior buccal soft tissue indicates a successful long buccal nerve and not inferior alveolar nerve block. The same blunt instrument must be applied in the gingival sulcus on the lingual side of the tooth to be extracted for lingual nerve anesthesia. The same can be done to check the buccal nerve anesthesia.

## 5.12.5 Complications (Table 5.6)

These were discussed very briefly as local complications of L.A in the earlier section. Specific complications after an Inferior Alveolar Nerve block include:

1. Failure to obtain anesthesia
2. Hematoma formation
3. Transient facial nerve palsy/weakness
4. Trismus
5. Breakage of the needle.

**Table 5.6** Complications with local anesthetics

| Local | Systemic |
|---|---|
| Needle breakage | Syncope |
| Paresthesia | Adverse drug reactions |
| Facial nerve paralysis | Overdose drug reactions |
| Trismus | Psychogenic reactions |
| Soft-tissue injury | |
| Hematoma | |
| Pain on injection | |
| Burning on injection | |
| Infection | |
| Edema | |
| Sloughing postanesthetic intraoral lesion | |

### 5.12.5.1 Failure to Obtain Anesthesia

It is the most common problem and usually due to the wrong technique. Repeating the block employing the right technique is usually the solution. However, this might be encountered in two other situations.

1. Failure to anesthetize the myolohyoid branch, which might occasionally innervate the site of the procedure.
2. Also as already mentioned, in an apprehensive patient, the symptoms of pressure may be interpreted as pain. In this situation, anxiety reduction techniques may be needed or alternately some other form of anesthesia, e.g., conscious sedation or General Anesthesia may have to be employed. The subjective symptom of numbness in the lower lip (same side) and tip of the tongue will be the distinguishing feature between a faulty technique and an apprehensive patient. In the former, it will be absent, and in the latter very much present.

### 5.12.5.2 Hematoma Formation

This may occur within the pterygo mandibular space as a result of bleeding induced by the needle prick. It may be a rare problem. The patient might have pain, swelling, & difficulty in opening the mouth. The treatment is symptomatic and possibly prophylactic antibiotic cover. It will resolve spontaneously.

### 5.12.5.3 Transient Facial Nerve Palsy

May occasionally occur as a result of a faulty technique where the needle is inserted farther posteriorly into the substance of the parotid gland (in this situation, the needle would have failed to encounter bony resistance) and paralyzes the facial nerve.

The patient will have typical signs of ipsilateral facial nerve palsy/weakness, which includes difficulty in closing the eye, absence of wrinkles on the forehead, and drooping of the corner of the mouth ipsilaterally with a possible asymmetry. This effect will be transient, till such time the local anesthetic effect persists (about 1–1½ h) and the patient needs to be reassured.

### 5.12.5.4 Trismus

Is a relatively more common complication and will be seen usually postoperatively. It could be due to a variety of causes, including:

1. Muscle spasm due to injury
2. Infection
3. Necrosis of tissue due to contact with contaminants, etc.

Most of the time it resolves spontaneously. But on occasion, this will require anti-inflammatory analgesics, muscle relaxants, and vigorous physiotherapy to overcome the problem. Wherever an infection is suspected, a suitable antibiotic cover may also be needed.

#### 5.12.5.5 Accidental Breakage of the Needle

Occurring within the tissues of the pterygo mandibular space, this is a very rare complication today where we use disposable needles for one use only. But when this happens, a radiographic guided exploration and removal of the broken piece may be needed. Gerbino G et al. [22] advocated use of brain LAB vector vision neuronavigation system for the retrieval of broken needle. This Intraoperative navigation system is very helpful in locating the broken needle fragment.

## 5.13 Vazirani–Akinosi (VA) Versus Inferior Alveolar Nerve Block

The closed mouth VA technique to anesthetize the IAN, lingual, and long buccal nerve simultaneously was described in 1977 [23]. VA is used only secondarily to conventional IAN block.

### 5.13.1 Indications for VA [24]

1. In patients with restricted mouth opening
2. In cases of failure of IAN blocks
3. Difficult-to-locate landmarks for IAN block

The percentage of Positive aspiration is much higher with IAN block in comparison to VA. This is because of the close proximity of the inferior alveolar artery, which enters the mandibular foramen just behind the nerve [25]. To avoid frequent aspiration, many surgeons prefer VA technique in normal patients also.

### 5.13.2 Akinosi–Vazirani Technique (Closed-Mouth Technique)

A 25-gauge long needle is used. The operator is in front of the patient on the right side (right-handed operator) for both sides on the patient.

With the left index finger or thumb, the coronoid notch is palpated and the soft tissues on the medial aspect of the ramus are pushed laterally. The needle is held parallel to the maxillary occlusal plane on the same side of the injection and is inserted adjacent to the maxillary third molar into the soft tissue overlying the medial border of the ramus, just adjacent to the maxillary tuberosity. This is now advanced posteriorly & slightly laterally. The bevel of the needle is away from the mandibular ramus and in an average-sized adult the needle is inserted about 25 mm into the tissue. At this point, the tip of the needle will be in the middle of the pterygo mandibular space close to the branches of the mandibular nerve. After aspiration, the LA solution is injected.

The areas anesthetized, signs and symptoms of anesthesia are similar to the open-mouth technique of mandibular nerve block.

Another viable alternative to the VA block is the technique of Gow-Gates described in 1973. In the Gow-Gates technique, anesthesia is administered more proximally, at the neck of the condyle and relies on extraoral landmark [26].

### 5.13.3 Technique

A 25-gauge long needle is used. The operator stands in front of the patient. It is very essential for the patient to extend his neck & open the mouth as wide as possible. Here the needle is inserted into the mucosa medial to the mandibular ramus on a line parallel to a line drawn from the intertragic notch to the corner of the mouth—just distal to the maxillary second molar. The needle is inserted from the corner of the mouth on the opposite side. The height of insertion is just at the level of the mesiolingual cusp of the maxillary second molar. Slowly advance the needle till the bone is contacted. (The needle here is in contact with the neck of the condyle. The position the patient is asked to assume, i.e., extend neck & open mouth wide, is to facilitate a more frontal position of the condyle closer to the mandibular nerve trunk). The average depth of insertion is about 25 mm. Aspirate & inject 2 ml of the solution slowly. Unlike with the classical method, injection is at one site only in this technique. This anesthetizes the inferior alveolar, lingual, long buccal branches of the mandibular here with similar effect as the classical block (Fig. 5.3a, b).

## 5.14 Mental/Incisive Nerve Block

These are two very similar blocks except that in a mental block the solution is deposited around the mental nerve as it exits the mandible at the mental foramen, whereas for an incisive nerve block, the solution is injected into the mandible through the mental foramen. This blocks the incisive nerve, which is the continuation of the inferior alveolar nerve anteriorly, up to the midline.

### 5.14.1 Technique

This may be carried out with the operator standing in front of the patient (can also be done easily with the operator standing behind).

With the left-hand thumb or index finger, palpate the mucobuccal fold on the mandible starting in the molar region moving anteriorly when depression will be felt. This is usually in relation to the apex of the premolar teeth where the mental foramen is present. The needle is now directed vertically to be inserted into this area with the bevel facing the bone. With the mental nerve block, the solution is deposited in the soft tissues, whereas for the incisive the needle is inserted into the foramen for a short distance before injection.

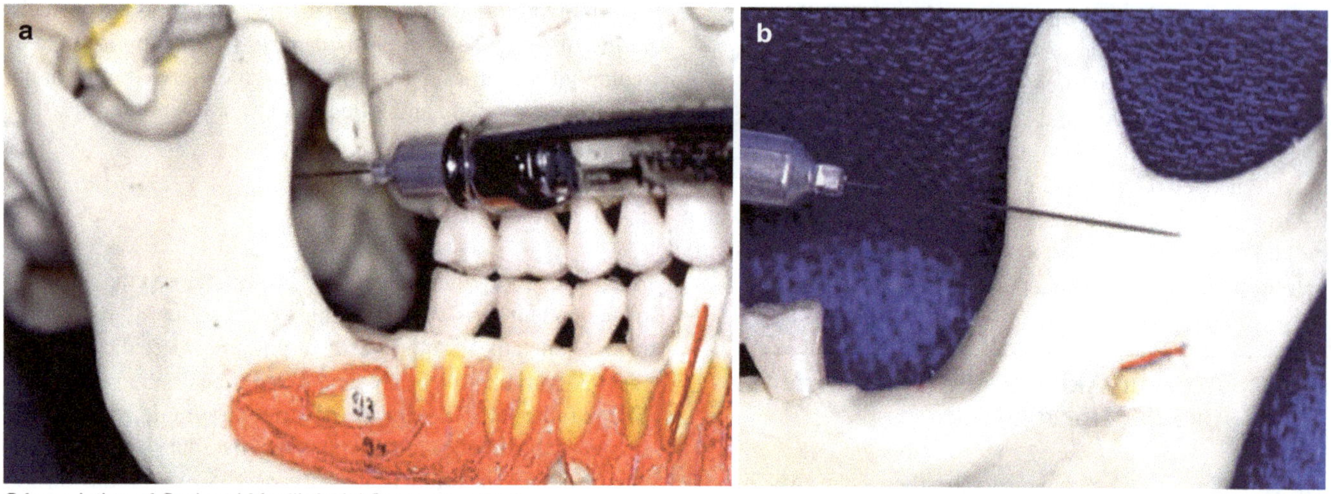




**Fig. 5.3** (**a**, **b**) Position of needle from medial and lateral aspect in case of closed-mouth technique

### 5.14.2 Areas Anesthetized

*Mental Nerve Block*: Buccal mucosa and gingiva in the mandible anterior to the premolar area, lower lip mucosa, and skin on the same side.

*Incisive Nerve Block*: In addition to the aforementioned structures, mandibular teeth anterior to the mental foramen, i.e., incisors, canine, and the premolars (which are anterior to the mental foramen).

### 5.14.3 Signs and Symptoms

*Subjective:* Tingling and numbness in the lower lip on the same side for both blocks as it is for the inferior alveolar block.

*Objective*: Lack of pain on probing with a blunt instrument over the buccal gingival/mucosa in the anterior Mandibular region.

*Complications:* Hematoma formation: If there is bleeding submucosally or subcutaneously, pressure application to stem the flow is all that is needed, with reassurance to the patient that it will resolve spontaneously in a short period of days.

## 5.15 Nerve Blocks in the Maxilla

As already mentioned, in maxilla buccal & palatal infiltration techniques are often followed because they are effective, particularly if the surgical area is limited, e.g., extraction of a single tooth. However nerve blocks are useful at times, particularly when anesthesia of a larger area is sought.

### 5.15.1 Posterior Superior Alveolar Nerve Block Technique

The position of the operator is on the front of the patient for both sides, on the right side, for a right-handed operator.

Palpate the maxillary mucobuccal fold after asking the patient to open mouth partially and retracting the buccal soft tissue with the index finger of the left hand. Insert the needle (25/27 gauge—20-mm length) into the height of the mucobuccal fold opposite the upper second (second) molar tooth. Advance the needle in inward, upward, backward direction with the needle at 45° angle to the maxillary plane for about 10–15 mm. The tip of the needle will now be close to the entry of the posterior superior alveolar nerve into the maxilla on its posterior surface. Inject 1–1.5 ml of the solution after aspiration (Fig. 5.4).

#### 5.15.1.1 Areas Anesthetized

1. Buccal alveolar mucosa and gingiva in relation to the maxillary molar teeth.
2. All the three maxillary molar teeth except the mesiobuccal root of the first molar in some instances. (This may be supplied by the middle superior alveolar nerve occasionally. In this case, to anesthetize the first molar tooth completely, a buccal infiltration has to be given in addition to the posterior superior alveolar nerve block if employed.)

Hence, this is a nerve block, which may be used if multiple extractions of molar teeth have to be done in the maxilla or any other procedure in this area.

#### 5.15.1.2 Signs and Symptoms

*Subjective*: The patient usually will not feel any tingling or numbness in this case.

*Objective*: Lack of pain on probing with the blunt instrument as with any other local anesthetic injection.

*Complications*: Most common problem is a swiftly developing hematoma particularly if the needle goes too far distally into the area of the pterygoid venous plexus.

As in earlier instances, pressure needs to be applied in this case, on the face above the area where the swelling is developing. The sudden swelling can be alarming but is of little consequence once the application of pressure stops flows.

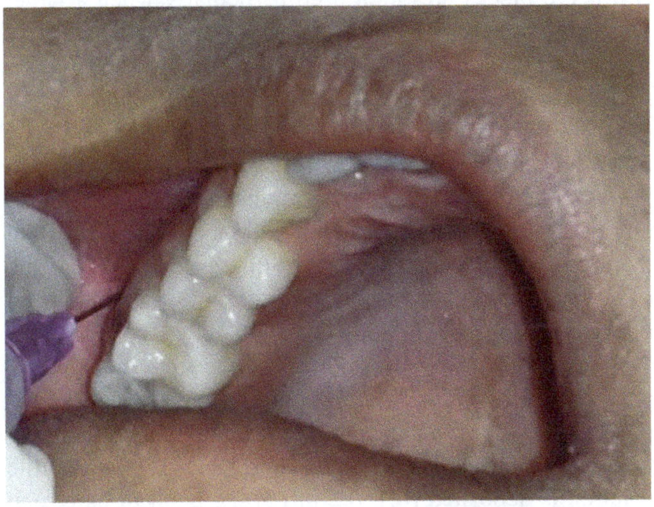



**Fig. 5.4** Needle insertion position in posterior superior alveolar nerve block

Once again, reassurance to the patient is needed. Prophylactic antibiotics to prevent secondary infection of the hematoma may be considered.

### 5.15.2 Infraorbital Nerve Block [Also Anterior and Middle Superior Nerve Blocks]

#### 5.15.2.1 Technique

The operator (right handed) is on the right side of the patient for both sides, i.e., left & right.

With the left index finger, the infraorbital rim on the face is palpated. A notch is felt on the medial third of this region, the finger is now slid down to feel for depression below this notch on the anterior surface of the maxilla. This is the position of the infraorbital foramen. With the left index finger over the infraorbital foramen, the cheek is retracted with the thumb and a 25-gauge needle is inserted intraorally into the height of the mucobuccal fold opposite the first premolar with the bevel of the needle directed toward the bone and the needle being parallel to the long axis of the tooth. The needle is advanced until gentle bone contact is made, and this will be the upper rim of the infraorbital foramen.

Aspirate and inject about 1–1.5 ml of the solution. As the solution is deposited, firm pressure is applied over the infraorbital foramen by the left-hand index finger so as to facilitate entry of the solution into the infraorbital canal through the foramen (Fig. 5.5a, b).

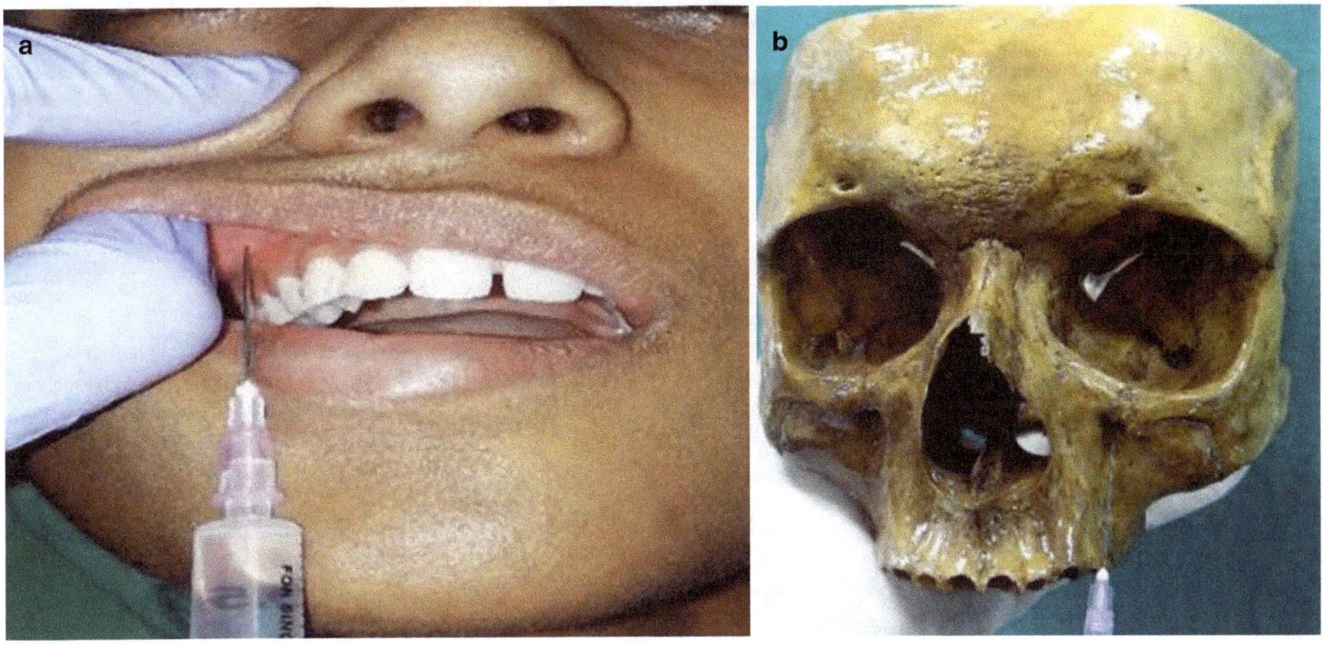





**Fig. 5.5** (**a**, **b**) Position of needle insertion and target point in dry skull in Infraorbital nerve block

#### 5.15.2.2 Areas Anesthetized

1. The lower eyelid, lateral side of the nose, and the upper lip on the same side (This is due to blockade of the terminal branches of the infraorbital nerve after it exits the foramen and will happen irrespective of whether the solution has entered into the foramen)
2. The buccal gingiva & mucosa, as well as the upper anterior and premolar teeth on the same side as well as the mesiobuccal root of the first molar if it is supplied by the middle superior alveolar nerve. (For this to happen, the anesthetic solution injected should diffuse into the infraorbital canal in the floor of the orbit from where the branches, anterior, & middle superior alveolar nerve are given off.)

#### 5.15.2.3 Signs and Symptoms of Anesthesia

*Subjective:* Tingling & numbness in the areas supplied by the terminal branches of the infraorbital nerve, i.e., the lower eyelid, lateral side of the nose, and the upper lip on the same side. (This symptom does not necessarily mean that the anterior & middle superior alveolar nerves have been anesthetized. This can be confirmed only objectively.)

*Objective*: Like always, lack of pain on probing with a blunt instrument in the area anesthetized.

*Complication*: Are few. Rarely a hematoma may develop.

### 5.15.3 Palatal Anesthesia

Injection into the palatal tissues, whether an infiltration or a nerve block, is the most painful. The reason is the palatal mucoperiostem is tightly adherent to the bone and there is no easy space for the solution to flow. This also makes the process of injection difficult as often there is backflow due to the resistance offered.

Most often, particularly when a single tooth is involved, infiltration anesthesia is preferred in the palate. However, two nerve blocks are often used particularly when a larger area is involved

1. Greater palatine nerve block
2. Nasopalatine or Anterior Palatine Nerve block.

#### 5.15.3.1 Greater Palatine Nerve Block

*Technique*: The greater palatine foramen in the adult is usually present on the palatal side of the second molar tooth at the junction of the alveolus and the horizontal palatine bone. (This may be palpated as a depression in this area but need not be done for the purpose of the nerve block.)

A 25/27-gauge short needle is inserted from the opposite side with the operator standing in front (for both sides of the patient) into the area palatal to the second molar at the junction of the alveolus & the palatine bone (Fig. 5.6a, b). A little solution is deposited (0.1–0.2 ml) at the point of entry and

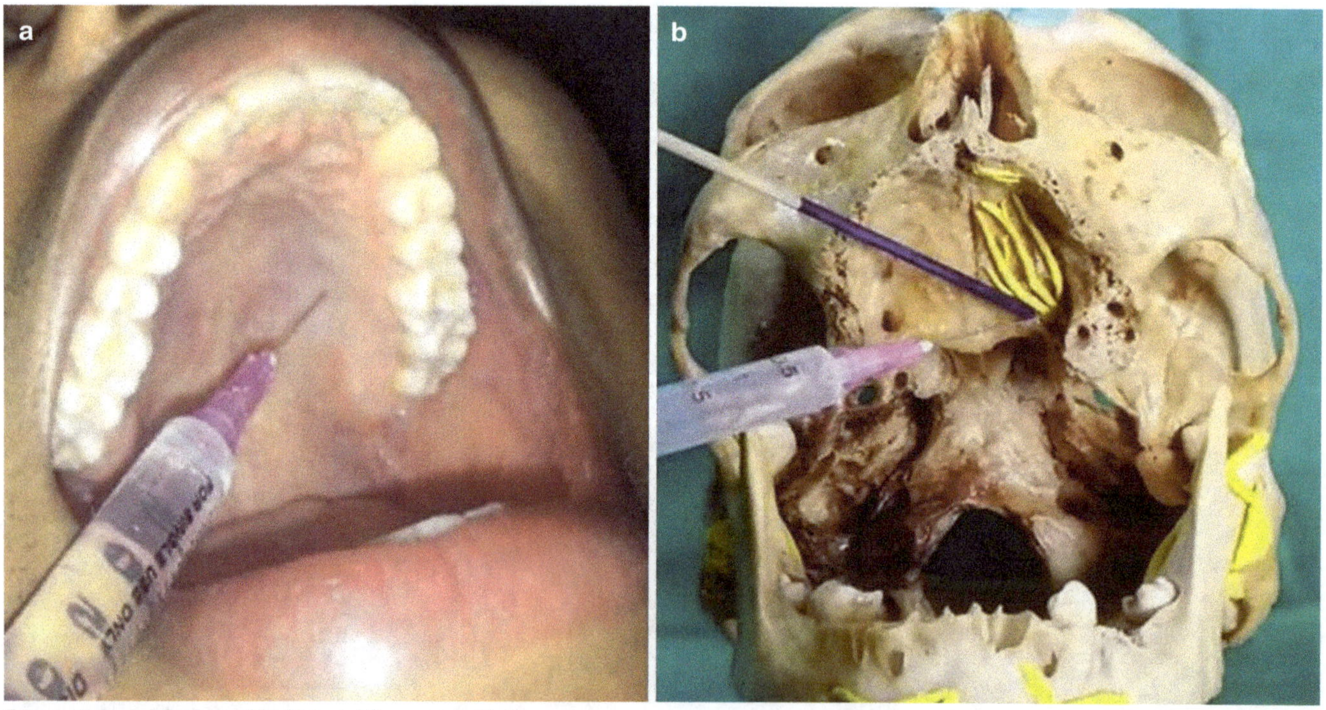




**Fig. 5.6** (**a**, **b**) Intraoral and in dry skull showing insertion of needle in greater palatine nerve block

the needle is advanced into the foramen for a variable distance (0.5–0.7 cm) and the rest, about 0.8 ml is deposited. As *usual, always aspirate* before depositing any solution.

*Areas Anesthetized*: The palatal gingiva of the maxillary teeth till the second premolar on the same side as well as the palatal mucosa & bone on the same side till the premolar region.

**Signs and Symptoms of Anesthesia**

*Subjective*: May not always be there. However, numbness in the posterior hard palate mucosa may be present.

*Objective*: Confirmation of anesthesia is always by lack of pain in the area and tested by probing with a blunt instrument.

#### 5.15.3.2 Nasopalatine Nerve Block

*Technique*: Operator in front with the patient mouth wide open, a 25/27 gauge needle is inserted into the palate just lateral to the incisive papilla. A small amount 0.1–0.2 ml of the solution is injected after aspiration. Now the needle is advanced further into the incisive foramen for a distance of about 0.5–0.75 cm and 1 ml of the solution is deposited as always after aspiration.

*Areas Anesthetized*: Probably the only nerve block, which anesthetizes bilaterally symmetrical areas and hence there is no separate right- & left-sided blocks. The palatal gingiva of the anterior teeth up to the first premolar on either side as well as the palatal mucosa and bone in the same anterior region.

**Signs and Symptoms**

*Subjective*: May be variable if present there is numbness of the anterior palate.

*Objective*: lack of pain in the anesthetized area on blunt probing.

The various nerve blocks discussed so far are the commonly used techniques. Usually this set of techniques is sufficient for all requirements of local anesthesia in the oral cavity. There are a number of alternative techniques, intraoral and extraoral, which are described in literature and may be popular in some parts of the world. However, a couple of them will be discussed here because they may have a specific indication or may be a popular technique.

## 5.16 Regional Blocks in Oral and Maxillofacial Surgery

Regional blocks are fast becoming popular in providing not only local anesthetic support for performing surgical procedures of the head and neck, but also as a method for perioperative pain control in the form of pre-emptive anesthetic techniques.

This section focuses on a few regional blocks, which can be added to the armamentarium of today's maxillofacial surgeon.

1. Maxillary nerve block
2. Mandibular nerve block
3. Greater auricular nerve block
4. Glossopharyngeal nerve block &
5. Sphenopalatine ganglion nerve block

### 5.16.1 Maxillary Nerve Block

There are numerous techniques for achieving total maxillary nerve anesthesia for dental and maxillofacial surgical procedures. These may be divided into intraoral and extraoral methods [27].

The intraoral techniques include:

1. *The "Greater Palatine Canal" Approach* where a 25-gauge needle is passed and manipulated through the greater palatine canal to reach the maxillary nerve trunk at the pterygopalatine fissure (PTM fissure) and
2. *The "High Tuberosity" Block Technique* where the maxillary nerve is anesthetized as it traverses the pterygomaxillary fissure. The technique involves the insertion of a 1.5-in. 25-gauge needle through the depth of the mucobuccal fold lateral to the maxillary tuberosity in a fashion similar to the posterior superior alveolar nerve block. The depth of penetration is about 30 mm and the target area is the pterygomaxillary (ptm) fissure posterolateral to the maxillary tuberosity.

*The extraoral technique* [28, 29]:

It involves a subzygomatic, technique. The clinical landmarks include the area below the zygomatic arch anterior to the articular eminence. This corresponds to the region above the midpoint of the sigmoid notch of the mandible. A 25-gauge 90-mm-long spinal needle is preferred for this method; the needle is inserted to a depth of about 45 mm till it contacts the lateral side of the lateral pterygoid plate. The needle is then withdrawn half-way and then angulated 15° in the forward and upward directions, which lead it to the region of the superior aspect of the ptm fissure, which corresponds to the exit of the maxillary nerve from the foramen rotundum across the ptm fissure. After negative aspiration, a volume of 2 ml is injected into the space, and the needle is withdrawn (Fig. 5.7).

### 5.16.2 Mandibular Nerve Block

The extraoral technique for the mandibular nerve block is very similar to the maxillary nerve block [30].

*Technique*—The surface landmarks and point of penetration for the block are the same and so is the armamentarium. The needle after penetrating the skin is advanced to

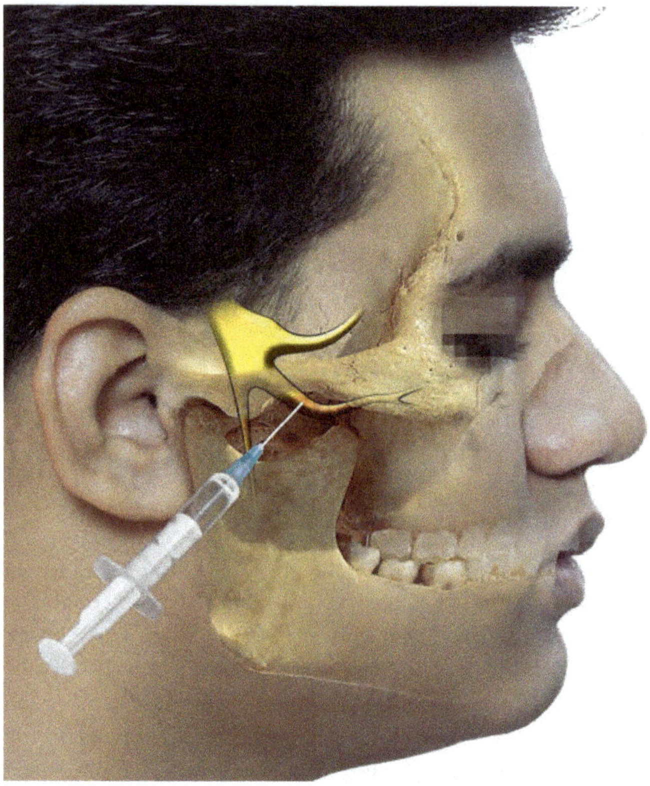



**Fig. 5.7** Representing pathway of needle in extraoral maxillary nerve block

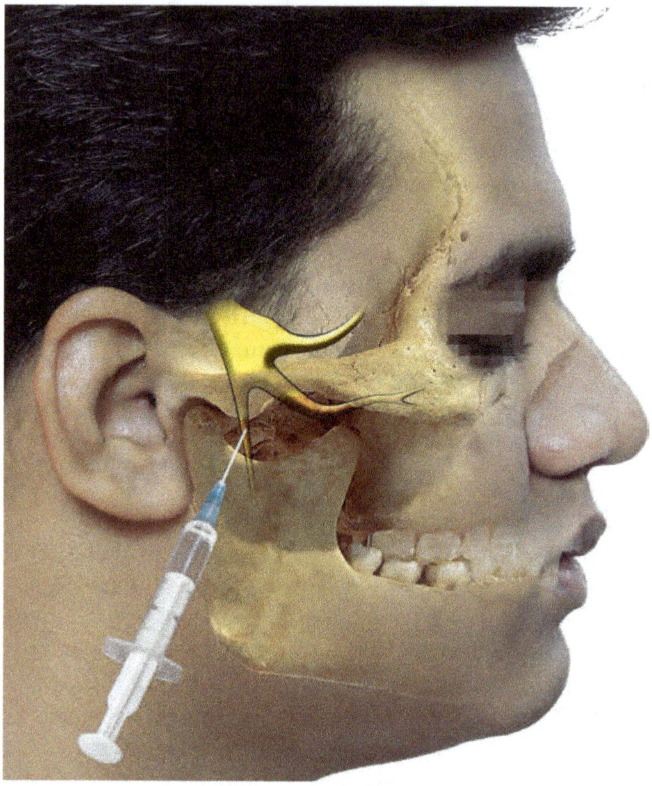



**Fig. 5.8** Showing position of needle insertion in extraoral mandibular nerve block

contact the lateral pterygoid plate as described earlier, following which the needle is withdrawn half way and turned posteriorly by 15° to the same depth of 45 mm. This area corresponds to the region just caudal to the foramen ovale through which the mandibular nerve trunk exits the skull base. After negative aspiration, a volume of 2.5–3 ml is injected to anesthetize the mandibular nerve.

The extraoral mandibular nerve block with suprazygomatic access can be safely and efficiently used with this unique approach for the mandibular nerve block to get relief in pain and Trismus. After local infiltration, an 18-gauge insulated and stimulating cannula is inserted into the retrozygomatic space just above the zygomatic arch and directed to the angle of mandible with medial and posterior inclination (Fig. 5.8) [31].

### 5.16.3 Greater Auricular Nerve Block

This nerve block is performed as an extraoral technique and provides good surface anesthesia to the periauricular skin and skin over the angle of the mandible [32].

*Technique*—The landmarks used for this technique include the cricoid cartilage and the posterior border of the sternocleidomastoid muscle. With the patient supine or semisupine, a line is drawn from the cricoid cartilage to intersect the posterior border of the sternomastoid muscle. This corresponds to the area where the superficial branches of the cervical plexus emerge from under the sternomastoid muscle, wrapping around the posterior border. A small subcutaneous injection of local anesthetic solution (around 2 ml) will anesthetize the greater auricular nerve and its area of distribution (Fig. 5.9).

### 5.16.4 Glossopharyngeal Nerve Block

The utility of the glossopharyngeal block has been studied in indications such as:

1. Excessive gag reflex during oral procedures
2. Excellent adjuvant for oropharyngeal anesthesia during awake endotracheal intubations (blind nasal or fibro-optic)
3. Management of pain due to glossopharyngeal neuralgias and atypical facial pain secondary to Eagle's syndrome [33–35]. The block can be administered both via an intraoral and an extraoral method. The intraoral technique is a relatively easy and simple technique to administer producing good outcomes.

*Technique*—A 25-gauge, 1 inch needle is chosen. The landmark for penetration is the base of the anterior tonsillar

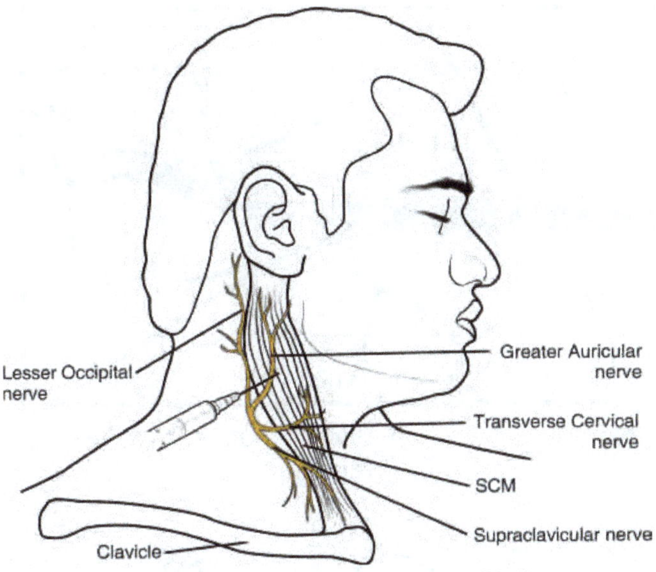


**Fig. 5.9** Showing position of needle for greater auricular nerve block

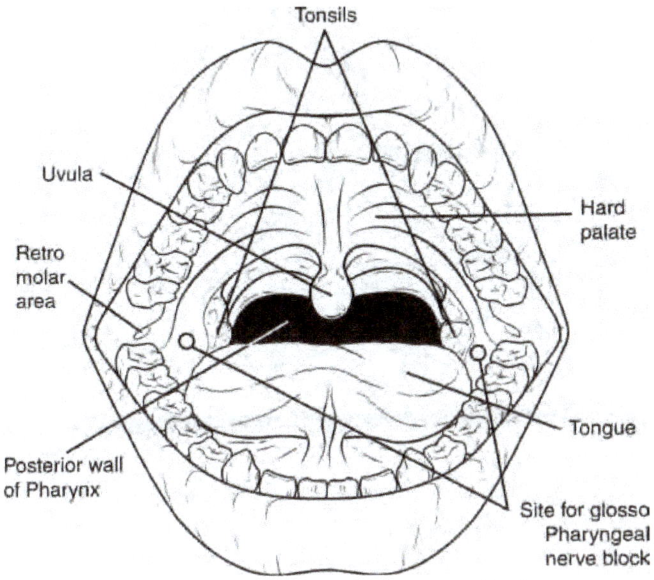


**Fig. 5.10** Target area for glossopharyngeal nerve block

pillar lateral to the base of the tongue. The syringe is positioned with the barrel near the maxillary premolar of the contralateral side with the needle facing the base of the anterior tonsillar pillar. The tongue is retracted medially to provide good visualization of the involved site. The needle is then made to pierce the mucosa and advance by 5 mm. This corresponds to the target site for the glossopharyngeal nerve in the submucosal space. After judicious aspiration, if found negative, a volume of 3 ml of anesthetic solution (2% lignocaine) is administered to block the nerve trunk (Fig. 5.10).

### 5.16.5 Sphenopalatine Ganglion Block

Indications for sphenopalatine ganglion block include:

1. Management of cluster headaches and migraine
2. Treatment for atypical facial pain
3. Palliative pain control for patients with maxillary malignancies and
4. Pre-Emptive nerve blockade for perioperative pain control in surgical procedures of the maxilla and palate [36, 37]

*Technique*—There are numerous techniques for the administration of sphenopalatine block, but the most commonly followed methods are the greater palatine approach and the transmucosal approach in the posterior aspect of the middle meatus. The greater palatine approach is the same as the maxillary nerve block via the greater palatine canal, which simultaneously blocks the sphenopalatine ganglion as well. The transmucosal method, which is most commonly followed, maybe done blind or using endoscopic guidance. A cotton pledget on a long application stick is dipped in anesthetic solution or gel and is advanced transnasally to the posterior aspect of the middle turbinate to reach the end of the middle meatus. This corresponds to the level of the sphenopalatine ganglion, which is a very superficial structure. The local anesthetic gel is then deposited, which produces anesthesia through transmucosal perfusion. Another recent technique involves the submucosal injection of the anesthetic solution into the posterior aspect of the middle meatus for achieving the block (Fig. 5.11) [37].

## 5.17 Recent Advances in Local Anesthesia

Research is ongoing to find newer modalities of pain management. In order to administer local anesthesia with less pain and adverse effects, newer technologies have been developed. Some of them are:

### 5.17.1 Vibrotactile Devices

This device is based on the Gate Control theory, which proposes that pain during injection can be decreased by simultaneous stimulation of nerve fibers by vibration.

#### 5.17.1.1 Vibraject [38]

An attachment, which is battery operated, is snapped on to the barrel to deliver strong vibrations, which is felt by the patient and therefore reducing the perception of pain.

#### 5.17.1.2 Dental Vibe [39]

It is a handheld device, which delivers pulsed percussive oscillations to the site of injection, thereby closing the pain

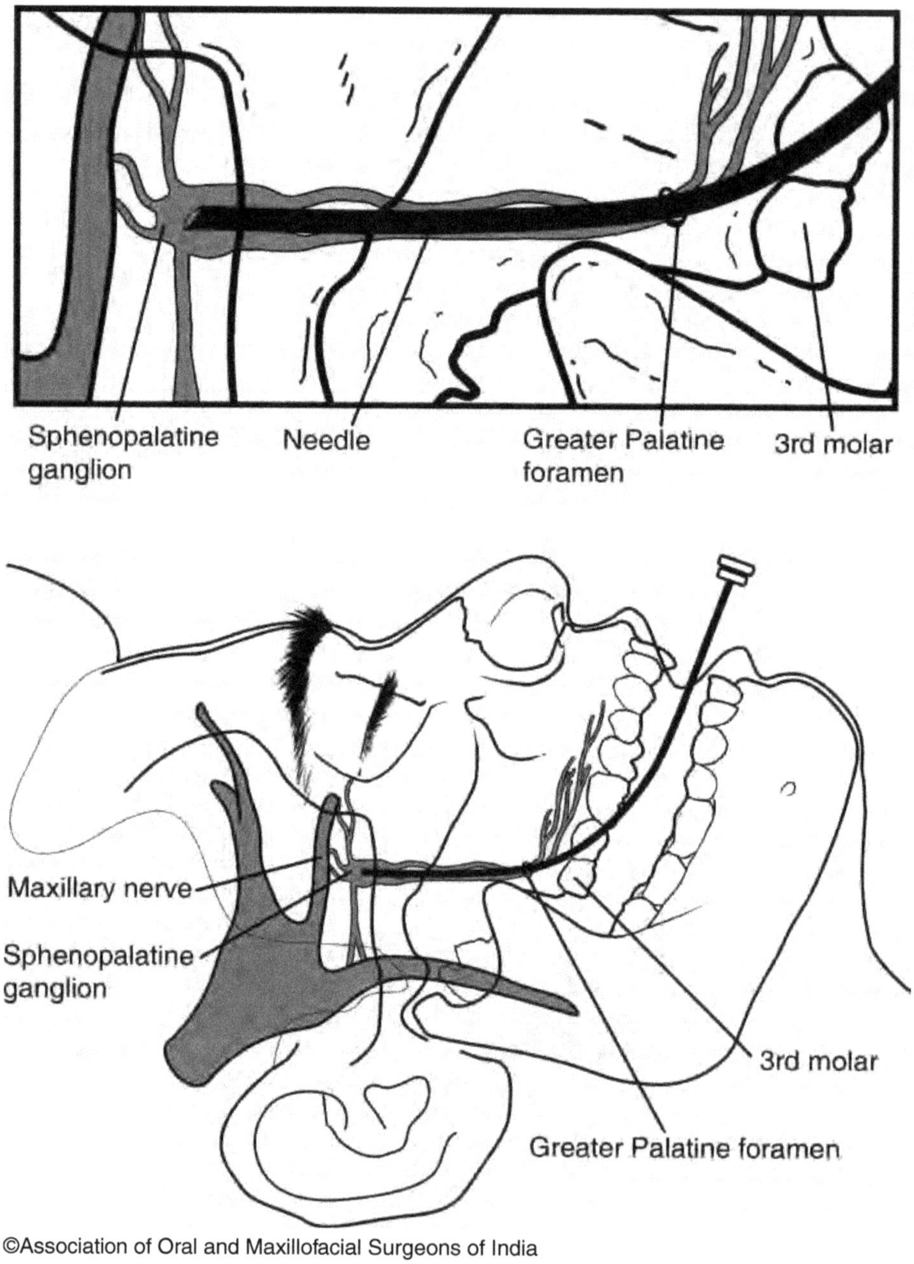


**Fig. 5.11** Showing technique of sphenopalatine ganglion block

gate. It does not have a cord and it can be recharged. Dental vibe significantly lowered the self-reported pain during local anesthesia injections compared to a conventional approach.

#### 5.17.1.3 Accupal

It is a cordless device, which shuts the pain gate by preconditioning the site of injection by pressure and vibration. To energize the dental tissue in and around the site to be punctured by the needle, Accupal incorporates the "Pain Gate theory" [40].

### 5.17.2 C-CLAD (Computer-Controlled Local Anesthetic Delivery)

With this device, there is a controlled delivery of the anesthetic and hence reduction of pain during injection. With this device, we can slowly administer anesthesia and control the injection speed [41].

**Advantages of C-CLAD device**

Higher success rates for single tooth anesthesia. The absence of pain especially in pediatric patient with disruptive behavior. More effective than a traditional syringe.

**Disadvantage**—Difficulty in locating the precise site for needle placement.

*C-CLAD* technology led to the development of an instrument for medical and dental injections capable of controlling all variables of subcutaneous injection event.

### 5.17.3 Compu-Flo

Allows instantaneous real-time measurement of fluid exit pressure at the tip of the needle. This approach to fluid exit pressure at the tip of the needle is called dynamic pressure-sensing technology (DPS) technology.

### 5.17.4 STA—single tooth anesthesia

More predictable, reliable, comfortable anesthesia than high-pressure mechanical syringe. The system incorporates the safety of using dynamic pressure-sensing technology allowing low-pressure administration of local anesthetic drugs. All patients receiving PDL with STA device reported subjective pain responses of minimal or no pain.

### 5.17.5 Jet Injection

The principle of Jet injection is that the mechanical energy is used to force a thin column of the local anesthetic solution through a small opening into the soft tissue under pressure without causing tissue damage. There is less or no pain during this procedure [42].

### 5.17.6 MED-JET H III

Local anesthetic solution in extremely small amount is administered under pressure through an orifice seven times smaller than the smallest available.

### 5.17.7 Safety Dental Syringes [43]

The protective sheath over the needle prevents accidental needle stick injury.

**Ultrasafety Plus XL Syringe**

The plunger, which is autoclavable and reusable, has a sterile disposable protective shield. It does not have to be disassembled prior to disposal.

**Ultrasafe Syringe**

Transparent disposable syringe with retractable needle sheath is helpful in aspiration and helps in seeing the aspirated contents in the syringe barrel.

**Hyposafety Syringe**

Disposable syringe and needle, which is translucent with a retractable needle into the barrel. Hence, less chance of needle stick injury. The main disadvantage is that the needle cannot be re-exposed to readminister the remaining solution.

**REV VAC Safety Syringe**

It is similar to the standard conventional syringe, the difference being that when the plunger reaches the bottom after all the medicine has been administered, further push on the plunger will cause breakage of the needle, which retracts into the plunger. It can be used only once.

### 5.17.8 Devices for Intraosseous Anesthesia [44]

**Stabident**

This device can be used with the armamentarium that is available in the clinic to administer the anesthetic solution. The main disadvantage is that inaccessible areas cannot be anesthetized with this equipment.

**X-Tip**

It is a single-step method. An initial drill is placed, which allows entry and withdrawal in one step during administration.

## 5.18 Conclusion

Pain is always a deterrent to seek treatment and hence local anesthesia is a boon to all clinicians and patients alike. Although the medication provides pain relief, its administration has always instilled fear in one and all. The advances in equipment and techniques of local anesthesia administration have undergone continuous research and development to make it as painless as possible.

## References

1. Ouchi K, Koga Y, Nakao S, Sugiyama K. Dexmedetomidine dose dependently enhances local anesthetic action of lidocaine. J Oral Maxillofac Surg. 2014;72:474.
2. Holmdahl MH. Xylocain (lidocaine, lignocaine), its discovery and Gordh's contribution to its clinical use. Acta Anaesthesiol Scand Suppl. 1998;113:8–12.
3. Howlader D, et al. Surgical management of mandibular subcondylar fractures under local anesthesia: a proposed protocol. J Oral Maxillofac Surg. 2019;77:1040.e1–9.
4. Burm AG, Van der Meer AD, Van Kleef JW. Pharmacokinetics of the enantiomers of bupivacaine following intravenous administration of the racemate. Br J Clin Pharmacol. 1994;38:125.
5. Chapman P. A controlled comparison of the effectiveness of bupivacaine for post-operative pain control. Aust Dent J. 1988;33:288.
6. Van Eeden SP, Patel MF. Prolonged paraesthesia following inferior alveolar nerve block using articaine. Br Oral Maxillofac Surg. 2002;40:519–20.

7. Da Silva CB, et al. Anaesthetic efficacy of unilamellar and multilamellar liposomal formulations of articaine in inflamed and uninflamed tissue. Br Oral Maxillofac Surg. 2016;54:295–300.
8. Neal JM. Effects of epinephrine in local anesthetics on the central and peripheral nervous systems: Neurotoxicity and neural blood flow. Reg Anesth Pain Med. 2003;28:124.
9. Vempaty S, et al. Is lignocaine with out adrenaline a better choice for lip wounds crossing vermillion border? Int J Oral Maxillofac Surg. 2017;46:90–1.
10. Haasio J, Jokinen T, Numminen M, Rosenberg PH. Topical anaesthesia of gingival mucosa by 5% eutectic mixture of lignocaine and prilocaine or by 10% lignocaine spray. Br J Oral Maxillofac Surg. 1990;28:99–101.
11. Pere P, Iizuka T, Rosenberg PH, Lindqvist C. Topical application of 5% eutectic mixture of lignocaine and prilocaine (Emla) before removal of arch bars. Br J Oral Maxillofac Surg. 1992;30:153–6.
12. Svensson P, Kolsen Petersen J, Svensson H. Efficacy of a topical anesthetic on pain and unpleasantness during scaling of gingival pockets. Anesth Prog. 1994;41:35–9.
13. Gow-Gates G, Watson JE. Gow-Gates mandibular block: applied anatomy and histology. Anesth Prog. 1989;36:193–5.
14. Gaum LI, Moon AC. The ART mandibular block. Can J Dent Assoc. 1997;63:454–9.
15. Aggarwal V, Singla M, Kabi D. Comparative evaluation of anesthetic efficacy of GowGates mandibular conduction anesthesia, Vazirani-Akinosi technique, buccal-plus-lingual infiltrations, and conventional inferior alveolar nerve anesthesia in patients with irreversible pulpitis. Oral Surg Oral Med Oral Pathol Oral Radiol Endod. 2010;109:303–8.
16. Frangiskos F, et al. Incidence of penetration of a blood vessel during inferior alveolar nerve block. Br Oral Maxillofac Surg. 2003;41:188–9.
17. Jabar J. Should we be giving bilateral inferior alveolar and lingual nerve blocks for third molar surgery? Br Oral Maxillofac Surg. 2014;52:16–7.
18. Singh B. Mandibular nerve block for the removal of dentures during trismus caused by tetanus. Anesth Analg. 2006;103:252–3.
19. Kashyap VM, et al. Effect of alkalinisation of lignocaine for intraoral nerve block on pain during injection, and speed of onset of anaesthesia. Br Oral Maxillofac Surg. 2011;49:e72–5.
20. Vinay M. Int J Oral Maxillofac Surg. 2007;36:1031.
21. Milner QJ, Guard BC, Allen JG. Alkalinization of amide local anaesthetics by addition of 1% sodium bicarbonate solution. Eur J Anaesthesiol. 2000;17:38–42.
22. Gerbino G, et al. Management of needle breakage using intraoperative navigation following inferior alveolar nerve block. J Oral Maxillofac Surg. 2013;71:1819–24.
23. Akinosi JO. A new approach to the mandibular nerve block. Br J Oral Surg Oral Med Oral Pathol Oral Radiol Endod. 1977;15:83.
24. Haas D. Alternative mandibular nerve block techniques. JAMA. 2011;142:8S.
25. Martinez Gonzalez J, Benito BP, Fernandez FC, et al. A comparative study of direct mandibular nerve block and the Akinosi technique. Med Oral. 2003;8:143.
26. Gow-Gates GA. Mandibular conduction anesthesia: a new technique using extraoral landmarks. Oral Surg Oral Med Oral Pathol. 1973;36:321.
27. Malamed SF. Techniques of regional anaesthesia in dentistry. Handbook of local anesthesia. St. Louis, MO: Elsevier; 2013.
28. Stojcev Stajcić L, Gacić B, Popović N, Stajcić Z. Anatomical study of the pterygopalatine fossa pertinent tothe maxillary nerve block at the foramen rotundum. Int J Oral Maxillofac Surg. 2010;39(5):493–6.
29. Stajcić Z, Todorović L. Blocks of the foramen rotundum and the oval foramen: a reappraisal of extraoralmaxillary and mandibular nerve injections. Br J Oral Maxillofac Surg. 1997;35:328–33.
30. Kampitak W, Tansatit T, Shibata Y. A novel technique of ultrasound-guided selective mandibular nerve block with a lateral pterygoid plate approach: a cadaveric study. Reg Anesth Pain Med. 2018;43:763–7.
31. Dziadzko MA, Heritier F. Suprazygomatic access for continuous bilateral mandibular nerve block for pain and trismus relief in the tetraplegic patient. J Oral Maxillofac Surg. 2016;74:1947.e1–5.
32. Suresh S, Barcelona SL, Young NM, Heffner CL, Coté CJ. Does a pre-emptive block ofthe great auricular nerve improve postoperativeanalgesia in children undergoing tympanomastoid surgery? Anesth Analg. 2004 Feb;98(2):330–3.
33. Garg R, Singhal A, Agrawal K, Agrawal N. Managing endodontic patients with severe gag reflex by glossopharyngeal nerveblock technique. J Endod. 2014 Sep;40(9):1498–500.
34. Rao S, Rao S. Glossopharyngeal nerve block: the premolar approach. Craniomaxillofac Trauma Reconstr. 2018 Dec;11(4):331–2.
35. Henthorn RW, et al. Which method for intraoral glossopharyngeal nerve block is better? Anesth Analg. 1995 Nov;81(5):1113–4.
36. Parameswaran A, Ganeshmurthy MV, Ashok Y, Ramanathan M, Markus AF, Sailer HF. Does sphenopalatine ganglion block improve pain control and intraoperative hemodynamics in children undergoing palatoplasty? A randomized controlled trial. J Oral Maxillofac Surg. 2018 Sep;76(9):1873–81.
37. Binfalah M, Alghawi E, Shosha E, Alhilly A, Bakhiet M. Sphenopalatine ganglion block for the treatment of acute migraine headache. Pain Res Treat. 2018;2018:2516953.
38. Roeber B, et al. Evaluation of the effects of the VibraJect attachment on pain in children receiving local anesthesia. Pediatr Dent. 2011;33(1):46–50.
39. Ching D, et al. Effect of the Dental Vibe injection system on pain during local anesthesia injections in adolescent patients. Pediatr Dent. 2014;36(1):51–5.
40. Melzack R, Wall PD. Pain mechanisms: a new theory. Science. 1965 Nov 19;150(699):971–9.
41. Kwak EJ, et al. Computer-controlled local anesthetic delivery for painless anesthesia: a literature review. J Dent Anesth Pain Med. 2016;16:81–8.
42. Lambrianidis T, et al. Dental analgesia by jet injection. Br J Oral Surg. 1979–80;17:227–31.
43. Zakrzewska JM, Boon EC. Use of safety dental syringes in British and Irish dental schools. Br Dent J. 2003;195:207–9.
44. Feridoz J, Raj JD. Intraosseous anesthesia in dentistry – a review. Drug Invention Today. 2018;10:3035–40.

# 6

# OMS: Office-Based Anesthesia

Payal Verma and Deepak G. Krishnan

## 6.1 Introduction

Anxiety and pain control has been the center of dental health provision from its inception. Dentists continue to practice some form of pain and anxiety control throughout the world. In the United States (US), Oral and maxillofacial surgery (OMS) has maintained a unique privilege where the surgeon is able to provide both anesthetic and surgical treatment for most of the procedures that are completed in a setting outside of the operation theater. The extensive, focused training received during OMS residency in the delivery of anesthesia, as well as continued education in anesthesia is central to this privilege. The art and science of alleviating pain and anxiety by providing office-based surgical treatment using various anesthetic techniques is associated with tremendous responsibility. Therefore, appropriate training along with local licensure, credentialing, and continuous education is of paramount importance.

While the Commission on Dental Accreditation (CODA) of the American Dental Association (ADA) stipulates standards in training OMS residents in anesthesia, American Association of Oral and Maxillofacial Surgeons (AAOMS) and state dental societies have developed parameters and protocols that are enforced among practicing OMSs, ensuring patient safety.

For the remainder of this chapter, the term ambulatory anesthesia would refer to the provision of anesthesia outside of a hospital operatory, such as a dental or an OMS office. Generally, this would entail provision of "open-airway" deep sedation with drugs delivered through an intra-venous (IV), intra-muscular (IM) or inhalational routes.

The American Society of Anesthesiology (ASA) recognizes four stages of anesthesia (Table 6.1) [1]. The most common forms of anesthesia used in an ambulatory office setting are mild-to-moderate sedation as well as deep sedation/general anesthesia with the use of inhalational and intravenous agents. As defined by ASA, moderate sedation/analgesia (replacing the term "Conscious Sedation," which has been condoned) is a medication-induced depression of consciousness during which patients respond purposefully to verbal commands, either alone or often accompanied by light tactile stimulation. Other interventions are not required to maintain a patent airway, while spontaneous ventilation is adequate, and cardiovascular function is usually maintained. Whereas deep sedation/analgesia is a drug-induced depression of consciousness during which patients cannot be easily aroused but respond purposefully following repeated or painful stimulation. The ability to independently maintain ventilatory function may be impaired and may require assistance in maintaining a patent airway. However, it is important that the cardiovascular function is maintained.

Given that the process of sedation is a continuum, the patient's response is unpredictable. Hence, practitioners should be able to rescue the patients whose level of sedation becomes deeper than initially intended. An oral and maxillofacial surgeon is well trained in airway management and advanced life support.

## 6.2 Brief History of Anesthesia in OMS

Over several decades, Oral and maxillofacial surgeons have been at the forefront of anesthesia and pain control among all dental specialties and have been providing safe outpatient anesthesia.

Nitrous oxide was produced by Joseph Priestly and was termed as "laughing gas" by Humphrey Davy in eighteenth

P. Verma (✉)
Oral & Maxillofacial Surgery, University of Cincinnati Medical Center, OH, Cincinnati, USA
e-mail: vermapl@ucmail.uc.edu

D. G. Krishnan
Oral & Maxillofacial Surgery, University of Cincinnati Medical Center, OH, Cincinnati, USA

Oral & Maxillofacial Surgery, Cincinnati Children's Hospital and Medical Center, OH, Cincinnati, USA

**Table 6.1** Continuum of depth of sedation: definition of general anesthesia and levels of sedation/analgesia

| | Minimal Sedation Anxiolysis | Moderate Sedation/ Analgesia ("Conscious Sedation") | Deep Sedation/ Analgesia | General Anesthesia |
|---|---|---|---|---|
| *Responsiveness* | Normal response to verbal stimulation | Purposeful response to verbal or tactile stimulation | Purposeful response following repeated or painful stimulation | Unarousable even with painful stimulus |
| *Airway* | Unaffected | No intervention required | Intervention may be required | Intervention often required |
| *Spontaneous ventilation* | Unaffected | Adequate | May be inadequate | Frequently inadequate |
| *Cardiovascular function* | Unaffected | Usually maintained | Usually maintained | May be impaired |

century [2, 3]. It was first used as an anesthetic agent in dental practice by Dr. Horace Wells [4] of Connecticut. He demonstrated the use of nitrous oxide for dental extractions that was aimed at the prevention of pain during surgery. Unfortunately, he was dismissed due to lack of medical background. His friend, William T G Morton [4], later demonstrated the use of ether vapors as anesthetic for the removal of a jaw tumor. Morton was therefore credited for the first anesthetic (October 16, 1846; also known as Ether Day). This solidified the foundation for the use of anesthetics in dental practice.

A prominent step forward in the provision of safe ambulatory anesthesia was the development and further refinement of the intravenous route of administration. It provided a safe route for rapid delivery and titration of medications along with giving the surgeon the ability to provide emergency medications. The practice of intravenous techniques allowed fast onset and recovery.

Adrian O. Hubbell [5] was critical in popularizing outpatient general anesthesia among OMS. He completed his training at Mayo Clinic and later demonstrated the safety of administering barbiturate anesthesia in an outpatient setting. He also advocated the utility and safety of recovering patients on their side or abdomen postoperatively to prevent aspiration of vomitus. Sylvan Shane [6] later reported on the use of intravenous drugs (benzodiazepines) for inducing sedation known as a "balanced" anesthetic. It was rapidly accepted due to its property of anxiolysis as a sole agent.

Another drug that became popular was methohexital [7] but was quickly overtaken by the introduction of Propofol [8], which is currently the most favored primary agent. In 1989, Propofol was officially approved for use, and its benefits related to the faster onset, improved recovery, and inherent antiemetic activity were soon recognized.

It became evident soon that to continue the privilege of administering outpatient anesthesia, it was important to receive adequate formal general anesthesia training and to maintain the highest standard of care. Today, Intravenous drug anesthesia is the mainstay of providing sedation in the outpatient setting of oral and maxillofacial surgery and has a history of safety [9].

## 6.3 The Anesthesia Team

A majority of the OMSs in the US work in private practice settings where ambulatory anesthesia is the mainstay of practice. This has led to the development of a unique office anesthesia model known as the Anesthesia Team model for OMS practice [10]. This was originally described as the operator-anesthetist model. That was a misnomer because in reality the entire team involved in patient care is trained to monitor and manage the patient under anesthesia in various capacities.

In a typical setting, it is the surgeon who performs the surgery and administers anesthesia. Apart from the surgeon, two or more other team members are present in the room (Fig. 6.1). At least one of these team members is required to be BLS (Basic life support) trained. Most commonly, one trained staff member observes the monitors, records drugs and vitals, and helps with i.v. drug administration, while another member acts as a surgical assistant. Assistant's job is to retract, suction, and irrigate during the surgery along with helping in supporting the airway (Fig. 6.2). Often surgeons employ a registered nurse with advanced cardiac life support (ACLS) training in their offices as well. The entire team is well versed with emergency equipment and is well trained to handle an airway emergency by providing positive pressure oxygen.

## 6.4 AAOMS Office Anesthesia Guidelines

AAOMS strives to ensure that its members throughout the country are in compliance with strict and mandated guidelines. It provides these guidelines through often-updated Office Anesthesia Evaluation document made available through the association. These guidelines are created by the Committee on Anesthesia (CAN) of the AAOMS. This committee uses the latest evidence-based recommendations and guidelines to make this document. This document is then vetted by the ASA to ensure that it gets the highest level of scrutiny and approval by that organization. This multilevel peer-review process of the guidelines is important for ensur-

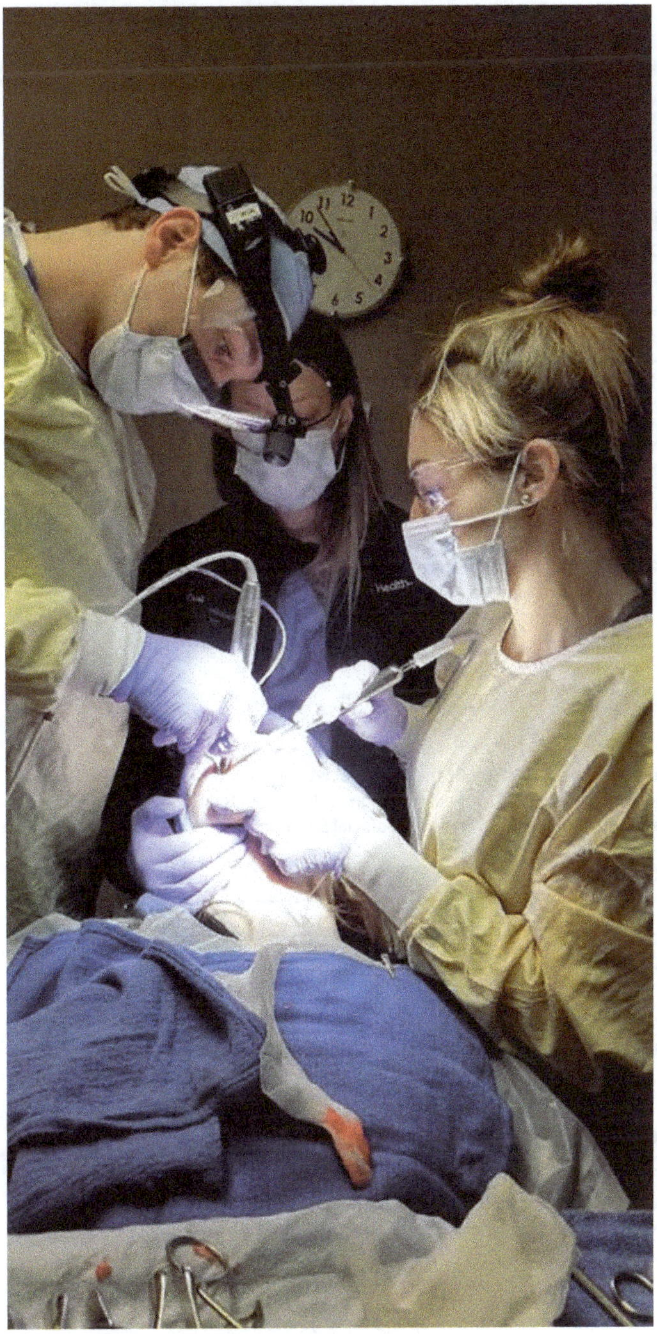



**Fig. 6.1** Example of the office anesthesia team. The surgeon provides the anesthesia and performs the procedure, one trained staff member supports the airway, and a second staff member is the surgical assistant

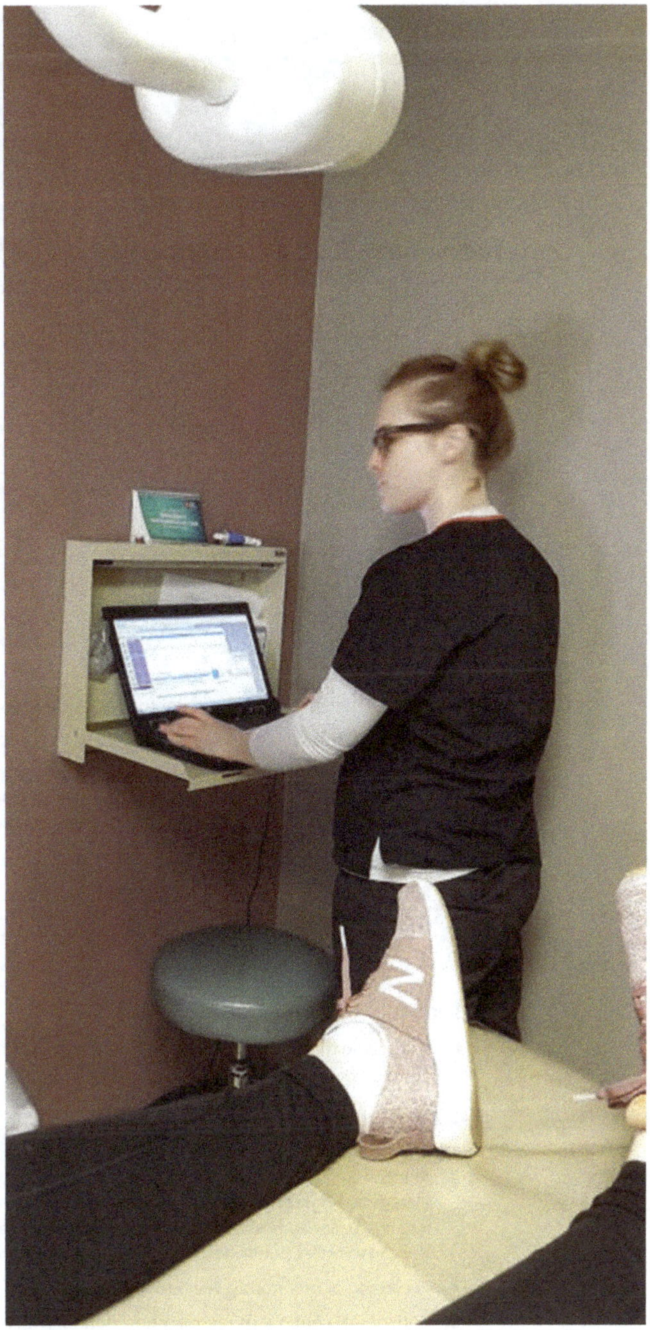



**Fig. 6.2** A dedicated registered nurse with ACLS training is often in charge of monitoring the patient under sedation

ing the safe delivery of anesthesia in the ambulatory OMS setting.

Every AAOMS member (close to 10,000 members) goes through a periodic office anesthesia evaluation process by peers to ensure that each office and team is current and well equipped to perform safe anesthetic practice in their setting (Fig. 6.3). Failure to pass such an evaluation leads to punitive action and inability to perform anesthesia in the office setting until corrective actions are taken. AAOMS, state dental societies, and third-party insurance carriers take this process seriously. Public safety cannot be compromised.

*Office Anesthesia Evaluation Manual: 9th Edition*

## Sample Anesthesia On-site Inspection and Evaluation Form

Date Sent to Society ______________________________

Name of Practitioner Evaluated ______________________ General Anesthesia Permit Number (if applicable) ______________________

Location(s) Inspected ______________________ Telephone Number ______________________

Date(s) of Evaluation ______________________ Time of Evaluation ______________________

Names of Evaluators ______________________________

______________________________

### A. Personnel

1. ACLS Certificate (Please have doctor's ACLS Certification available)
2. PALS Certificate (if appropriate)
3. Evidence of: one year advanced training in anesthesiology, Fellow of the American Dental Society of Anesthesiology, Diplomate of the American Board of Oral and Maxillofacial Surgery, eligible for examination by American Board of Oral and Maxillofacial Surgery, or Fellow of the American Association of Oral and Maxillofacial Surgeons
4. List of assisting staff's credentials/CV/training:
   a. ______________________________
   b. ______________________________
   c. ______________________________

### B. Records

Have available three charts of patients who have been treated in your office with intravenous sedation or general anesthesia.

1. An adequate medical history of the patient.
2. An adequate physical evaluation of the patient.
3. Anesthesia records showing: continuous monitoring of heart rate, blood pressure, and respiration using electrocardiographic monitoring and pulse oximetry, and ventilation by capnography. In patients undergoing inhalational anesthesia, preoperative and postoperative temperature monitoring, and if the procedure is longer than 30 minutes, continuous temperature monitoring.
4. Recording of monitoring every five minutes.
5. Evidence of continuous recovery monitoring, with notation of patient's condition upon discharge and person to whom the patient was discharged.
6. Accurate recording of medications administered, including amounts and time administered.
7. Records illustrating length of procedure.
8. Records reflecting any complications of anesthesia.

### C. Office Facility and Equipment

1. ***Noninvasive Blood Pressure Monitor***
2. ***Electrocardiograph***

8

**Fig. 6.3** Sample on site form for periodic office anesthesia evaluation. Available at www.aaoms.org

Chapter 1 The OAE Program Component Society Guidelines and Evaluation Guidelines

3. ***Defibrillator/Automated External Defibrillator***
4. ***Pulse Oximeter***
5. ***Capnography equipment***
6. ***Operating Theater***
   a. Is the operating theater large enough to accommodate the patient on a table or in an operating chair adequately?
   b. Does the operating theater permit an operating team consisting of at least three individuals to move freely about the patient?
   c. Does the operating theater allow easy access for emergency personnel and transportation equipment?
7. ***Operating Chair or Table***
   a. Does the operating chair or table permit the patient to be positioned so the operating team can maintain the airway?
   b. Does the operating chair or table permit the team to alter the patient's position quickly in an emergency?
   c. Does the operating chair or table provide a firm platform for the management of cardiopulmonary resuscitation?
8. ***Lighting System***
   a. Does the lighting system permit evaluation of the patient's skin and mucosal color?
   b. Is there a battery-powered backup lighting system?
   c. Is the backup lighting system of sufficient intensity and power for an adequate period of time to permit completion of any operation underway at the time of general power failure?
9. ***Suction Equipment***
   a. Does the suction equipment permit aspiration of the oral and pharyngeal cavities?
   b. Is there a backup suction device available?
10. ***Oxygen Delivery System***
   a. Does the oxygen delivery system have adequate full-face masks and appropriate connectors, and is it capable of delivering oxygen to the patient under positive pressure?
   b. Is there an adequate backup oxygen delivery system?
11. ***Recovery Area (recovery area can be the operating theater)***
   a. Does the recovery area have available oxygen?
   b. Does the recovery area have available adequate suction?
   c. Does the recovery area have adequate lighting?
   d. Does the recovery area have adequate electrical outlets?
   e. Can the patient be observed by a member of the staff at all times during the recovery period?
12. ***Ancillary Equipment***
   a. Is there a working laryngoscope complete with an adequate selection of blades, spare batteries and bulbs?
   b. Are there endotracheal tubes and appropriate connectors?
   c. Are there oral airways?
   d. Are there any supraglottic airway devices?
   e. Is there a tonsillar or pharyngeal type suction tip adaptable to all office outlets?
   f. Are there endotracheal tube forceps?
   g. Is there a sphygmomanometer and stethoscope?
   h. Are there an electrocardioscope and defibrillator/automated external defibrillator?

9

**Fig. 6.3** (continued)

i. Is there a pulse oximeter?
j. Is there a capnography monitor?
k. Is there adequate equipment for the establishment of an intravenous infusion?

## D. Drugs

1. Vasopressor drug available?
2. Corticosteroid drug available?
3. Bronchodilator drug available?
4. Muscle-relaxant drug available?
5. Intravenous medication for treatment of cardiopulmonary arrest available?
6. Narcotic antagonist drug available?
7. Benzodiazepine antagonist drug available?
8. Antihistamine drug available?
9. Antiarrhythmic drug available?
10. Anticholinergic drug available?
11. Coronary artery vasodilator drug available?
12. Antihypertensive drug available?
13. Mechanism of response for dantrolene (Dantrium)?

**Overall Equipment – Facility** ________ **Adequate** ________ **Inadequate**

Comments ____________________________________________

____________________________________________

____________________________________________

____________________________________________

Recommendations ____________________________________________

____________________________________________

____________________________________________

____________________________________________

Signature(s) of Evaluators ____________________________________________

____________________________________________

**Printed Name(s) of Evaluators** ____________________________________________

____________________________________________

10

**Fig. 6.3** (continued)

## 6.5 Office Requirements

The facilities where ambulatory anesthesia is provided in OMS practices are subject to stringent guidelines [11]. Specific building codes and local fire department regulations have to be followed for installation of remote gases. Proximity to a larger healthcare facility and access to emergency personnel are of paramount importance. Recommendations per Centers for Disease Control (CDC) and prevention on controls for exposure to anesthetic gases and other potential chemical hazards, as well as sterilization of the instruments and facilities are enforced. Office's fire safety and emergency protocols should be known by all staff and easily accessible for reference. Telephone numbers of the local ambulance service and nearest hospital should be clearly displayed and their location known to all office staff.

## 6.6 Record Keeping

Medical record keeping is paramount in current OMS practice. For the purpose of OMS procedures, proper electronic records have to be maintained. This includes preanesthesia assessment forms, i.e., history and physical evaluation, consent forms, intraoperative anesthesia records, operative notes as well as recovery records (Fig. 6.4). Anesthesia records typically consist of vital signs (recorded every 5 min), type and amount of drugs administered with time of administration, start and end times of anesthesia and surgery, surgeon and other team members' names, and details of complications and management, if any.

## 6.7 Office Anesthesia Evaluation Program and Parameters of Care

Every practicing AAOMS member agrees to a uniform peer inspection of their properly equipped office and their techniques and preparation for managing emergencies and complications of anesthesia in the treatment of the OMS patient in their office or outpatient setting.

In 1975, the AAOMS established the Office Anesthesia Evaluation Program. This program was conceived, developed, and implemented by the AAOMS through its component state societies to benefit the public, whom its members serve. This ensures a level of safety to the practice of anesthesia in the OMS office, which is often outside a hospital or other healthcare facility. Since 1990, AAOMS Bylaws require official component societies' constitutions and bylaws to include provision for the fulfillment of an onsite office evaluation based on the AAOMS Office Anesthesia Evaluation Program as a prerequisite for active membership. The office anesthesia evaluation is now required every 5–6 years for every AAOMS member.

AAOMS periodically offers an Office Anesthesia Evaluation Manual [12] with the following intent—"AAOMS Committee on Anesthesia developed the Office Anesthesia Evaluation Manual to provide information that could aid oral and maxillofacial surgeons in preparing themselves and their offices for the management of anesthetic complications. It presents scientific and clinical information and can serve as a reference for the practitioner." The most recent evaluation manual is available for purchase by the members in 2019.

In addition, a separate document called "AAOMS Parameters of Care" [13, 14] is intended to reflect practice considerations for 11 designated areas of oral and maxillofacial surgery and is an additional guide for AAOMS members to establish parameters of care for anesthesia in outpatient facilities. The most recent version of this document was published in 2017. The document provides complementary recommendations for the provision of safe sedation and anesthesia in the office. Members are encouraged to review both documents, which provide essential information on contemporary OMS office anesthesia practice and practice accordingly.

## 6.8 AAOMS National Simulation Program

AAOMS recognizes that the provision of anesthesia at an OMS office is a team effort. It expects each member of the team—from the surgeon to the assistants—to be highly trained and qualified to address every anesthesia-related situation that may occur during a surgical procedure. This training is initiated in OMS residencies but is continuous throughout the surgeon's career, mandated by continuing education and team exercised. Similar to professional sports teams, successful oral and maxillofacial surgery teams train as a unit to ensure they can seamlessly and quickly manage an unexpected airway emergency. The most recent AAOMS offering to help the office anesthesia team partners with advanced simulation technology making it possible to train surgeons and staff by simulating a full range of real-life emergency airway situations [15]. This program allows participants to practice and master critical techniques for administering and monitoring office-based anesthesia; a standardized approach that ensures that every participant experiences the same simulated events. The program allows for evaluation of each participant's performance and can pinpoint those areas that may benefit from additional training. The three-module program offers oral and maxillofacial surgeons and their staff an effective method of assessing their readiness to meet an office anesthesia emergency situation by practicing these in a low-risk, high-stake simulation scenario.

## Sedation and Anesthesia Record

Patient ______________________________

ID # ______________________________

☐ Premed ______________________________

☐ Equipment Check Dx: ______________________

☐ Time Out Tx: ______________________

Preoperative start time: ______________

| Date | Age | NPO | ASA | Surgeon | Anesthetist |
|---|---|---|---|---|---|
| | | | 1 2 3 | | |
| Weight | Height | BMI | Airway | Surgeon Asst. | Anesthetist Asst. |
| | | | Mallampati 1 2 3 4 | | |

| Agents/Drugs | 0 | 5 | 10 | 15 | 20 | 25 | 30 | 35 | 40 | 45 | 50 | 55 | 60 | 65 | 70 | 75 | TOTAL |
|---|---|---|---|---|---|---|---|---|---|---|---|---|---|---|---|---|---|
| Midazolam | | | | | | | | | | | | | | | | | |
| Fentanyl 50 mcg/ml | | | | | | | | | | | | | | | | | |
| Propofol 10 mg/ml | | | | | | | | | | | | | | | | | |
| Methohexital 10 mg/mL | | | | | | | | | | | | | | | | | |
| Ketamine | | | | | | | | | | | | | | | | | |
| Dexamethasone 4 mg/mL | | | | | | | | | | | | | | | | | |
| Remifentanil mcg/cc | | | | | | | | | | | | | | | | | |
| Zofran mg | | | | | | | | | | | | | | | | | |
| Exparel mg | | | | | | | | | | | | | | | | | |
| Sevoflurane % | | | | | | | | | | | | | | | | | |
| Lidocaine 2% 1:100 k epi | | | | | | | | | | | | | | | | | |
| Articaine 4% 1:100 200k epi | | | | | | | | | | | | | | | | | |
| Mepivacaine 3% | | | | | | | | | | | | | | | | | |
| Fluids NS RL | | | | | | | | | | | | | | | | | |
| Nitrous Oxide L/min | | | | | | | | | | | | | | | | | |
| Oxygen L/min % | | | | | | | | | | | | | | | | | |

| MONITORS |
|---|
| ☐ Auto BP R L |
| ☐ ECG (Lead II) |
| ☐ Pulse Oximeter |
| ☐ Stethoscope |
| ☐ Capnograph |
| ☐ BIS |
| ☐ Temp |
| **SYMBOLS** |
| SBP ∨ |
| DBP ∧ |
| Pulse • |
| Resp ❍ |
| Anes x |
| Anes x̲ |
| Surg ⊙ |
| Surg ⊙̲ |
| **POSITION** |
| ☐ Reclined |
| ☐ Supine |

| | 0 | 5 | 10 | 15 | 20 | 25 | 30 | 35 | 40 | 45 | 50 | 55 | 60 | 65 | 70 | 75 |
|---|---|---|---|---|---|---|---|---|---|---|---|---|---|---|---|---|
| ECG | | | | | | | | | | | | | | | | |
| SpO2 | | | | | | | | | | | | | | | | |
| mmHg | | | | | | | | | | | | | | | | |
| Temp | | | | | | | | | | | | | | | | |
| 200 | | | | | | | | | | | | | | | | |
| | | | | | | | | | | | | | | | | |
| 180 | | | | | | | | | | | | | | | | |
| | | | | | | | | | | | | | | | | |
| 160 | | | | | | | | | | | | | | | | |
| | | | | | | | | | | | | | | | | |
| 140 | | | | | | | | | | | | | | | | |
| | | | | | | | | | | | | | | | | |
| 120 | | | | | | | | | | | | | | | | |
| | | | | | | | | | | | | | | | | |
| 100 | | | | | | | | | | | | | | | | |
| | | | | | | | | | | | | | | | | |
| 80 | | | | | | | | | | | | | | | | |
| | | | | | | | | | | | | | | | | |
| 60 | | | | | | | | | | | | | | | | |
| | | | | | | | | | | | | | | | | |
| 40 | | | | | | | | | | | | | | | | |
| | | | | | | | | | | | | | | | | |
| 20 | | | | | | | | | | | | | | | | |
| | | | | | | | | | | | | | | | | |
| 0 | | | | | | | | | | | | | | | | |

| IV | |
|---|---|
| ☐ 22G Catheter | x___ |
| ☐ 20G Catheter | x___ |
| ☐ __________ | x___ |
| R ☐ Antecubital | x___ |
| ☐ Radial | x___ |
| L ☐ Dorsum hand | x___ |
| ☐ __________ | x___ |
| **AIRWAY** | |
| ☐ Nasal Cannula | |
| ☐ Nasal Mask | |
| ☐ Mask | |
| ☐ Nasopharyngeal | |
| ☐ Oral | |
| ☐ LMA | |
| ☐ ET Tube | |

Comments ______________________________ Dr. Signature ______________________________

______________________________

17

**Fig. 6.4** Sample sedation and anesthesia record form. Available at www.aaoms.org

## 6.9 Dental Anesthesia Assistant National Certification Examination (DAANCE)

The practice of office-based anesthesia depends largely on the skillset of the assistants in the office as much as it does on the surgeon leading the team. In an effort to elevate the education and knowledge base of the other team members, a program called the Dental Anesthesia Assistant National Certification Examination (DAANCE) was implemented nationwide. This is a continuing education program that comprises 36 h of self-education and a computerized exam to be completed in 6 months. This course is designed primarily for OMS assistants. Upon successful completion of the final examination, certification is provided.

The course is designed to cover important topics, including general review of basic sciences, patient's medical history evaluation, basic knowledge on anesthetic drugs and techniques, role of anesthesia equipment and monitoring, and covers basic maneuvers to handle office anesthesia emergencies.

This course is available to allied staff all year round to register and complete. More and more states in the US are now mandating courses like DAANCE or others to all team members in an effort to keep the practice of ambulatory anesthesia team model safe and viable in the OMS office.

## 6.10 Anesthesia Training during OMS Residency

OMS trainees in the US have a rigorous curriculum in anesthesia. The Commission on Dental Accreditation (CODA) of the American Dental Association (ADA) is the independent body that accredits all residency training programs. This accreditation is based on a peer-review process that enforces adherence to training standards created and vetted by the CODA. The educational standards for anesthesia read as follows:

> 4-3.1… Anesthesia Service: The assignment must be for a minimum of 5 months, should be consecutive, and one of these months should be dedicated to pediatric anesthesia. The resident must function as an anesthesia resident with commensurate level of responsibility.
> *Intent: The pediatric portion could include Pediatric intensive care unit (PICU), Neonatal intensive care unit (NICU), pediatric anesthesia service, or ambulatory pediatric anesthesia. Oral and maxillofacial surgery residents rotating on the anesthesia service have levels of responsibility identical to those of the anesthesia residents, and abide by the anesthesia department's assignments and schedules. Part of this time can be during medical school as long as oral and maxillofacial surgery trainee functions at the anesthesia resident level.*
>
> 4-9… The off-service rotation in anesthesia must be supplemented by longitudinal and progressive experience throughout the training program in all aspects of pain and anxiety control. The ambulatory oral and maxillofacial anesthetic experience must include the administration of general anesthesia/deep sedation for oral and maxillofacial surgery procedures to pediatric, adult, and geriatric populations, including the demonstration of competency in airway management. Examples of evidence to demonstrate compliance may include:
>
> - Resident's anesthetic log.
> - Clinical tracking system.
> - Anesthesia records.
> - Oral and Maxillofacial Surgery Benchmarks.
>
> 4-9.1… The cumulative anesthetic experience of each graduating resident must include administration of general anesthesia/deep sedation for a minimum of 300 cases. This experience must involve care for 50 patients younger than 13. A minimum of 150 of the 300 cases must be ambulatory anesthetics for oral and maxillofacial surgery outside of the operating room. Intent: The cumulative experience includes time on the anesthesia rotation as well as anesthetics administered while on the oral and maxillofacial surgery service. Locations for ambulatory anesthesia may include dental school clinics, hospital clinics, emergency rooms, and oral and maxillofacial surgery offices.
> Examples of evidence to demonstrate compliance may include:
>
> - Resident's anesthetic log.
> - Clinical tracking system.
> - Anesthesia records.
> - Oral and Maxillofacial Surgery Benchmarks.
>
> 4-9.2 …In addition to general anesthesia/deep sedation, the residents must obtain extensive training and experience in all sedation techniques.
> Examples of evidence to demonstrate compliance may include:
>
> - Detailed curriculum plans
> - Patient charts
> - Simulation experience
>
> 4-9.3 …The clinical program must be supported in part by a core comprehensive didactic program on general anesthesia, deep sedation, and other methods of pain and anxiety control. The didactic program must include lectures and seminars emphasizing:
>
> - Patient evaluation
> - Risk assessment
> - Anesthesia and sedation techniques
> - Monitoring and
> - The diagnosis and management of complications
>
> 4-9.4 …Advanced Cardiac Life Support (ACLS) must be obtained in the first year of residency and must be maintained throughout residency training and thereafter.

Examples of evidence to demonstrate compliance may include:

- ACLS certification records and cards

4-9.5… Each resident must be certified in Pediatric Advanced Life Support (PALS) prior to completion of training.
Examples of evidence to demonstrate compliance may include:

- PALS certification records and cards

Adherence to these standards is strictly enforced ensuring a standardized education in anesthesia to each OMS resident in training in the US.

## 6.11 Preanesthetic Evaluation of the Patient

The OMS planning an office-based anesthetic is trained to do a thorough preoperative evaluation of the patient to deem them fit for office anesthesia. Just as an anesthesiologist would evaluate the patient for systemic disease, functional capacity and medications along with a detailed anesthetic history and physical examination to classify every patient into an American Society of Anesthesiologists (ASA) status (Table 6.2) [16], every OMS would do the same for formulating an anesthetic plan for the patient.

Ideally, ASA I and II patients are best suited for office-based anesthetics. Careful preanesthetic patient evaluation is critical in choosing the type and venue for the anesthetic. This evaluation has the following essential steps:

- Reviewing and understanding patient's medical, family, social, surgical, and anesthetic history through questionnaire and interview.
- Full physical examination of all systems.

This detailed preop evaluation gives the OMS the knowledge to classify all according to the ASA classification and adequately plan for an appropriate anesthesia technique.

## 6.12 Monitoring

Provision of anesthesia in the OMS office requires that monitoring is done according to the ASA standards and more.

This includes the following minimal time-stamped monitoring and documentation [17].

1. Noninvasive monitoring of blood pressure every 5 min
2. Continuous ECG monitoring
3. Continuous pulse oximetry
4. Continuous end-tidal CO2 monitoring of ventilatory effort

**Table 6.2** ASA physical status classification system.

| | | |
|---|---|---|
| *ASA I* | A normal healthy patient | Healthy, nonsmoking, no or minimal alcohol use |
| *ASA II* | A patient with mild systemic disease | Mild diseases only without substantive functional limitations. Examples include (but not limited to): Current smoker, social alcohol drinker, pregnancy, obesity (30 < BMI < 40), well-controlled DM/HTN, mild lung disease |
| *ASA III* | A patient with severe systemic disease | Substantive functional limitations; one or more moderate-to-severe diseases. Examples include (but not limited to): Poorly controlled DM or HTN, COPD, morbid obesity (BMI ≥40), active hepatitis, alcohol dependence or abuse, implanted pacemaker, moderate reduction of ejection fraction, ESRD undergoing regularly scheduled dialysis, premature infant PCA < 60 weeks, history (>3 months) of MI, CVA, TIA, or CAD/stents. |
| *ASA IV* | A patient with severe systemic disease that is a constant threat to life | Examples include (but not limited to): Recent (< 3 months) MI, CVA, TIA, or CAD/stents, ongoing cardiac ischemia or severe valve dysfunction, severe reduction of ejection fraction, sepsis, DIC, ARD or ESRD not undergoing regularly scheduled dialysis |
| *ASA V* | A moribund patient who is not expected to survive without the operation | Examples include (but not limited to): Ruptured abdominal/thoracic aneurysm, massive trauma, intracranial bleed with mass effect, ischemic bowel in the face of significant cardiac pathology or multiple organ/system dysfunction |
| *ASA VI* | A declared brain-dead patient whose organs are being removed for donor purposes | |

Developed By: ASA House of Delegates/Executive Committee

5. Ability to measure temperature, i.e., very essential in a setting where Malignant Hyperthermia (MH) triggering agents are in use.

Majority of OMS offices now use monitor units (Fig. 6.5) that interface directly with an electronic health record. The entire team is clued into monitoring with a staff member often dedicated to only monitoring the patient.

All patients receive supplemental oxygen before, during, and after the procedure. Most facilities have a separate recovery area with the same monitors, although there are several offices that recover in the operatory. The goal is the improvement of efficacious monitoring to establish the safe performance of anesthetic without the need for a separate anesthesia provider. It is imperative to have a meticulously trained team to allow for continuous monitoring, thus facilitating immediate recognition of changes in patient's vital signs. A properly evaluated and selected patient is unlikely to have a catastrophe in the OMS anesthetic, but when an untoward event does occur, it is often a respiratory event.

### 6.12.1 Methods for Monitoring Ventilation

Data available from closed claims cases from the OMS National Insurance Corporation (OMSNIC) allow us as a specialty to audit the near-misses and tragic outcomes from our offices. The data suggest a strong correlation between airway-related failure and adverse events in the open-airway anesthetic techniques. The emphasis is on monitoring of both ventilation and oxygenation to allow adequate monitoring of the respiratory system during anesthesia. This can be achieved by using a pulse oximeter, which is a device that measures oxygen saturation and provides an indirect indication of oxygenation. Recently, AAOMS recommended a newer ASA standard monitoring of ventilation with continuous capnography. Although chest movements are a reliable method but are least exact, hence the addition of capnography. Most OMSs use a pretracheal/precordial stethoscope (Fig. 6.6) to auscultate while the patient is sedated.

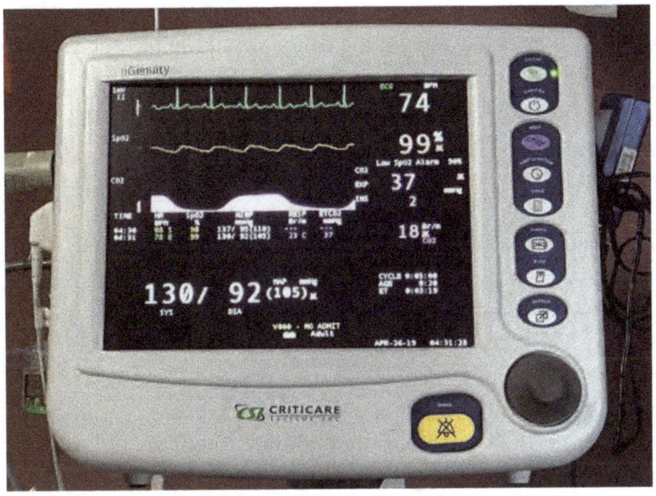




**Fig. 6.5** Example of monitor commonly used in oral and maxillofacial surgery anesthetic administration. The single unit clearly displays the electrocardiogram, noninvasive blood pressure monitor, oxygen saturation, and end-tidal carbon dioxide

Historically, pulse oximetry has been used for respiratory monitoring. But due to its limitation in lacking real-time responsiveness to major respiratory events like airway obstruction or respiratory depression, there was an imminent need to incorporate a different parameter to provide a real-time assessment. Thus was developed capnography [18], which is the noninvasive measurement of the partial pressure of carbon dioxide (CO2) from the airway during inspiration and expiration. It can provide real-time sensitivity to early changes in ventilation and is reliable even in low-perfusion states.

Although, in the nonintubated sedated patient, there is loss of CO2 through the nose and mouth, and thus requires modification of the collection cannula, it still provides valuable clinical information on patient's ventilation during sedation.

It cannot be stressed enough how critical it is to manage intraoperative airway and monitor respiratory status. Ventilation is monitored by inspection of chest movement by the assistants, monitoring of capnography as well as auscul-

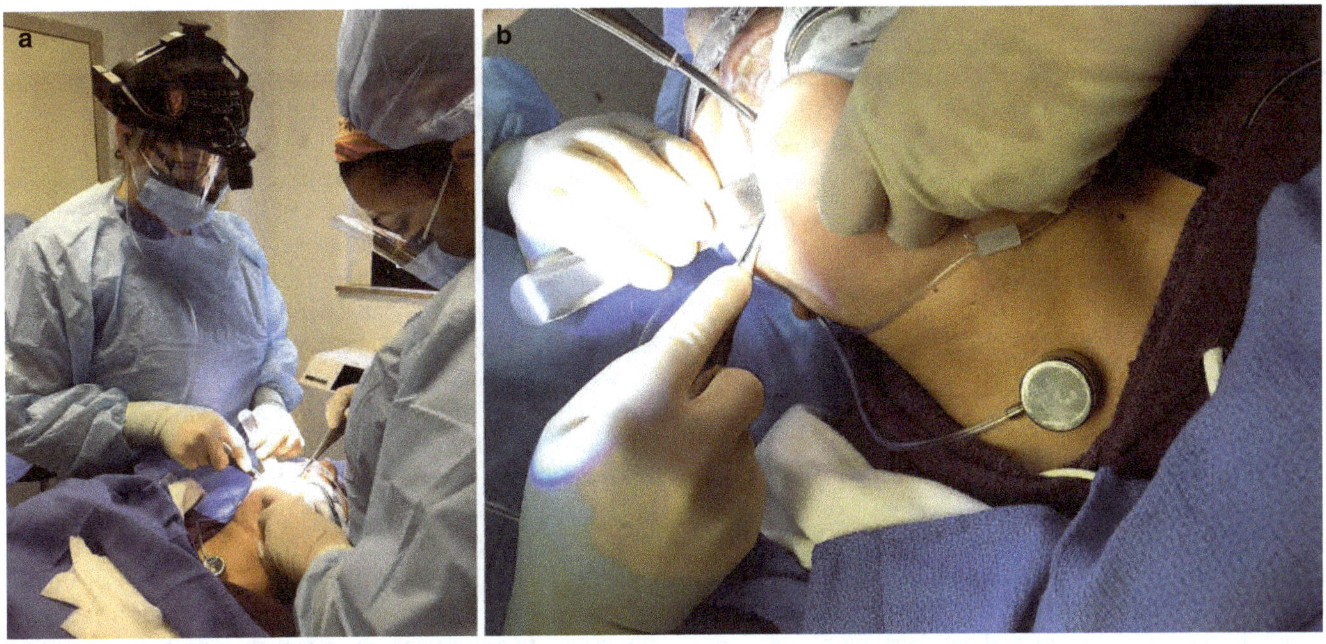




**Fig. 6.6** (**a**, **b**) Pretracheal/precordial stethoscope used by the surgeon to auscultate while the patient is sedated

tation with a precordial stethoscope. The newer Bluetooth models of the precordial stethoscope allow wireless speakers that allow the entire team to listen to the patient's respiratory patterns.

Now with multiple modalities such as a real-time capnography tracing, listening to breath sounds with high fidelity, OMS team has an opportunity to assess and act promptly on potential airway threats even before the adverse respiratory event comes to light. With these available modalities, along with surgeon's experience and developed senses, anticipation and prediction of an impending laryngospasm or bronchospasm prompts the team to act preemptively. Even before a drop in oxygen saturation or loss of waveform on capnography becomes apparent, both the depth and rate of breathing as well as the cessation of breathing can be promptly recognized.

## 6.13 Airway Armamentarium

Despite several preventive modalities available to the OMS performing anesthesia, emergencies are bound to happen. The unit must be prepared to handle airway and other emergencies. All the anesthesia providers should be exceptionally familiar with emergency airway equipment that must be readily accessible in both the operating suites and the recovery area [11].

Emergency airway equipment must include full face mask, bag-valve-mask device capable of providing positive pressure ventilation, oral and nasopharyngeal airways, supraglottic airway devices, endotracheal tubes, and laryngoscope and cricothyrotomy kit. All these equipment should be available in both pediatric and adult sizes. The entire staff should have periodic in-office training to familiarize themselves with the equipment and their use. Apart from emergency airway instruments, all offices are required to have either a basic monophasic defibrillator or automated external defibrillator.

## 6.14 Oxygen and Supplemental Gas Delivery System

In addition to oxygen, most OMS offices utilize other gases such as nitrous oxide and inhalational anesthetics as well as air. The oxygen delivery system should be able to deliver metered oxygen to the patient under positive pressure. A standard fail-safe mechanism along with scavenging system should be part of all gas delivery machines installed in the office. This prevents delivery of any hypoxic amount of gases. To prevent the accidental administration of an incorrect gas, the gas outlets used should be pin-indexed. The gas delivery machines also are mandated to have periodic calibration records, which should be maintained with proper documentation stored at a known location. Anesthesia equipment, including ventilators, are similarly required to have a periodic inspection by biomedical engineers. The OMS office is responsible for ensuring this happens and the office anesthesia evaluation is a mechanism to keep a check on this.

## 6.15 Suction Equipment

As trivial as it may seem, the office suction unit (central and portable) is an integral part of both the normal and emergency functions of that office. A portable suction unit must be readily accessible in the operatory and recovery area in case of unanticipated power failure or central suction pump failure. Again, routine maintenance of the suction system and its documentation is required.

## 6.16 Recovery Room

Most OMS offices have a postoperative recovery unit separate from the operatory that allows unobstructed patient observation. The design of this area must allow resuscitation and management of the patient during an emergency. The recovery area should have a suction system, oxygen delivery system, all appropriate monitors and emergency equipment as detailed earlier. It is also the responsibility of the recovery nurse to document the patient's recovery from anesthetic to deem their fitness to leave the office. A recovery checklist such as the Modified Aldrete Scale is useful in making this determination.

## 6.17 Techniques in Anesthesia

Training in anesthesia exposes the oral and maxillofacial surgeon to the different modalities of anesthesia from light to deep sedation. As described before, levels of anesthesia are a continuum (Table 6.1). The effects of different drugs and techniques may vary between individuals. Patients may achieve deeper or lighter levels of anesthesia than anticipated based on their unique metabolic responses to the different anesthetics administration. The OMS team is prepared to anticipate these differences in responses and intervene accordingly.

The techniques utilized to get to different levels of anesthesia include inhalational anesthesia, oral anesthetic technique, parenteral anesthesia, and local anesthesia. Regardless of the technique employed, the goals of each of these techniques are to reduce anxiety, establish cooperation, amnesia and analgesia, ensuring comfort and hemodynamic stability. In order to choose the level of anesthesia, one should consider the age of the patient, level of anxiety and ability to cooperate, detailed medical history, and prior anesthesia experience.

### 6.17.1 Enteral Anesthesia

Oral or nasal route of delivery of drugs is the least threatening route of administration of anesthesia. While some anxiolysis is achieved via this modality, it is rarely used to achieve deeper levels of anesthesia. Often the oral route of sedation is used as a premedication prior to IV access in an uncooperative patient. Various ingestives such as syrups, popsicles, needleless syringes, other creative methods are employed to get the patient to consume the medication. Dosing is adjusted in such a way that a higher dose of the drug may be administered in a limited volume to prevent the likelihood of aspiration. Despite that, a crying child or a coughing adult may end up aspirating the medication. The other disadvantages of this technique include a slow onset and variable response to the action of the drug as well as an unpredictable recovery pattern. In an uncooperative patient, patient compliance will limit oral or nasal administration of any drug. Additionally, oral dosing is often empiric with almost predictable erratic absorption. Titration of the drug is difficult via this route.

Yet, it remains a convenient mode of administration, requiring very little training to deliver, and any adverse reactions are slow to the onset and usually less severe and manageable. In the US, a medical provider providing oral sedation in the office does not have an increase in their malpractice premiums because of this practice. In contrast, practitioners of general anesthesia have higher malpractice coverage due to the inherent risks of that practice.

An ideal oral medication must be able to provide rapid absorption, must have a rapid onset, and must have a high therapeutic index allowing rapid and predictable recovery.

The following are the drugs most commonly used in oral sedation techniques:

- Benzodiazepines
- Histamine blockers
- Opioids
- Scopolamine
- Chloral hydrate
- Barbiturates
- Alpha agonists—Dexmedetomadine, Clonidine

Oral sedation techniques are primarily useful in the OMS as a premedication tool. An orally sedated patient is likely to accept a mask or an IV for further induction of anesthesia. Several minor procedures, however, can be performed with oral sedation and good local anesthesia alone.

### 6.17.2 Parenteral Anesthesia: Intravenous Anesthesia and Inhalational Anesthesia

Hubbell [5] was known to promote the use of intravenous thiopental anesthesia. It was eventually replaced by the shorter-acting barbiturate methohexital. This became the primary agent used for office-based anesthesia for multiple decades. A shortage in supply of methohexital and an increased use of Propofol [8] in the operating theater setting prompted an adaptation of the use of that drug in the office-based anesthetic technique. The basic technique for deep sedation and general anesthetic in the nonintubated patient in the OMS office typically employs a cocktail of medications under strict ASA-mandated guidelines for monitoring with the personnel as described earlier.

These medications include, but are not limited to, the following:

- A benzodiazepine such as Midazolam for anxiolysis, amnesia, sedation, and hypnosis
- A potent narcotic analgesic such as Fentanyl or Remifentanil
- A potent non-narcotic analgesic such as Ketamine
- A sedative hypnotic such as Propofol. It also acts as an adjunct antiemetic agent.
- Adjuvant drugs such as dexamethasone for prevention of postoperative edema and nausea and vomiting.
- Toradol or i.v. Tylenol for adjunct pain control

Most of these medications are characterized by their ability to have a rapid onset and offset. Medications such as Propofol rapidly redistribute and metabolize and are eliminated from the system. The combination of these medications often results in a cumulative effect of sedation and hypnosis in addition to central analgesia. Discomfort from the administration of local anesthesia is often obtunded by this level of sedation. Patients maintain their ventilation and careful monitoring of their vital signs and protection of their airway allows for smooth sedation. The surgeon who is performing the procedure is in close proximity to the patient's airway understanding its minute undulations and sensing the level of the patient's sedation and acting preemptively to either prolong or discontinue the sedation. It is an art and science that is built on years of training and experience.

The dosing of these medications is based on the patient's ideal body weight. The administration of these medications is through a continuous intravenous catheter infusion with an appropriate IV fluid. Typically, a 20- or a 22-gauge catheter is inserted into a peripheral vein in the upper extremity. Most OMSs practice the bolus technique, which introduces incremental doses of each medication, titrated to effect. Infusion pumps are often utilized in longer cases, while shorter cases of sedation seldom require infusion.

Using a continuous infusion has the following tangible advantages:

- Minimize fluctuations in drug serum concentration
- Smoother intraoperative course
- Enhanced cardiovascular stability
- Enhanced respiratory stability
- Less patient movement
- More rapid recovery
- Minimal drug utilization

## 6.18 Emergency Drugs

The ninth edition of the AAOMS Office Anesthesia Evaluation Manual [12] provides a detailed list of medications that can be used during anesthetic emergency. OMS offices are recommended to have a refrigerator designated for medications requiring cold storage. Pharmacy boards of different states control the storage and distribution of these drugs.

Listed are suggested drugs used in the event of anesthetic emergencies:

- Intravenous fluids: normal saline, lactated Ringer, etc.
- Cardiovascular medications: Oxygen, Atropine, Nitroglycerin, Dopamine, Epinephrine, Dobutamine, Ephedrine, Phenylephrine, Lidocaine, Propranolol, Procainamide, Verapamil, Amiodarone, Adenosine
- Antihypertensive medications: Diazoxide, Hydralazine, Esmolol, Labetalol
- Diuretics: Furosemide (Lasix)
- Antiemetics: Prochlorperazine, Ondansetron
- Reversal agents: Naloxone (Narcan), Flumazenil (Romazicon)

**Additional Drugs**

- Dextrose 50%, Dexamethasone (Decadron), Hydrocortisone sodium succinate or Methyl prednisolone sodium succinate (Solu-Medrol), Glycopyrolate (Robinul), Diazepam (Valium), Midazolam (Versed), Albuterol inhaler, Succinylcholine (Anectine), Morphine sulfate, Dantrolene (Dantrium), Lidocaine, Nonenteric-coated aspirin, Famotidine (Pepcid), Diphenhydramine (Benadryl)

## 6.19 Activism and Leadership in Office-Based Anesthesia

Dental anesthesia is an ADA-recognized specialty in the US as of 2019. Several dental practitioners, including OMSs, practice anxiolysis and sedation in their offices, outside a hospital operating suite and without a separate anesthesia provider. The concerted efforts by various interested parties to politically organize and better protect our intellectual and political interests in the discipline make this practice a reality in the US.

To ensure the commitment to patient safety, the AAOMS and its Board of Trustees have embraced a multipronged approach:

- undiluted enforcement of educational standards that requires resident rotation on the medical anesthesia service
- a self-imposed mandatory AAOMS Office Anesthesia Evaluation Program
- a devotion to the anesthesia team approach and development of the DAANCE program for the assistants
- the development of anesthesia and emergency management simulation programs such as Basic Emergency Airway Management [BEAM] and Office-Based Crisis Management [OBCM] are some examples of some of this commitment.

The AAOMS developed an Anesthesia Safety Conference for our own specialty that was held on April 27, 2017, at the American Society of Anesthesiologists headquarters in Schaumburg, Illinois. Representatives of the ASA as well as representatives of the appropriate disciplines of dentistry attended this meeting. In April 2019, a second patient safety conference focusing on pediatric sedation was organized at the AAOMS headquarters in Rosemont, Illinois.

By staying on the forefront of office-based anesthesia and by enforcing the highest standards of safety in patient care, OMS as a specialty has become stalwart in this arena. Continued positive momentum with nationwide simulation workshops and a mobile application supporting the office anesthesia evaluation will enhance our role as leaders in ambulatory anesthesia in our offices. The rapid response and emergency system and the healthcare infrastructure in the US allows for OMSs in this country to adapt this technique and methodology into their practices almost effortlessly. In other parts of the world, this may not be a model that is easy to replicate.

## References

1. American Society of Anesthesiologists (ASA). Continuum of depth of sedation: definition of general anesthesia and levels of sedation/analgesia. (Approved by the ASA House of Delegates on October 13, 1999 and last amended on October 15, 2014). Available at: https://www.asahq.org/standards-and-guidelines/continuum-of-

depth-of-sedation-definition-of-general-anesthesia-and-levels-of-sedationanalgesia
2. Bicentenary of nitrous oxide. Br Med J. 1972 May 13;2(5810):367-368. PubMed PMID: 4554156; PubMed Central PMCID: PMC1788276.
3. West JB. Humphry Davy, nitrous oxide, the pneumatic institution, and the royal institution. Am J Physiol Lung Cell Mol Physiol 2014 Nov 1;307(9):L661-L667.
4. Desai MS, Desai SP. Discovery of modern anesthesia: a counterfactual narrative about Crawford W. long, Horace Wells, Charles T. Jackson, and William T. G. Morton. AANA J 2015 Dec;83(6):410-415. PubMed PMID: 26742335.
5. Hubbell AO, Adams CR. Intravenous anesthesia for dental surgery with sodium ethyl (1-Methylbutyl) Thiobarbituric acid. J ADA. 1940;27(8):1186–91.
6. Shane SM. Intravenous amnesia for total dentistry in one sitting. J Oral Surg 1966 Jan;24(1):27-32. PubMed PMID: 5214559.
7. Lieblich SE. Methohexital versus propofol for outpatient anesthesia. Part I: Methohexital is superior. J Oral Maxillofac Surg 1995 Jul;53(7):811-815. Review. PubMed PMID: 7595796.
8. Dembo JB. Methohexital versus propofol for outpatient anesthesia. Part II: Propofol is superior. J Oral Maxillofac Surg 1995 Jul;53(7):816-820. Review. PubMed PMID: 7595797.
9. Lieblich S. Providing anesthesia in the Oral and maxillofacial surgery office: a look Back, where we are now and a look ahead. J Oral Maxillofac Surg 2018 May;76(5):917-925. Review.
10. Drew SJ. Oral and maxillofacial surgery team anesthesia model and anesthesia assistant training. Oral Maxillofac Surg Clin North Am 2018 May;30(2):145-153. Review.
11. Chung WL. Anesthesia equipment for the oral and maxillofacial surgery practice. Oral Maxillofac Surg Clin North Am 2013 Aug;25(3):373-383.
12. American Association of Oral and Maxillofacial Surgeons (AAOMS). Office anesthesia evaluation manual. 9th edition. 2018. Available at: http://www.aaoms.org.
13. American Association of Oral and Maxillofacial Surgeons (AAOMS). Parameters of Care: AAOMS Clinical Practice Guidelines for Oral and Maxillofacial Surgery (AAOMS ParCare) Sixth Edition 2017. Patient assessment. Available at: https://www.aaoms.org/images/uploads/pdfs/parcare_assessment.pdf
14. American Association of Oral and Maxillofacial Surgeons (AAOMS). Parameters of Care: AAOMS Clinical Practice Guidelines for Oral and Maxillofacial Surgery (AAOMS ParCare) Sixth Edition 2017. Anesthesia in outpatient facilities. Available at: https://www.joms.org/article/S0278-2391(17)30488-3/pdf
15. Todd DW, Schaefer JJ 3rd. The American Association of Oral and Maxillofacial Surgeons Simulation Program. Oral Maxillofac Surg Clin North Am 2018 May;30(2):195-206. Review.
16. ASA Physical Status Classification System. Developed By: ASA House of Delegates/Executive Committee, Last Amended: October 15, 2014 (original approval: October 15, 2014). Available at: https://www.asahq.org/standards-and-guidelines/asa-physical-status-classification-system.
17. American Society of Anesthesiologists (ASA). Standards for basic anesthetic monitoring. Developed By: Committee on Standards and Practice Parameters (CSPP) Last Amended: October 28, 2015 (original approval: October 21, 1986). Available at: https://www.asahq.org/standards-and-guidelines/standards-for-basic-anesthetic-monitoring.
18. Farish SE, Garcia PS. Capnography primer for Oral and maxillofacial surgery: review and technical considerations. J Anesth Clin Res 2013 Mar 18;4(3):295. PubMed PMID: 24459603; PubMed Central PMCID: PMC3897173.

# 7

# Maxillofacial Surgery: Application and Issues with Anesthesia

Rebecca Jacob, Subramanyam S. Mahankali,
Renita Maria, Suman Ananathanarayana, Garima Sharma,
and Mary Thomas

## 7.1 Introduction

Maxillofacial surgery encompasses a wide range of procedures on the head and neck, combining oral and facial procedures with the ear, nose and throat (ENT), plastic surgery, neurosurgery and base of skull specialities. It ranges from simple dental extractions to complex reconstructive and free flap surgery.

Patients of all age groups may present for maxillofacial surgery. The main issues involve managing a shared airway; providing good access to head, neck and oral cavity. The management of difficult airways and measures to reduce tissue bleeding and oedema, both intra- and post-operatively pose a unique challenge to the anaesthetist. Good communication between all members of the team is essential [1].

## 7.2 Preoperative Assessment

All patients should be assessed preoperatively and an anaesthetic plan should be formulated as these patients may have a suspected or a known difficult airway or are undergoing complex or prolonged surgery. Patients may give the history of poor oral intake and nutritional state due to pain, dysphagia and odynophagia. If dyspnoea is present, it should be evaluated as to whether it is cardiac or respiratory in origin.

R. Jacob (✉) · S. S. Mahankali · R. Maria · S. Ananathanarayana · G. Sharma
Department of Anesthesiology, Columbia Asia Referral Hospital, Yeshwantpur, Bangalore, Karnataka, India

M. Thomas
Department of Anesthesiology, Regional Cancer Centre, Medical College Campus, Thiruvananthapuram, Kerala, India

Previous surgeries, medication history and comorbidities diagnosed earlier should be noted. Medication history is important in all patients, especially elderly patients with cardiac, respiratory or renal involvement. It is also important to ascertain whether the patients have any comorbid ailments like hypertension, diabetes, thyrotoxicosis or myxoedema, a history of epistaxis or bleeding tendency and use of anticoagulants [2, 3].

### 7.2.1 Patients on anticoagulants

Patients on anticoagulants may present for emergency or elective surgery. The type of anticoagulant the patient is on should be noted during pre-operative assessment. Risk of peri-operative bleeding versus thrombosis on discontinuation of anticoagulants should be stratified and accordingly discontinued or bridged with preferably unfractionated heparin or low-molecular-weight heparin prior to elective surgery. Usually, three half-lives ($T_{1/2}$) discontinuation of anticoagulants prior to surgery is considered optimal to prevent blood loss (Table 7.1) [3].

In emergency situations, the main goals are discontinuation of anticoagulation, delaying semi-urgent procedures as appropriate and employment of reversal strategies like plate-

**Table 7.1** Recommendations for discontinuation of anticoagulation prior to elective surgery

| Drug | Time of discontinuation |
|---|---|
| Warfarin | 5 days |
| Factor Xa inhibitors | > 24 h |
| Rivaroxaban | ROCKET AF ≥ 3 days |
| Apixaban | Low bleed risk ≥24 h |
| | High bleed risk ≥48 h |
| Low-molecular-weight heparin | 12 h |
| Prophylactic | 24 h |
| Therapeutic dose | |

American College of Chest Physician 2012 Guidelines published in Chest, the RE-LY trial published in Circulation 2014, the ROCKET AF trial, and the manufacturer's recommendations let transfusions, fresh frozen plasma, vitamin K antagonists, and prothrombin complex concentrates.

The previous anaesthetic charts should be reviewed for the techniques used, ease of mask ventilation, best direct laryngoscopy grade, Endotracheal tube (ETT) size used, and any difficulties encountered and should be noted. The airway of previously operated patients may be altered due to previous surgeries and/or oedema, so this should be taken into account while reviewing the anaesthetic and follow-up records of the patient. If nasal intubation is required, one should enquire about nostril patency (history of nasal polyps or deviated septum). Contraindications to the use of controlled hypotension, e.g. cerebrovascular, reno-vascular and moderate-to-severe coronary artery disease should also be assessed. Specific attention should be given to the needs of each class of patient.

### 7.2.2 Oncology Patients

Patients with head and neck cancer sometimes constitute the most challenging patients. Their upper airway may be seriously distorted, and they may have tracheal stenosis or hardening and fixation of the soft tissues due to radiotherapy.

In these patients, documents concerning previous surgeries, radiation and chemotherapy should be studied. The difficult airway may have been encountered, tracheostomy and residual tracheal stenosis, limited mouth opening, and neck extension may have been recorded [4].

Symptoms such as hoarse voice, stridor, and dyspnoea will indicate whether there is airway compromise due to stenosis, tumour, nerve damage or oedema. Post radiation, the patients may have tissue fibrosis with limited mouth opening or neck extension. Make a note of chemotherapy drugs, duration and interval since the last cycle of chemotherapy.

### 7.2.3 Trauma Patients

Trauma patients require a thorough history of the mechanism of injury, which would indicate intracerebral or spinal injury. Drug and/or alcohol ingestion is often a contributory factor, and 15% have other injuries. There is also potential for injuries to other organs and massive blood loss. Cervical spine injury occurs in 5–10% of patients with blunt trauma to the head and face. Therefore, the patient should be evaluated from 'head to toe' [5].

### 7.2.4 Paediatric Patients

Consider age, weight, prematurity, feeding, nutritional status and position during sleep. In patients with craniofacial abnormalities, look for associated syndromes such as Pierre Robin sequence or Treacher Collins syndrome as in addition to a difficult airway these patients may have involvement of other systems, such as cardiac, as a part of the syndrome, which will require specialist consultation [6].

### 7.2.5 Toxic Airway/Infections

Infection of dental and facial structures commonly leads to erythema and swelling of tissues. This can result in obstruction of airway and difficulty in airway management. Toxic airways (e.g. Ludwig's angina, dental cysts and osteomyelitis) with spreading infection often present as acute emergencies and may pose an extreme airway maintenance challenge. Direct laryngoscopy due to trismus, tissue distortion, oedema or abscess cavity and pus may not be possible and other means of securing the airway must be considered [4] (Fig. 7.1a, b).

**Examination Table 7.2**

## 7.3 Airway Assessment

A detailed airway assessment based on criteria in the 'L-E-M-O-N' method would help to stratify the risk of difficult intubation. The 'LEMON Law' can be used to quickly assess for potentially difficult airways [7]. A total score of 10 can be given as per the criteria and higher scores are associated with poor glottic visualization and difficult intubation.

Please refer the Fig. 2.2 on LEMON in Chap. 2 on preoperative evaluation and investigations.

In paediatric patients, the Mallampati score does not accurately predict a poor view of the glottis and there are no standard values for the thyromental and horizontal length of the mandible. Thus, an adaptation is required, and this is found in the 'COPUR SCALE' (Table 7.3) [7, 8].

Once the airway assessment is done, check

- Whether mask ventilation would be possible after induction of General Anaesthesia (GA).
- Anticipated view during direct laryngoscopy.
- Whether it would be possible to use a supraglottic airway as a rescue device.
- Possibility and accessibility of a surgical airway in case of a dire emergency.

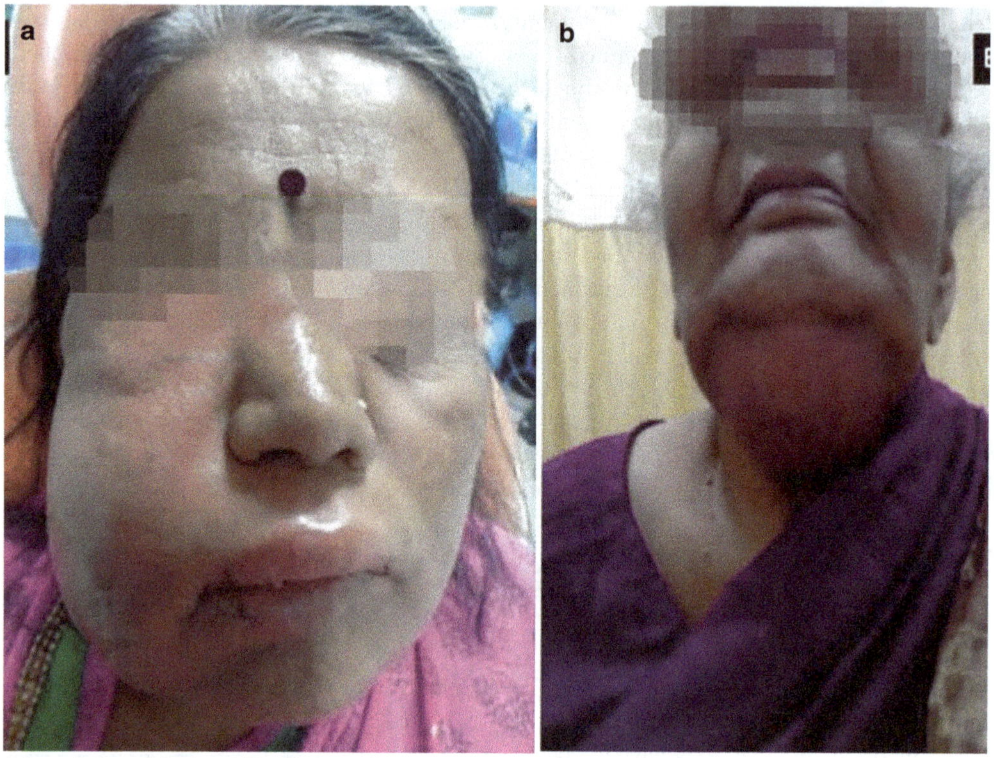


**Fig. 7.1** (**a**) Buccal abscess (**b**) ludwigs angina



**Table 7.2** Checklist of things for a safe surgery

| Pre-Anaesthesia Checklist |
|---|
| • Age and weight of the patient |
| • Type of maxillofacial surgery |
| • Previous surgeries/ associated complications |
| • Comorbidities and detailed medication list |
| • Known drug allergies |
| • CVS, RS, abdomen examination |
| • Detailed airway examination |
| • Venous access |
| • Adequate blood and blood products |

## 7.4 General Physical Examination

Look for pallor, icterus, cyanosis, clubbing, lymphadenopathy and oedema as well as the general nutritional status. Follow this up with pulse rate, blood pressure, respiratory rate, oxygen saturation, signs of dehydration, and responses denoted as AVPU–Alert, Verbal, Pain, Unresponsive.

AVPU is a simplified version of the Glasgow Coma Scale (GCS), which is easy to remember and apply to patients (Table 7.4) [9, 10]. It consists of four possible stages. When recording AVPU, it is important to document the time the observation was taken and to track any changes over time as this will help monitor the progress of the patient (Table 7.4).

Apart from these, specific systemic examination, including cardiovascular, respiratory, per-abdomen and central nervous system, should be done and if in any doubt a specialist should be consulted.

There are various scales used to record a patient's level of consciousness. One of the most detailed is the GCS, which is used worldwide (Table 7.5) [9, 10]. The GCS is a reasonably complicated system, which, unless you use regularly, can be difficult to remember and apply correctly.

### 7.4.1 Investigations

In addition to routine blood tests like complete blood counts, kidney function tests, blood sugars, coagulation profile, serology, blood grouping and cross-matching is required for major surgery.

Chest X-ray helps in visualising any pathology in the lungs. It may also reveal tracheal deviation. X-ray soft-tissue neck, airway ultrasound, computerized tomography (CT), and magnetic resonance imaging (MRI) scans may be helpful in cancer, infections, abscesses or trauma cases.

For cancer surgery, a nasoendoscopy & indirect laryngoscopy provides valuable information about the upper airway anatomy.

Electrocardiogram (ECG), echocardiogram, cardiopulmonary exercise testing or pulmonary function tests are required if there are symptoms or signs of cardiorespiratory disease.

**Table 7.3** Description of COPUR scale

| COPUR SCALE | |
|---|---|
| *C = Chin* | Normal – 1<br>Small, moderately hypoplastic - 2<br>Markedly recessive – 3<br>Extremely hypoplastic – 4 |
| *O – Opening*<br>Interdental space between front teeth | > 40 mm – 1<br>20-40 mm – 2<br>10-20 mm – 3<br>< 10 mm – 4 |
| *P – Previous intubation or OSA* | Previous easy – 1<br>No attempt/no h/o OSA – 2<br>OSA, previous difficult intubation – 3<br>Extremely difficult intubation/ tracheostomy/can't lie down supine – 4 |
| *U – Uvula*<br>Mouth open tongue out | Tip of uvula visible – 1<br>Uvula partially visible – 2<br>Uvula concealed/soft palate visible – 3<br>Soft palate not visible – 4 |
| *R – Range*<br>Line from eye to orbit, range of motion looking up & down | >120°– 1<br>60–120° –2<br>30–60°–3<br>< 30°– 4 |
| *Prediction points for ease of intubation*<br>5–7: Easy normal intubation<br>8–10: Laryngeal help may be required<br>12: More difficult, may be less traumatic<br>14: Difficult intubation, fibre optic or other advanced technique may be required<br>16: Dangerous airway, consider awake intubation/potential tracheostomy | |

**Table 7.4** AVPU scale described with examples

| | | Adult Behaviour | Paediatric Behaviour |
|---|---|---|---|
| A | ALERT | Eyes open spontaneously.<br>Appears aware of and responsive to the environment.<br>Follows commands, eyes track people and objects | Child is active and responds appropriately to parents and other external stimuli |
| V | VOICE | Eyes do not open spontaneously but open to verbal stimuli.<br>Able to respond in some meaningful way when spoken to | Responds only when his or her name is called |
| P | PAIN | Does not respond to questions but moves or cries out in response to painful stimuli such as pinching the skin or earlobe | Responds only when painful stimuli are received such as pinching the nail bed |
| U | UNRESPONSIVE | Patient does not respond to any stimuli | No response at all |

**Table 7.5** Glasgow Coma Scale described in detail

| Glasgow Coma Scale | | |
|---|---|---|
| Behaviour | Response | Score |
| Eye opening (E) | Spontaneous | 4 |
| | To speech | 3 |
| | To pressure | 2 |
| | None | 1 |
| Verbal response (V) | Orientated | 5 |
| | Confused | 4 |
| | Words, but not coherent | 3 |
| | Sounds, but no words | 2 |
| | None | 1 |
| Motor response (M) | Obeys command | 6 |
| | Moves to localised pain | 5 |
| | Flexion withdrawal to pain | 4 |
| | Abnormal flexion (decorticate) | 3 |
| | Abnormal extension (Decerebrate) | 2 |
| | No response | 1 |
| Total score | Best response | 15 |
| | Comatose | </=6 |
| | Totally unresponsive | 3 |

### 7.4.2 Counselling and Reassurance

This is essential in all cases but especially so in patients who may have dramatic cosmetic changes or are undergoing cancer surgery like hemi-mandibulectomy. The possibility of tracheostomy and loss of voice must also be discussed with empathy. Video counselling may be resorted to in case of need.

### 7.4.3 Informed Consent

Any patient above the age of 18 years may give consent for surgery and anaesthesia. In the case of patients younger than 18 years, consent must be obtained from a parent or guardian after full explanation of procedures. The consent must be documented and signed by both the person taking the consent and the person giving the consent.

### 7.4.4 Transport to Operation Theatre (OT)

Should be with a trained health care worker especially if the patient has been given a sedative premedication. It is advisable for a parent or guardian to accompany younger children to the OT.

### 7.4.5 Handover Documents

All documents pertaining to the case must be handed over to the OT personnel and the handover documented.

## 7.5 Intraoperative Considerations

### 7.5.1 Before Induction (Figs. 7.2, 7.3, 7.4, 7.5, 7.6, 7.7, and 7.8) [6]

- Discuss the procedure and options with the lead surgeon
- Ensure patients vitals are stable
- Check anaesthetic machine and all equipment, including the 'Difficult Airway' cart and 'rescue devices' like Laryngeal Mask Airway (LMA) and tracheostomy tubes.
- If an 'uncommon' ETT like a flexometallic or (RAE) Ring-Adair-Elwyn tube is to be used, ensure that a regular tube of the appropriate size and one size smaller are available
- Ensure you have adequate help and each one knows what is expected of him/her
- Check intravenous (IV) access and all drugs available in the OT—drawn up and labelled.
- Check that blood is available if deemed necessary
- If intubation is difficult do not try more than 2–3 times with any one method (you will precipitate oedema and make matters worse)
- *CALL FOR HELP EARLY*

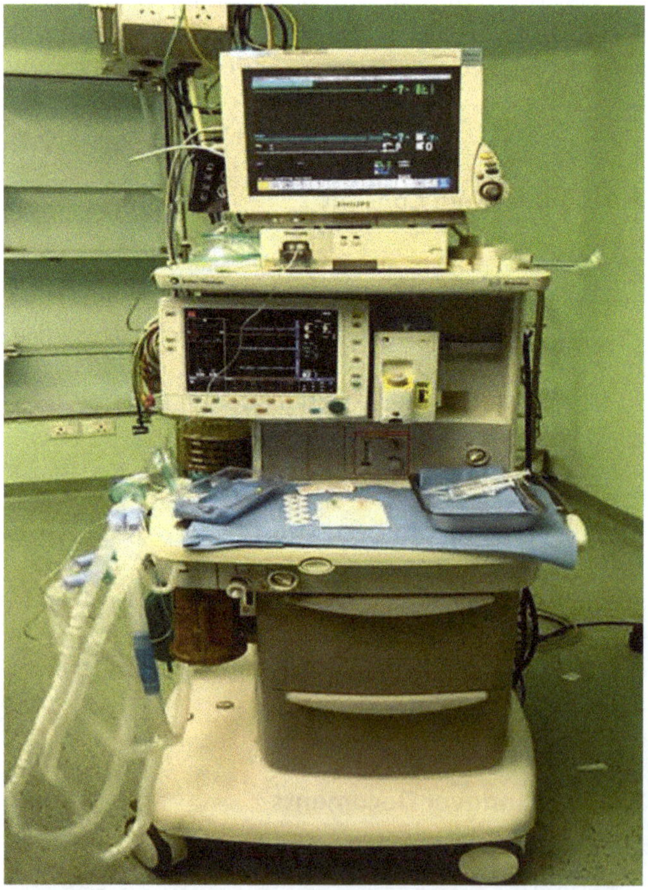



**Fig. 7.2** Anaesthetic apparatus

- Continue oxygenation with spontaneous respiration and wake up the patient if intubation is unsuccessful

*More patients have died from lack of oxygen than from lack of an endotracheal tube!*

*Please see Chap. 42 in this book to read about avoidable human errors for a safer patient care. (A case of loss of airway is discussed in Chap. 42).*

### 7.5.2 Induction

Anaesthesia may be induced either intravenously or with an inhalational agent. The choice of technique depends on:

- *Airway factors:* For example, an anticipated 'difficult airway' or limited mouth opening
- *Patient factors:*
  Paediatrics
  Post radiation
  Trauma
- *Associated comorbidities:* e.g. ischemic heart disease or emphysema.
  Nil-per-oral status
- *Surgical factors:*
  Trauma
  Cancer surgery
  Cosmetic
  Infective
  Vascular malformation

### 7.5.3 Monitoring

In young patients belonging to ASA (American Society of Anesthesiologists) Grade I and II, standard monitoring will suffice. Invasive arterial blood pressure monitoring may be required if controlled hypotension is planned or if comorbidities warrant. Monitoring of temperature is required in children and those undergoing prolonged surgeries like corrective LeFort osteotomies. Urinary catheterization may be required during prolonged surgeries.

### 7.5.4 *Airway management:* (Flow Chart 1)

The method of securing the airway should be discussed with the surgeon. This depends on:

- Patient factors, such as age, obesity, pan-facial trauma or anticipated difficult airway
- Site of operation may require oral or nasal intubation with specially configured tubes.
- Anaesthetists'/surgeons' preferences.

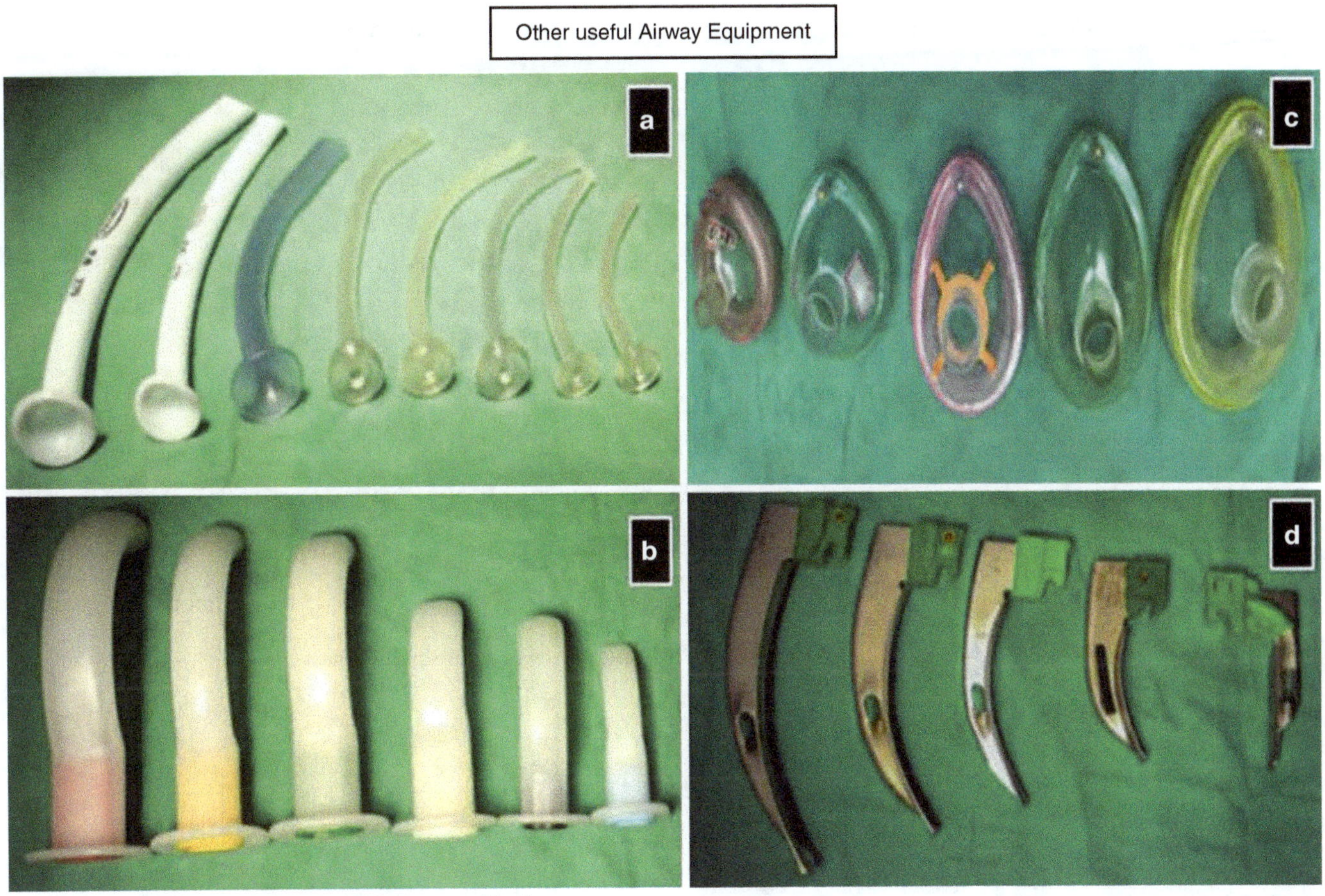


©Association of Oral and Maxillofacial Surgeons of India

**Fig. 7.3** (**a**) Nasal airway, (**b**) Oral airway, (**c**) Ventilation mask and (**d**) Laryngoscope blades

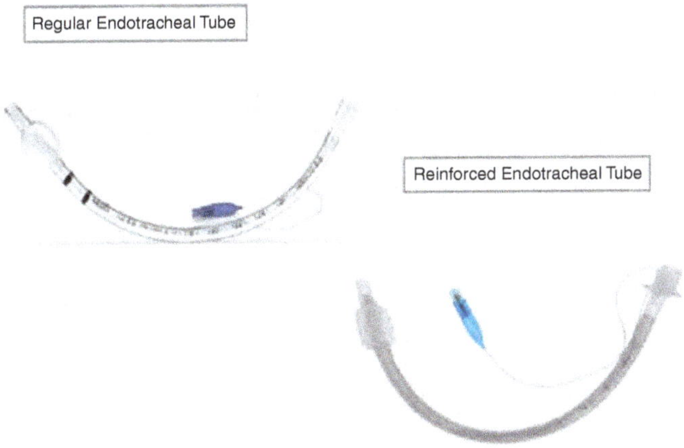


**Fig. 7.4** Endotracheal tubes

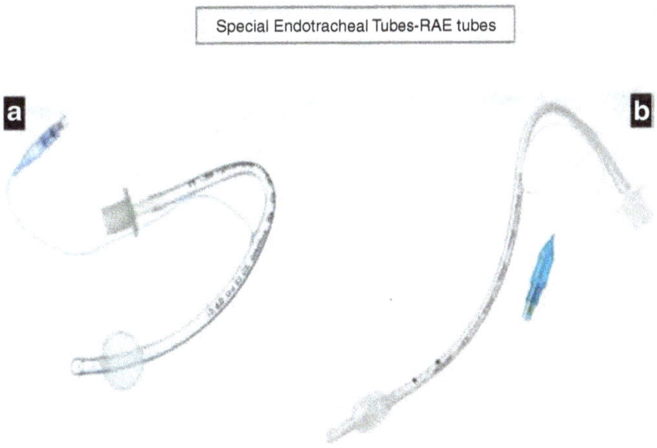


**Fig. 7.5** RAE tubes

Simple intraoral operations with no anticipated difficult airways can be done with standard nasal intubation or oral intubation under general anaesthesia with endotracheal tube pushed to the side opposite of surgery. Use of specially preformed tubes like RAE tubes and Reinforced/Armoured tube can be used to give good access to the surgical area (Figs. 7.4 and 7.5). However, major corrective surgeries will require the oral cavity to be empty and hence warrant nasal intubation, submental intubation or a tracheostomy. Anticipated non-obstructed difficult airway as assessed by history and/or examination or suspected (cervical) C-spine injury should be managed with awake fibre optic bronchoscopy or blind nasal

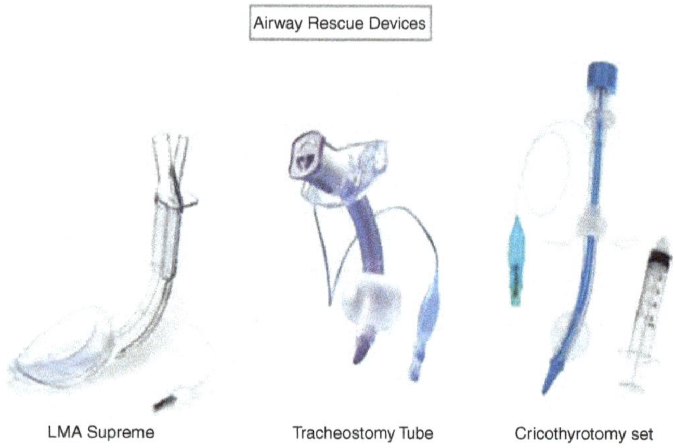


**Fig. 7.6** Airway rescue devices

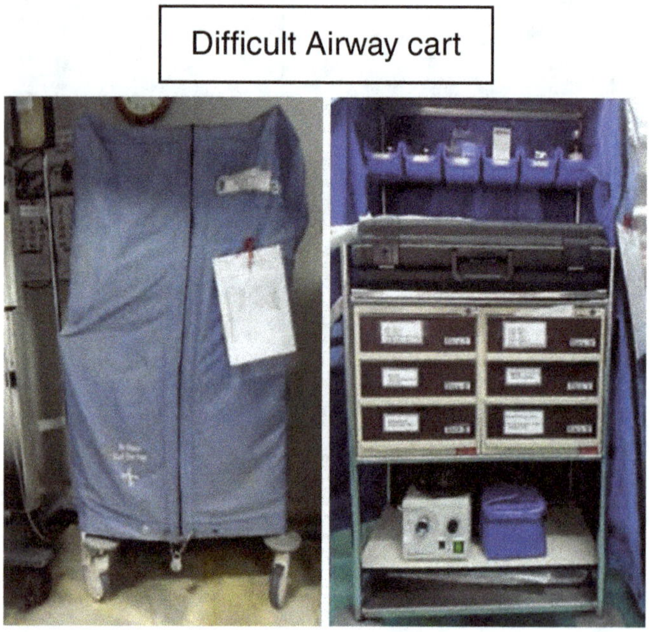


©Association of Oral and Maxillofacial Surgeons of India

**Fig. 7.7** Difficult airway cart

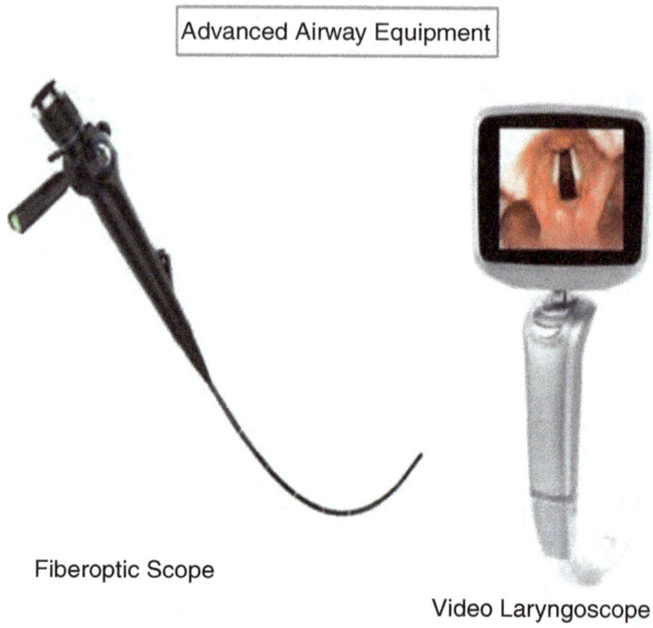


**Fig. 7.8** Advanced airway equipment

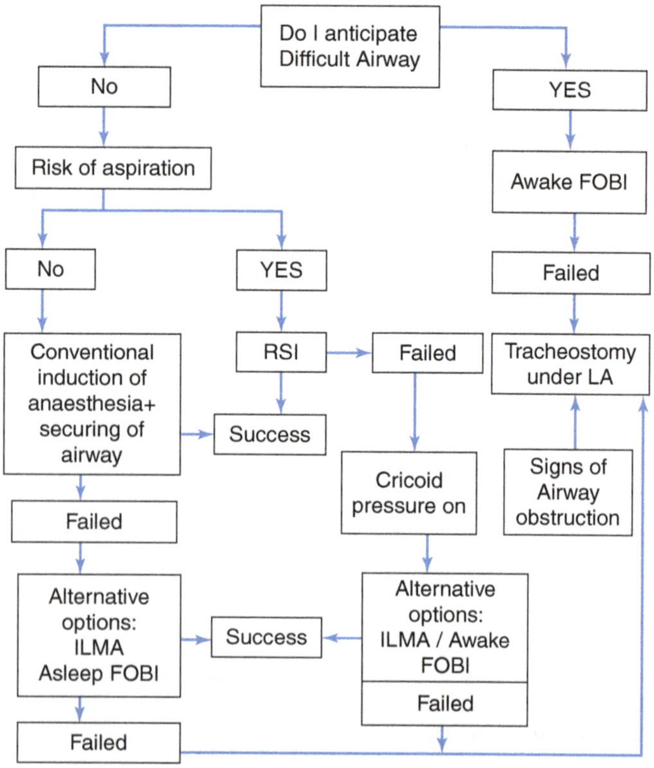


**Flow Chart 1** Airway management in oro-maxillo-facial surgery

intubation. The safety of awake intubation relies on the maintenance of spontaneous breathing, and the ability to stop and perform a different technique, such as awake tracheostomy, if intubation is unsuccessful. Most anaesthesiologists prefer the nasal route for fibre optic intubation, as it is technically easier. For this, the patency of the nostril should be assessed preoperatively, and roomier nostril should be chosen and prepared with vasoconstrictor drops like oxymetazoline hydrochloride.

Sedation may enhance the acceptability of awake fibre optic intubation. Dexmedetomidine infusion [11] serves this purpose very well. Airway instrumentation can be facilitated by local anaesthetic topicalisation of airway either by means of lignocaine nebulisation or 'spray as you go' technique and/airway blocks (glossopharyngeal, superior laryngeal and recurrent laryngeal nerve blocks) [12]. An antisialogoguelike glycopyrrolate administered 30–45 min prior will reduce the secretions and will facili-

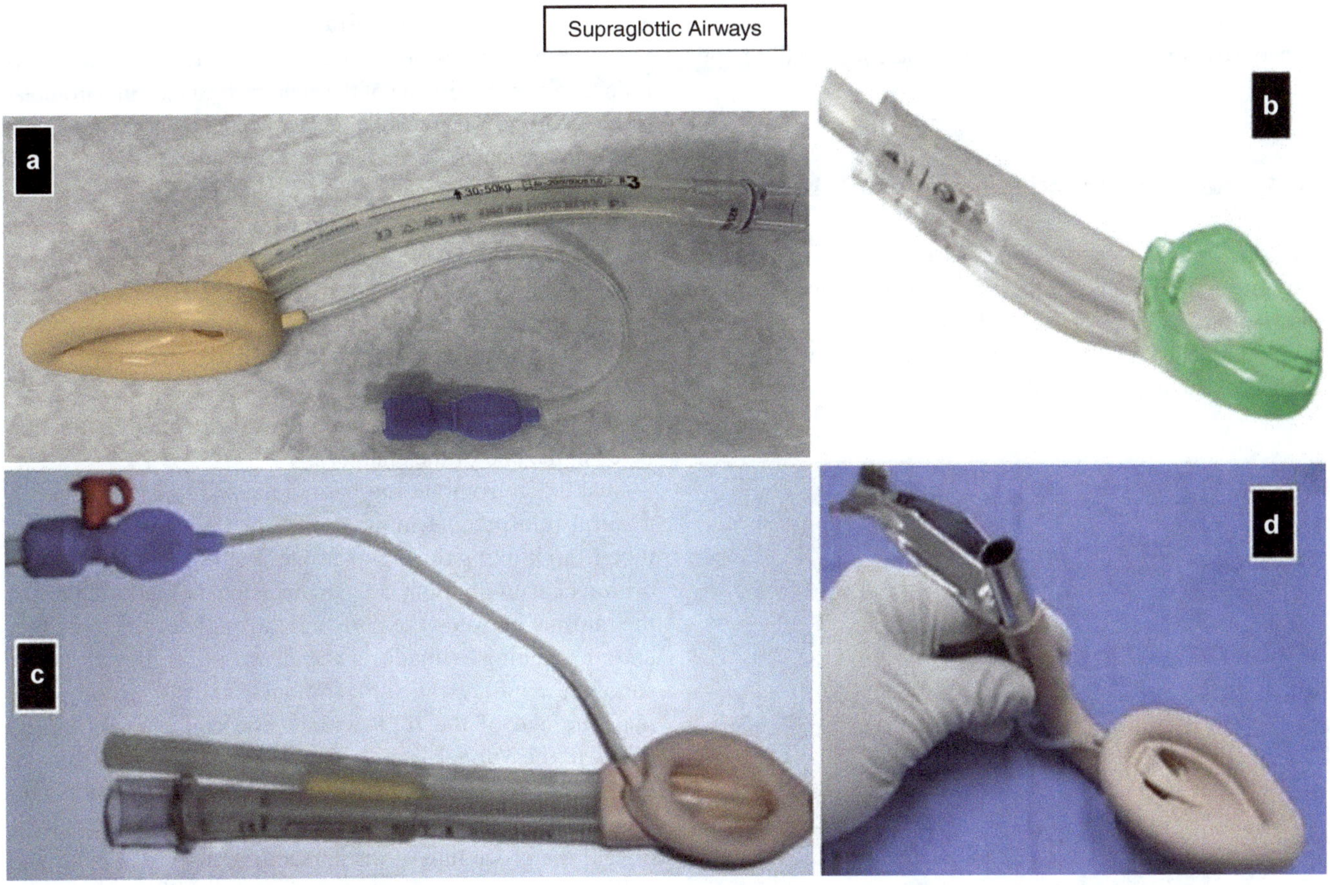




**Fig. 7.9** (**a**,**b**,**c**,**d**) Supraglottic airways

tate awake fibre optic intubation. Airway blocks may not be an option to facilitate awake intubation in cases such as extensive pan-facial fractures or post-radiation fibrosis of the neck. Fibre optic intubation may be impractical in case of oro-maxillofacial trauma if associated with severe airway bleeding that can obscure visibility and other options such as tracheostomy under local anaesthesia (LA) should be considered.

The traditional 'blind nasal intubation' is rarely employed these days but may be used if a fibre optic scope is not available or not possible (Video 7.1).

A 'plan B' should always be present if intubation by one method is unsuccessful.

During long surgery and if ventilated in the post-operative period, the Endotracheal (or tracheostomy) cuff pressure should be measured using an aneroid manometer. A pressure of 20–30 cm of $H_2O$ is considered as standard in adults.

In supraglottic obstruction—associated with stridor and respiratory distress, as in case of upper airway trauma, rapidly expanding infections like epiglottitis, Ludwig's angina, etc. awake fibre optic bronchoscopy and intubation may not be the right choice. In such a situation, an awake tracheostomy under local anaesthesia must be considered.

### 7.5.5 Supraglottic Airway Devices

Several varieties of supraglottic airway devices are available (Fig. 7.9). However, these are not ideal devices for oro-maxillofacial surgeries requiring the oral cavity to be empty, but can be lifesaving as rescue devices in 'cannot ventilate, cannot intubate' situations to ventilate a patient until the definitive airway is secured. However, a flexible reinforced LMA can be used for simple dental extractions and nasal, zygomatic and superficial facial surgery. However, obstruction and dislodgement can occur, especially when the mandible is moved.

## 7.6 Special Considerations

*Paediatrics:* [6] Children will not co-operate for awake fibre optic intubation. Hence, in such cases, the airway can be secured after inhalational induction without relaxation after establishing IV access. A nasopharyngeal airway may be passed gently into one nostril and connected to a breathing circuit while monitoring the end-tidal carbon dioxide ($EtCO_2$) and continuing the anaesthetic and oxygenation via the airway. The other nostril may now be prepared with a vasoconstrictor and local anaesthetic and used for fibre optic intubation (Fig. 7.10).

## 7.6.1 Retromolar and Submental Intubation

These techniques were developed as alternatives to tracheostomy in maxillofacial surgeries requiring intra-operative inter-dental fixation for malocclusion correction like comminuted fracture of the mid-face or the nose, where nasal intubation is contraindicated.

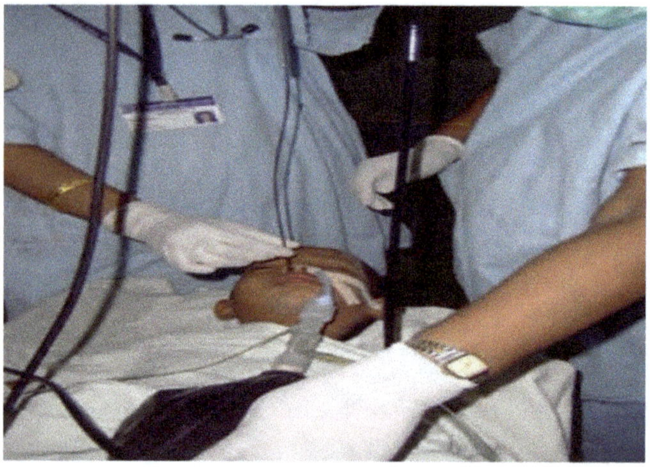



**Fig. 7.10** Fibre optic intubation in children

### 7.6.1.1 Retromolar Intubation

Pre-operatively check the adequacy of the retromolar space. This is done to prevent kinking of the endotracheal tube in retromolar space by insinuating the index finger behind the third molar and asking the patient to clench his teeth. The patients' airway is then intubated by the conventional method and the ETT is pushed in the retromolar space and brought out from the angle of the mouth and connected to the ventilator. The spiral reinforced/armoured ETT is preferred as it is kink resistant (Fig. 7.11).

### 7.6.1.2 Submental Orotracheal Intubation: [13] (Fig. 7.12a–f)

(See additional reading material on submental intubation given at the end of the chapter).

Just like retromolar intubation, it also requires the use of a spiral reinforced/armoured ETT in order to prevent the tube from kinking during its usage. Following conventional orotracheal intubation, a 2-cm incision is made lateral to the midline between the chin and the angle of the mandible and an opening is made in the floor of the mouth by the surgeon, avoiding the submandibular salivary glands. The machine end of the ETT without the connector is pulled through the tunnel, using gentle rotational movements. Following this manoeuvre, the tube is connected to the ventilating machine and sutures are used to fix the tube in position. If the procedure of disconnecting the ETT is long and pulling it out is prolonged, there is a possibility of hypoxia. So monitor oximetry closely and use high oxygen concentrations immediately before and after the placement of the submental tube (Video 7.2).

**Fig. 7.11** Retromolar intubation

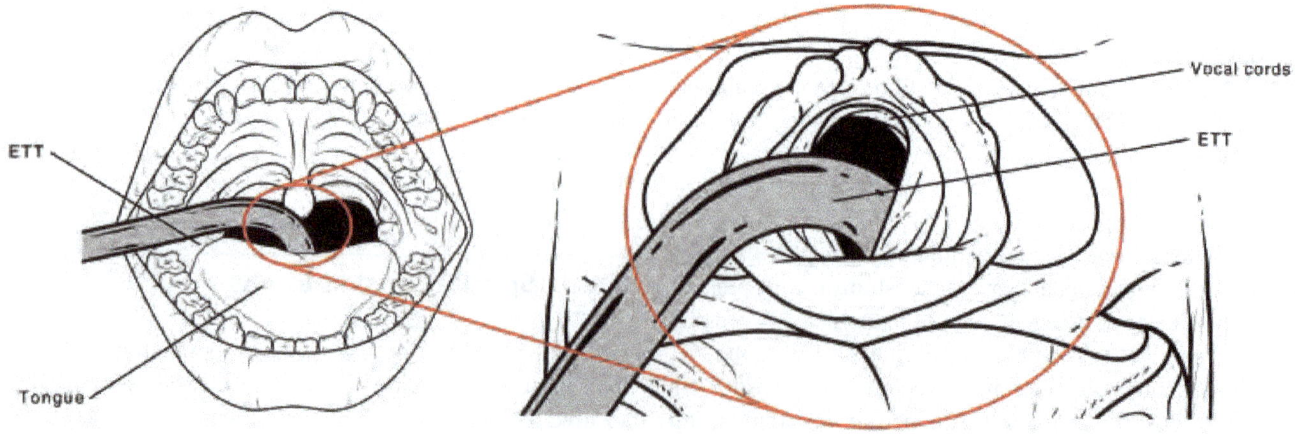

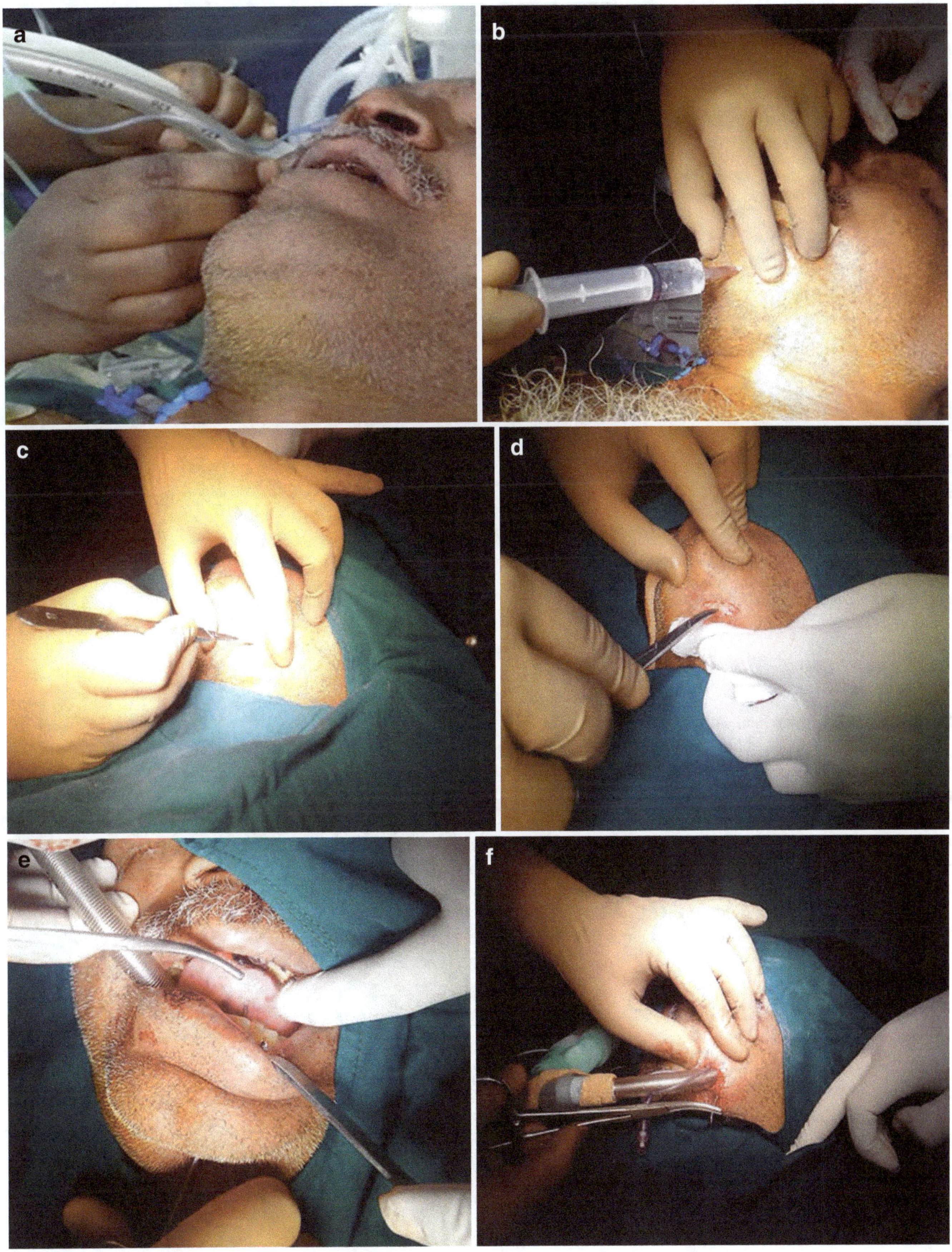

©Association of Oral and Maxillofacial Surgeons of India

**Fig. 7.12** (**a**–**f**) Various steps in submental intubation

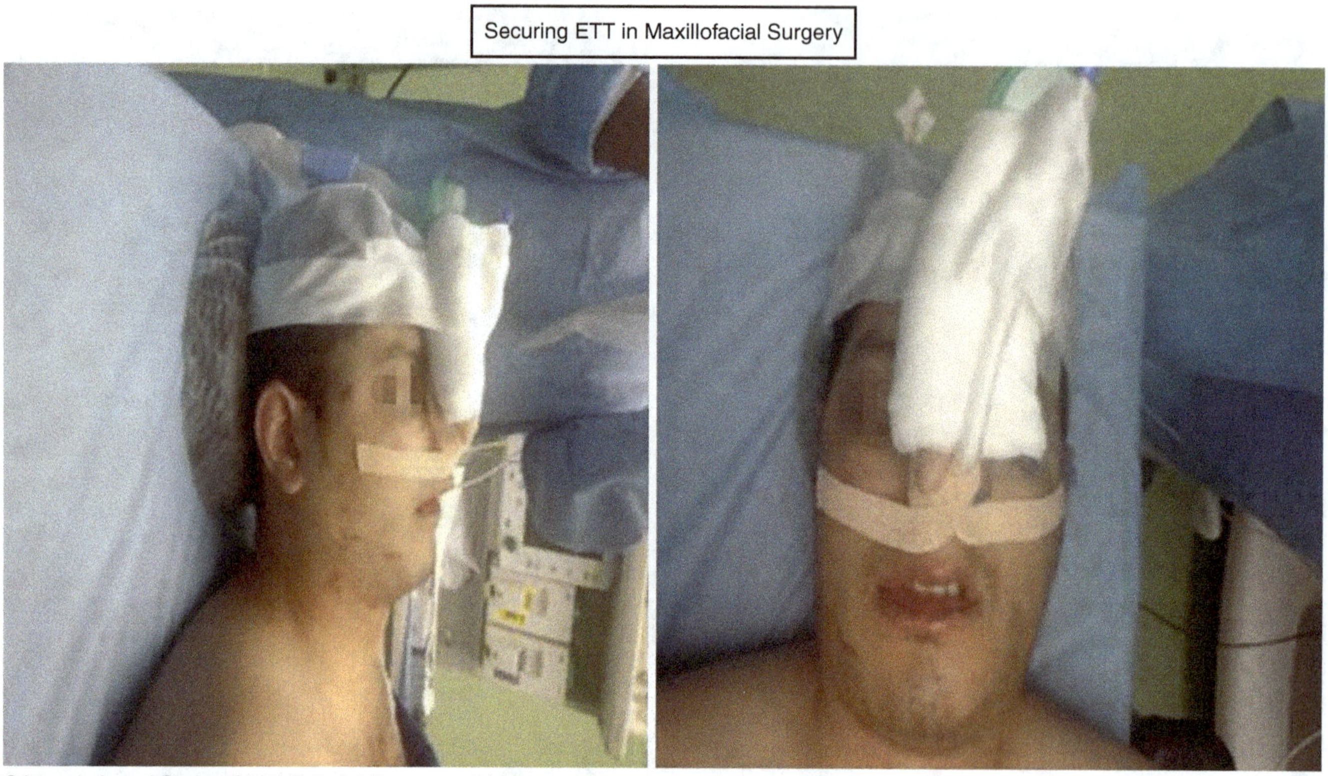


©Association of Oral and Maxillofacial Surgeons of India

**Fig. 7.13** Securing ETT in maxillofacial surgery

**Securing the Endotracheal Tube**

The ETT may dislodge intra-operatively as the airway is shared between the surgeon and anaesthetist; hence, special attention should be paid to securing the ETT. Preformed nasal RAE tubes, if used, should be supported on the nasal bridge and forehead with the help of preformed supports or pads and secured on the forehead with tapes in addition to securing at the nostril (Fig. 7.13). Submental tubes can be secured with sutures (Fig. 7.14) South Pole oral RAE tubes are usually fixed in the middle of the lower jaw with tapes (Fig. 7.15).

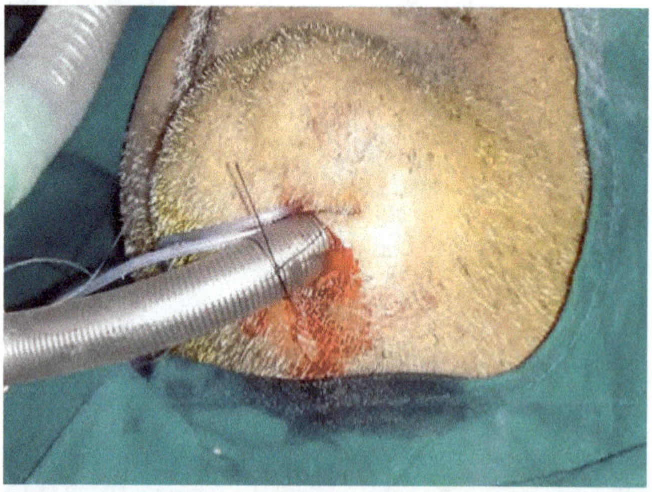

©Association of Oral and Maxillofacial Surgeons of India

**Fig. 7.14** Securing submental tube with sutures

## 7.6.2 Eyes

Preferably taped with transparent dressing or specialized eye pads to capture moisture and prevent drying especially during prolonged surgeries (Fig. 7.15).

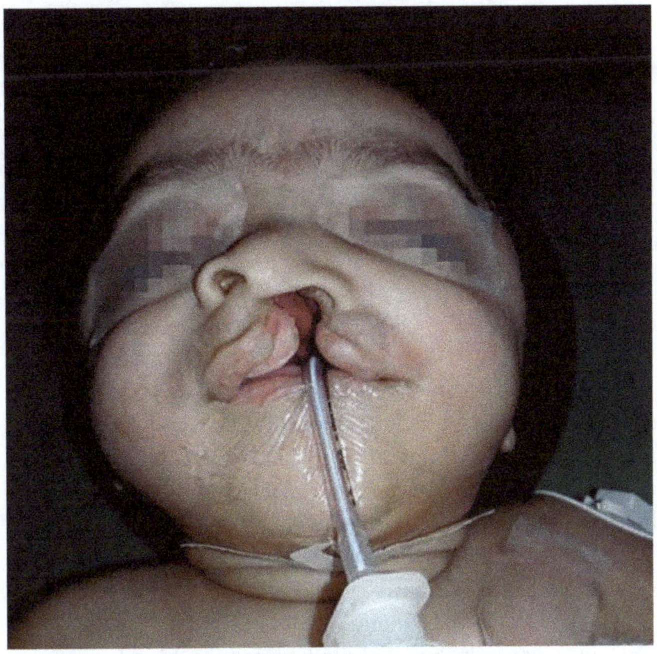



**Fig. 7.15** Securing oral south pole tubes/protection of the eyes with tapes

### 7.6.3 Positioning

Reverse Trendelenburg (anti-gravity) position with shoulder roll for adequate surgical exposure is preferred. Further, the operation table may be turned away from the anaesthetist and the anaesthesia machine by 90° or 180°. Hence, long breathing circuits, IV extensions and long cables for monitoring will be required.

### 7.6.4 Throat Pack

Saline-soaked throat packs will be required to protect the airway from blood, debris and saliva. It is advised to fix the tail end of the throat pack to the oral endotracheal tube whenever feasible to prevent accidental leaving behind of the throat pack at the end of surgery. Time of insertion and removal of the throat pack should be documented and carefully checked before extubation. If interdental wiring is planned at the end of surgery, then prior to doing so all throat packs should be removed and gauze counts should be confirmed.

## 7.7 Maintenance of Anaesthesia

Once the airway is secured, anaesthesia can be maintained with total intravenous anaesthesia (TIVA) or with volatile anaesthetics or combination of both as described earlier. Controlled ventilation with an intermediate-acting muscle relaxant such as atracurium or vecuronium is used.

Intra-operative analgesia is preferably provided with short-acting opioids such as fentanyl. Dexamethasone can be administered intra-operatively to reduce post-operative swelling, for its analgesic properties and as a prophylactic against post-operative nausea and vomiting (PONV) [14]. Orthognathic surgeries are associated with a high incidence of PONV; hence, additional antiemetics such as ondansetron should be administered prior to extubation especially if interdental wires are planned. Hypothermia can be a potential complication of prolonged orthognathic surgeries. Hence, temperature should be monitored and warming measures like intra-operative warm I.V fluids, forced air mattresses should be used. If there is a fear of airway compromise post-extubation, a tracheostomy should be done electively.

### 7.7.1 Deep Vein Thrombosis (DVT) Prophylaxis

Cancer patients and patients undergoing long surgery are at risk of developing thromboembolic complications. One or more of the following methods may be used to reduce its incidence.

Mechanical—Thromboembolic deterrent/Compression stockings (TEDS), pneumatic calf compression boots.

Pharmacological—Low-molecular-weight heparin such as Clexane could be used in patients at high risk for venous thromboembolism (VTE).

### 7.7.2 Control of Bleeding

The head and neck region receives rich blood supply from the branches of the carotid artery, and hence there is a tendency to bleed profusely during maxillofacial surgeries. Major bleeding can occur from branches of the maxillary artery or from pterygoid venous plexuses, leading to significant blood loss, warranting blood transfusion. Further, some of these procedures especially corrective osteotomies are extensive and time consuming. Surgical haemostasis is hampered by limited access. Risks involved in allogeneic blood transfusion have also been well documented and hence it is important to institute measures to reduce intra-operative blood loss and blood transfusion.

**Methods to control intra-operative blood loss include:**

Reverse Trendelenburg (anti-gravity) positioning.

Ensuring adequate venous drainage.

Antifibrinolytics, e.g. Tranexamic acid.

Infiltration of the tissues with vasoconstrictors like adrenaline.

Controlled hypotension.

Intermittent positive pressure ventilation and maintenance of mild hypocarbia.

1&2. *Positioning and venous drainage*: Reverse Trendelenburg (anti-gravity) positioning by 30° is recommended as it decreases bleeding by causing mild postural hypotension. Neck should be preferably positioned in the neutral position or turned slightly towards the surgeon. Extreme flexion or rotation of the neck to one side should be avoided to prevent venous engorgement. A minimum of 2-finger breadth space is recommended between chin and chest if flexion of neck is required.

3. *Antifibrinolytics:* A number of clinical trials have shown that the use of antifibrinolytics like tranexamic acid (TXA) reduces the peri-operative blood loss and the need for blood transfusion significantly. In 2011 World Health Organization added tranexamic acid (TXA) to its list of essential drugs [15]. The European guidelines on management of major bleeding and coagulopathy following trauma suggests a 1A recommendation for the use of TXA in the case of traumatic and perioperative bleeding [16]. Dose reduction is required in renal impairment. Also, caution should be exercised while administering to patients with history of seizures.
4. *Infiltration of the tissues with lignocaine + adrenaline:* Usually the surgeons infiltrate the tissues with lignocaine, a local anaesthetic (LA), and adrenaline, a vasoconstrictor, prior to incision so as to reduce bleeding. Before doing so, the maximum allowable dose of local anaesthetic and adrenaline must be calculated and not exceeded to avoid toxicity and arrhythmias. A dilution of 1:200000 adrenaline is considered safe. If a local anaesthetic drug has been used for securing the airway, the dose of LA used must be considered in total calculation. ECG should always be monitored during and after infiltration.
5. *Controlled hypotension:* is defined as iatrogenic reversible reduction of the patients mean arterial blood pressure. Controlled hypotension can be achieved either by decreasing peripheral vascular resistance and/or cardiac output [17]. However, hypotension induced by decreasing cardiac output may not be ideal as it decreases tissue perfusion. A reduction by 30% from the baseline mean arterial pressure (MAP) level is generally considered to be safe. But it may be unsafe in some patients such as those with chronic kidney disease, ischemic heart disease and carotid artery disease [17]. Therefore, their suitability for controlled hypotension should be assessed and recorded during the pre-anaesthetic workup.

Over the years, several protocols have been developed. The main strategies are

- Standard anaesthesia with non-pharmacological measures.
- Deep anaesthesia with analgesia.
- Standard anaesthesia with hypotensive drugs.

Standard anaesthesia with Non-pharmacological measures: This relies on

- Optimal anti-Trendelenburg positioning to achieve postural hypotension.
- Intermittent positive pressure ventilation with mild hypocarbia.

*Pharmacological measures:* It relies on drugs used to either deepen the plane of anaesthesia and/or produce vasodilatation.

The ideal drug used for controlled hypotension should be easy to administer, quick in onset and recovery with predictable effect, no toxic metabolites and should preserve organ perfusion [17]. At present, no such drug is available and hence a combination of drugs is often used.

Deep anaesthesia can be achieved either with volatile anaesthetics or with intravenous agents.

Most volatile anaesthetic agents are potent vasodilators. This property can be exploited to reduce blood pressure. However, when used alone, the minimum alveolar concentration (MAC) values required to achieve this are high and can result in hepatic and renal injury and also delay awakening. They are therefore used at lower concentrations with other pharmacological agents. Most commonly used volatile agents include isoflurane, sevoflurane and desflurane. Halothane is preferably avoided due to its arrhythmogenic potential with adrenaline.

*Propofol Infusions:* This has been extensively used in neuro anaesthesia for controlled hypotension as part of total intravenous anaesthesia (TIVA). It can be used either as part of TIVA or combined with volatile anaesthetics.

*Opioids:* Opioids decrease the doses of agents required to produce anaesthesia and hypotension by decreasing pain. Most commonly used short-acting opioids include fentanyl and remifentanil.

#### 7.7.2.1 Hypotensive Drugs: (Appendix II)

Hypotension should be carried out only to that level needed to reduce bleeding and only for that time of the surgery where it is of benefit in reducing significant blood loss. A number of drugs have been tried either alone or in combination to reduce blood pressure. While using them, one needs to be aware of their potential complications and contraindications. Drugs commonly used are beta-blockers, glyceryl trinitrate and sodium nitroprusside. Newer drugs like dexmedetomidine along with a propofol/remifentanil combination are gaining popularity [18, 19].

Invasive arterial blood pressure monitoring is recommended if infusions of hypotensive drugs are used for controlled hypotension. Intra-op serial monitoring of ABG (arterial blood gases), acid–base balance and lactate levels

**Table 7.6** Potential complications in specific maxillofacial procedures

| Complications | Surgery | Pathogenesis | Management |
|---|---|---|---|
| Bradycardia [21] | Levering of zygomatic fractures.<br>Manipulation of midface | Oculocardiac reflex | 1. Cessation of stimulus.<br>2. Anticholinergics: Atropine/ glycopyrrolate |
| Intra-operative bleeding:<br>Occurs due to high vascularity of the area not amenable to cauterization. | Maxillary osteotomies.<br>LeFort-I osteotomies | Bleeding from Pterygoid venous plexuses.<br>Sphenopalatine artery<br>Descending palatine artery<br>Internal maxillary artery | 1. Large bore I.V. cannula.<br>2. Intraoperative tranexamic acid.<br>3. Controlled hypotension.<br>4. Autologous blood donation.<br>5. Blood transfusion may be needed. |
| Tracheal tube damage | Lateral nasal osteotomies [20]<br>Le fort surgeries | Direct damage.<br>Bubbling of gas from the nose-Anaesthesia circuit leak with inability to ventilate. | 1. Immediate tube change.<br>2. Laryngeal packing may be attempted.<br>3. Precautions – Careful surgery<br>4. Unilateral: Intubate via contralateral nare. |
| Wiring of tracheal tube to maxilla<br>Wide haemodynamic swings – Bradyarrythmias/ asystole | Radical neck dissections | Carotid sinus stimulation/ stellate ganglion stimulation. | 1. Cessation of stimulus<br>2. Carotid sinus block with LA<br>3. Stellate ganglion block.<br>4. Vagolysis. |

with hourly urine-output measurement should help to prevent organ dysfunction.

*Isovolaemic haemodilution* was once considered an adjunct in orthognathic surgeries to induce hypotension to reduce blood transfusion. It has become less common these days. The technique involves preoperative blood donation with IV fluids replacement of circulating volume followed by autologous whole blood transfusion as needed in the intra- or post-operative period.

*Intra-op Analgesia* can be achieved with NSAIDs, Paracetamol, opioids, intraoral LA infiltration and by mandibular or maxillary nerve blocks performed intra-op by the surgeon.

*Intra-operative complications:* The anaesthetist must be aware of and prepared for potential intra-operative complications [20, 21] (Table 7.6).

### 7.7.3 Elective Tracheostomy

Indications for elective tracheostomy are:

- Airway obstruction above the glottis - consider tracheostomy under LA.
- After extubation, Known or anticipated presence of an obstructed airway.
- Other general conditions requiring tracheostomy:
  - Certain head injuries
  - Massive chest injuries
  - Incidental pre-existing disease

  Inadequate postoperative nursing care.

## 7.8 Post-Operative

*Emergence and extubation* [22] Flow Chart 2—AIDAA (All India Difficult Airway Association) Guidelines for the management of anticipated difficult extubation and Table 7.7.

(flow chart 2 re-used with permission from IJA and AIDAA)

- After discussion with the surgeon, the decision of extubation post-surgery should be taken on a case-by-case basis.
- Before completion of the surgery, the induced hypotension should be ceased and time should be given to the surgeon to check for haemostasis. To check haemostasis, few surgeons prefer to increase mean blood pressure by 20–30% above pre-op level.
- At the end of the surgery, throat packs should be removed and clots or debris should be suctioned from the oropharynx.
- Prior to extubation cuff leak test may be performed to check for no airway oedema.
- A smooth emergence and extubation with less coughing and bucking is desirable. With the risk of the possibility of ongoing bleeding in the upper airway it is usual for patients to be extubated awake. Confirm that the patient is awake and breathing spontaneously.
- The Endotracheal tube should be left in situ, until the patient is fully conscious when the jaws are wired together, or any other airway obstruction is anticipated. Two types of maxillomandibular fixation (MMF) are available: Rigid MMF with jaw wiring, i.e. patients would be extubated with no ability to open their mouths and

**Table 7.7** Guidelines for extubation

| | |
|---|---|
| Decision based on | Individual case |
| | AIDAA guidelines Flow Chart 2 |
| | Cuff leak test |
| | Jaws wired - awake extubation |
| | Jaws not immobilized > Guedel airway/ nasopharyngeal airway |
| Stop | Induced hypotension |
| Keep ready | Difficult airway cart |
| | Appropriate anaesthetic drug drawn up |
| | Surgical team for tracheostomy |
| | Post op ICU bed |
| Avoid | Tight face mask ventilation |

MMF with elastics often applied, albeit later (from hours to 1 or 2 days) into the recovery phase where mouth opening will not be a problem.

- Guedel's airway or nasopharyngeal tube should be used to maintain the airway if jaws are not immobilized. A nasopharyngeal tube provides an extra dimension of safety in recovery.
- Nasal Endotracheal tubes removal should be gentle. To avoid passing of fresh tube through the vulnerable nasal mucosa, the ETT can be withdrawn into and left in oro pharynx to serve as a nasopharyngeal airway. Submental ETT should be removed back from the oral cavity and closure of the submental incision done before the extubation.
- Consider extubation over a tube changer in case of difficult intubation or surgery.
- Avoid applying tight facemask to protect surgical correc tion after extubation.
- For reintubation, airway equipment / difficult airway chart should be available on standby and in case of failed extubation appropriate anaesthetic drugs drawn up in the required doses.
- In case of MMF, wire cutters or scissors should be available immediately for release of elastics band fixation.
- Until successful extubation and stabilization of patient, the surgical team should remain in the operating theatre.
- Before transfer to recovery, a short period of observation in the theatre should be followed.
- Handover and transfer to recovery should be done by the anaesthetist.
- Careful documentation of surgery details, vital signs, sta tus at transfer, blood loss and replacement, drugs given, analgesia planned and expected problems should be done.

### 7.8.1 Handover from OT to Recovery Room/ICU

**Clinical Criteria for Shifting:**

- Patient should be awake and moving all 4 limbs
- Respiration should be regular with adequate depth
- Stable vital parameters
  - SpO2 > 95% on room air
  - Pulse rate optimum for age
  - Respiratory rate < 30/min
  - Normothermic
- No active bleeding from surgical site

Anaesthesiologist should accompany patient to recovery

- Give handover to responsible personnel
- Handover should include
  - Name and age of patient
  - Surgery done
  - Any positive history and examination
  - Type of anaesthesia and drugs (time and dose) given, including analgesics.
  - Any intraoperative event
  - Clear postoperative orders
- Complete anaesthesia form and sign and name
- Nursing in the postoperative period should be in the reverse Trendelenburg position to decrease oedema and bleeding.
- In cases of Le Fort II and III fractures, one should be aware that the degree of oedema could worsen in the first 48 h.
- For close observation, some patients need to be admitted to a high dependency unit. Patients sent to ICU are those who remain intubated or ventilated.

In case of inadequate postoperative care facilities like an ICU, the patient may be required to be sent to another hospital (see appendix III and 1V).

## 7.9 Post-Operative Complications and Management

- Immediate
  - Airway Problems
  - Postoperative bleeding and haematoma
- Delayed
  - Nausea and Vomiting
  - Post-operative pain

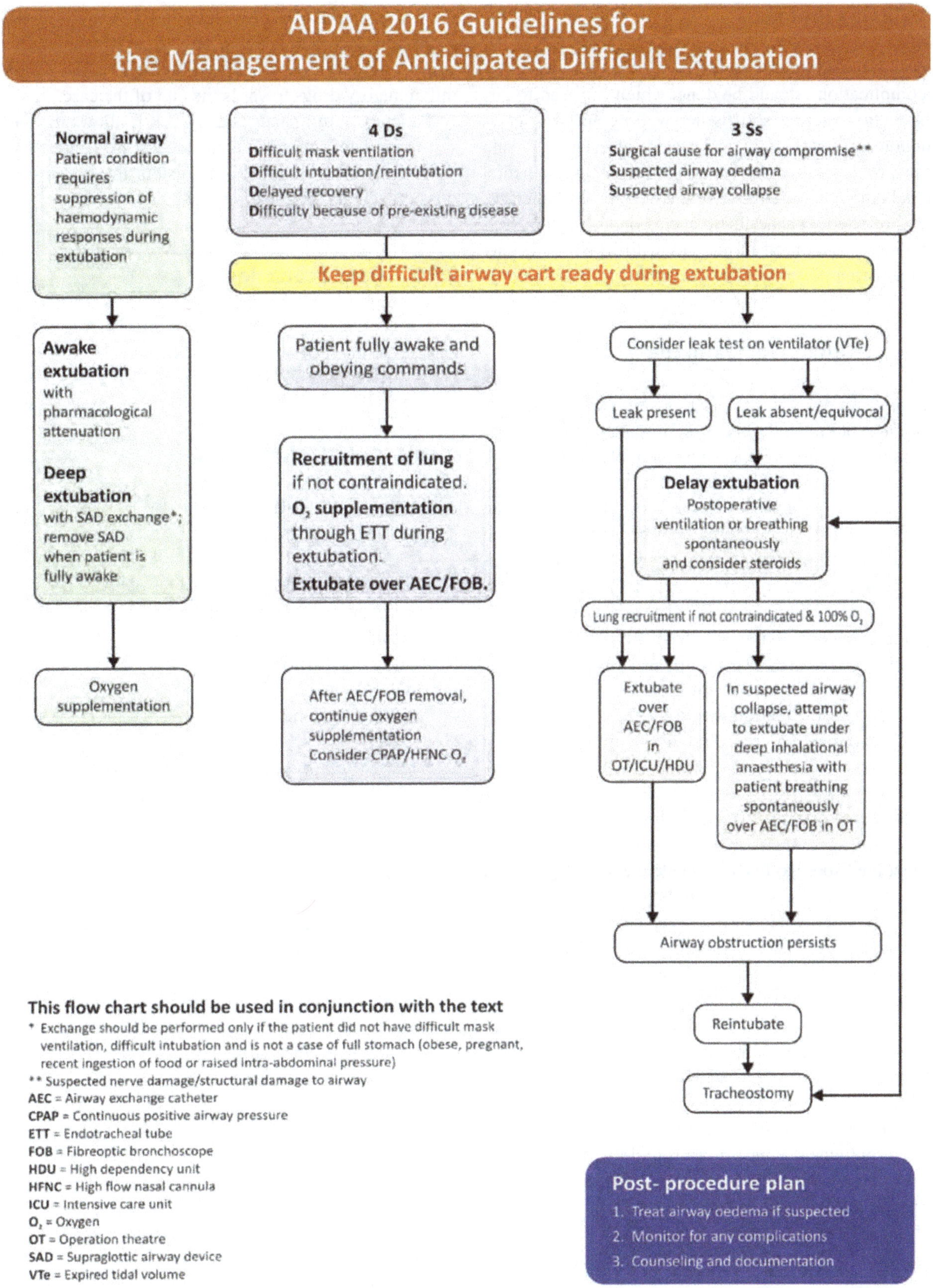


**Flow Chart 2** AIDAA Guidelines for the management of anticipated difficult extubation [22]

### 7.9.1 Airway Problems

In the post-anaesthesia care unit (PACU) the close monitoring of complications should be done, which can lead to airway obstruction such as soft-tissue swelling and formation of haematoma. Capnography may provide an earlier warning of serious problems than pulse oximetry when supplemental oxygen is being administered. Even in uncomplicated cases, the effects of residual anaesthetic agents on airway physiology are more pronounced in patients with MMF who may experience increased resistance to breathing.

### 7.9.2 Post-Operative Haematoma

Haematoma formation in the early postoperative period is an uncommon but potentially airway-threatening complication of some maxillofacial operations, notably neck surgery, thyroid resections and floor of mouth surgery. The rate at which airway compromise occurs is variable. Emergency decompression of the haematoma may be even done at the bedside. It involves removing the clips/sutures and manually evacuating the haematoma with a Yankaur sucker. However, this may not alleviate the airway obstruction adequately due to oedema that results from venous congestion. The airway needs to be secured urgently. The method of securing the airway should take into consideration information from the initial operation, but it is expected to be more challenging and may require expert airway management.

### 7.9.3 *Nausea and vomiting* [23]

Factors that predispose to PONV include the female gender, a history of motion sickness, a low threshold for nausea, preoperative anxiety, obesity and gastric distension. Volatile anaesthetic agents, nitrous oxide, opioid usage and intubation have also been implicated as has prolonged surgery, early oral intake and certain types of surgery, including maxillofacial surgery.

Vomiting in patients with MMF is dangerous as it may predispose to aspiration. If the jaws are wired together, there must be wire cutters immediately available, which accompany the patient from theatre, to the PACU, and also to the ward.

Elastics in MMF can be cut easily with ordinary scissors.

PONV prophylaxis is best given round the clock for the first 24 h and longer if opioids continue to be used. If treatment for PONV is required within 6 h of PONV prophylaxis, it should ideally be with a different class of anti-emetic drug to that used initially *(See Appendix I).*

### 7.9.4 *Analgesia* [23–25]

After orthognathic surgery immediate postoperative pain is often not severe, and this is contributed to by the generous intra-operative use of local anaesthesia. A multi-modal analgesia approach should also be utilized perioperatively by combining opioids with paracetamol and non-steroidal anti-inflammatory drugs towards the end of the case.

Patient Control Analgesia (PCA): It allows the patient to self-administer intravenous analgesics by means of a computer-controlled pump. It administers the pre-programmed dose on demand by the individual.

## 7.10 Case Scenarios

Case 1: Problem-Based Learning Tool
Case 2: Multiple choice questions

### 7.10.1 Case 1: Cleft Palate

A 10-month-old child presents for surgery with a cleft palate

1. *What are the problems special for cleft babies*

- Regurgitation and repeated aspiration
- Repeated respiratory infections
- Airway obstruction
- Malnutrition/anaemia
- Associated syndromes

2. *What are the important features to look for during the pre- anaesthetic/presurgical evaluation?*

History–

- Feeding—Type of food, difficulty in swallowing, nasal regurgitation
- Repeated respiratory infections and/or hospitalization
- Airway obstruction especially during sleep (snoring or sleep apnoea)—position adopted when asleep
- Previous surgery as for repair of the cleft lip
- Episodes of cyanosis or referral to a cardiologist
- Birth history with details of ventilator requirements or neonatal ICU admission,
- Milestones and immunization

Examination

- Body weight, signs of malnutrition, dehydration or anaemia
- Pulse, BP and Room air saturation, temperature to be recorded
- Mouth opening, neck extension
- Respiratory system—signs of respiratory infection
- Rule out cardiovascular involvement
- Look for associated syndromes the most common of which are Pierre Robin Sequence, Treacher Collins syndrome and Down syndrome.

Investigations

- Hb,- nutritional anaemia is common
- Complete blood picture—white blood counts may be elevated due to repeated infections
- Bleeding parameters—to rule out coagulopathies
- Chest x-ray if repeated chest infections or respiratory signs present on clinical examination
- Cardiology consult: ECG and ECHO cardiogram if cardiac involvement suspected

In addition:

- Meet the parents, allay their anxiety and give full explanation of procedure.
- Explain fasting guidelines with details of timing of feeds
- Solids and milk feeds 6 h prior to surgery and clear fluids, especially with glucose/sugar, 2 h prior to surgery
- Document informed consent form.
- Discuss procedure and requirements with primary surgeon

3. *What preparations are necessary on day of surgery?*
   Preparation: On day of surgery
- Ensure adequate help
- Ensure operating room temperature is not too cold
- Check Equipment and Drugs: Suction, Oxygen, Airway, Pharmacy (the pneumonic SOAP helps)
- Check anaesthesia machine
- Ensure that the difficult airway cart with rescue devices is available

*Monitors*: ECG, NIBP, Pulse Oximeter, $EtCO_2$, and airway pressure (once intubated)

4. *What are the problems that can present during anaesthesia?*
- Induction—intravenous or inhalational?
- Mask ventilation may be difficult especially in cases of facial cleft
- Laryngoscopy. The larynx is anterior, the tongue relatively large and laryngoscope tends to slip into the cleft
- Position of the patient in this case the trunk of the baby should be supported on a large pillow with the neck hyperextended and head stabilized within a head ring.
- Sharing the airway with the surgeon
  - kinking of tube when the gag is placed
  - accidental extubation during positioning of the baby or removal of the gag
  - tube may be pushed endobronchially resulting in one lung ventilation when gag is applied
  - throat pack/other packs may be left behind after surgery causing airway obstruction
- Intraoperative monitoring + access to the monitors difficult—so ensure they are fixed well and working well before patient is draped
- Access to the patient difficult, so make sure that intravenous access is good and fixed well before draping
- Analgesics like paracetamol and short-acting opioids like fentanyl may be used.
- Extubation is often more difficult than intubation. If there is any query regarding obstruction to the airway, place a nasopharyngeal airway and a tongue stitch prior to extubation.

5. *Could there be any problems post operatively? If so enumerate them.*
- Bleeding.
- Airway obstruction.
- Laryngospasm or post extubation stridor due to oedema of the upper airway: Treat with CPAP, humidified oxygen, aerosolized adrenaline, intravenous dexamethasone and nebulized steroids.
- Bronchospasm: Bronchodilators, oxygen and adrenaline, if severe.
- Aspiration: Suck out the mouth, nurse laterally, start antibiotics and chest.
- Physiotherapy along with nebulized bronchodilators.
- Electrolyte imbalance/hypoglycaemia: Send blood for investigations and correct
- Hypothermia/hyperthermia
- Seizures/Anticonvulsants: Rule out hyperthermia (tepid sponging and paracetamol) and hyponatraemia (intravenous normal saline).

### 7.10.2 Case–2: Polytrauma with Facial Injuries

A 27-year-old male presented with the history of polytrauma following a road traffic accident. He gives a history of brief period of loss of consciousness following injury. No history of seizures, or other comorbidities. On examination, his GCS was 15/15, and he was haemodynamically stable. Airway examination revealed restricted mouth opening of just one finger breadth, a short neck and a lacerated wound on the lower lip and chin with emphysema on the left side of the face extending into submandibular region. Cardiovascular, respiratory, abdominal and central nervous system examination was unremarkable. Blood investigations revealed increased CPK.

CT brain and spine showed a 3.5-mm extra-dural haemorrhage in the right temporal region, right frontal haemorrhagic contusion, an undisplaced fracture of the body of the mandible in bilateral parasymphyseal region with a displaced right zygomatic arch, a comminuted, mildly displaced fracture of right squamous temporal bone and undisplaced fracture of superior facet of C5 vertebra (Fig. 7.16).

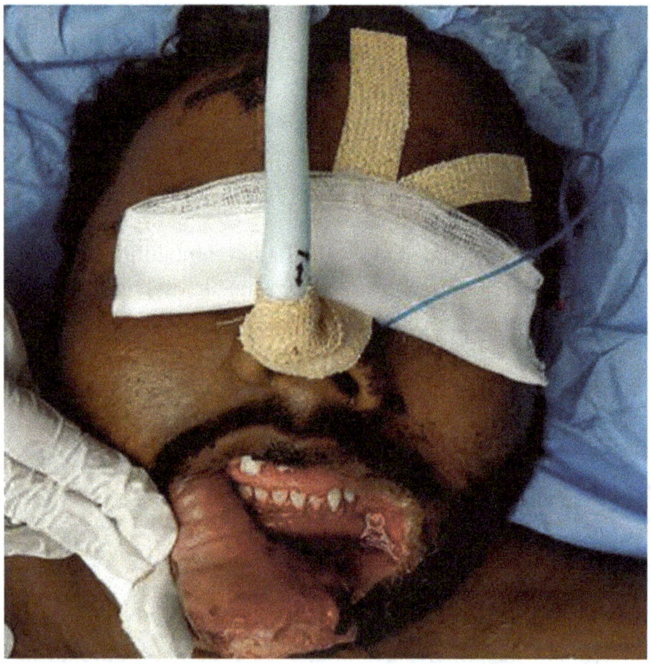



**Fig. 7.16** Photograph of a patient with polytrauma & facial injuries

*Questions*:

1. Following things are true about blunt trauma to face EXCEPT
   a. Cervical spine injury occurs in up to 10% of cases
   b. Drugs and alcohol could be a contributing factor
   c. Potential for injuries to other organs & massive blood loss
   d. Injuries in children are less severe than in adults

Answer: d) Injuries in children are usually more severe than in adults

2. In this patient, following could be cause of restricted mouth opening EXCEPT:
   a. Fracture Mandible
   b. Presence of trismus
   c. Cervical collar
   d. # of superior facet of C5 vertebra

Answer: d) Fracture of Cervical vertebra usually does not restrict mouth opening

3. What is the reason for the presence of subcutaneous emphysema of the face in this patient?
   a. Pneumothorax
   b. Tracheal injury
   c. Soft-tissue injury
   d. # involving sinuses

Answer: d) Fractures involving air-filled sinuses around face can cause subcutaneous emphysema

4. What is the EXCEPTION to the bedside predictors of difficult intubation in a case like this?
   a. Receding mandible
   b. Facial injury
   c. Edentulous
   d. Cervical collar

Answer: c) Absence of teeth usually causes difficulty in ventilation rather than difficulty in intubation

5. Which of the following is most useful for detection of Extradural haematoma?
   a. CT scan of head
   b. MRI scan of head
   c. X-Ray Skull
   d. Careful clinical examination

Answer: a) A CT scan is more appropriate investigation in an emergency

6. What would be your preferred method for securing the airway?
   a. Conventional laryngoscopy with oral endotracheal intubation.
   b. Conventional laryngoscopy with nasal endotracheal intubation.
   c. Fibre optic bronchoscopy with nasal intubation.
   d. Conventional laryngoscopy with manual in line stabilization with nasal endotracheal intubation.

Answer: b) Conventional laryngoscopy with nasal endotracheal intubation

7. What would be your preferred airway device for securing the airway?
   a. Regular endotracheal tube
   b. Nasal RAE tube
   c. Oral RAE tube
   d. Reinforced cuffed endotracheal tube

Answer: b) Nasal RAE tube.

8. What do you anticipate with respect to airway in this case?
   a. Difficult mask ventilation
   b. Difficult laryngoscopy
   c. Both a) and b)
   d. Normal ventilation and laryngoscopy.

Answer: c) Both difficult mask ventilation and laryngoscopy.

9. The following monitoring would be useful during surgery in a case like this EXCEPT:
   a. Invasive arterial pressure
   b. Urine output
   c. Central venous pressure monitoring
   d. BIS monitoring

Answer: c) Central venous pressure monitoring would not add any additional value in a case like this

10. Where would you shift this patient after the surgery?
    a. General ward
    b. Special ward

c. ICU
d. HDU

Answer: d). HDU will be an appropriate place to monitor this patient post operatively

11. What is the most suitable method for pain relief in this patient?
a. NSAIDs
b. Nerve blocks
c. Tramadol
d. PCA Fentanyl

Answer: d) PCA fentanyl will be an appropriate choice as patient has multiple injuries and is being monitored in HDU.

12. Which intravenous fluid is appropriate during the surgery for this patient?
a. Dextrose-containing solutions
b. Balanced salt solutions
c. Hypertonic saline
d. Colloids

Answer: b) Balanced salt solutions

## Appendix I: Dosage of common Drugs

| Drug | Action/group | Dosage |
|---|---|---|
| Dexmedetomidine[11] | $\alpha_2$-adrenergic-agonists | Bolus: 1 mcg/kg over 10 mins followed by continuous infusion of 0.2-1mcgs/kg/h |
| Atropine | Anticholinergic | 0.5 mg I. V |
| Glycopyrrolate | Anticholinergic | Antisialagogue: 3-4 µ/kg I. M 30–60 min prior.<br>Bradycardia: 0.1 mg I.V repeated every 2 to 3 mins. |
| Topical Lignocaine | Local anaesthetic | Maximum safe dose: Adults: 9-10 mg/kg lean body weight.<br>Paediatrics: 4.5 mg/ kg |
| Dexamethasone | Adrenocortical steroid:<br>Anti-inflammatory dose<br>Antiemetic [14] | <br>0.1–0.2 mg/ kg<br>4–5 mg I.V |
| Ondansetron | Antiemetic—Serotonin antagonist | 0.1–0.2 mg/ kg |
| Prochlorperazine (Stemetil) | Antiemetic—Dopamine receptor antagonist | 0.25 mg/kg |
| Tranexamic acid [15] | Antifibrinolytic | 1. Bolus dose: 15 mg/kg can be repeated every 6–8 h (prior to incision) or<br>2. Continuous infusion during the surgery: 1 g over 10 mins followed by 1 gm over 8 h or 20–25 mg/kg followed by 1–2 mg/kg/h). |

## Appendix II: Commonly Used Drugs for Controlled Hypotension

| Drug | Administration and Dose | Advantages | Disadvantages |
|---|---|---|---|
| Vasodilators:<br>SNP | Infusion:<br>Up to 1.5mcgs/kg/min | Potent venous and arteriolar dilatation. | Reflex tachycardia.<br>Rebound hypertension.<br>Tachyphylaxis.<br>Cyanide toxicity. |
| NTG | Infusion: - 0.5–2 mcgs/kg/min | Venodilator | Reflex tachycardia.<br>Tachyphylaxis. |
| Adreno-receptor antagonists:<br>Selective:<br>∂ -selective:<br>Phentolamine | <br><br>Intermittent boluses: 2–5 mg. | <br><br>Vasodilatation. | |
| ß-selective:<br>Metoprolol | Intermittent boluses: 0.1 mg/kg. | Heart rate control | Bronchospasm.<br>Negatively inotropic |
| Esmolol | Loading: 1 mg/kg over 1 min followed by Infusion: 0.5–1 mg/kg/h. | | |
| Non-selective:<br>Labetolol | Boluses: 0.25 mg/kg followed by infusion: 0.5–2 mg/min | Vasodilatation + heart rate control | Bronchospasm |
| $\alpha_2$-adrenergic-agonists:<br>Clonidine | Infusion/boluses: 1mcgs/kg | Vasodilatation with heart rate control.<br>Analgesic properties | Post op sedation.<br>Rebound hypertension. |
| Dexmedetomidine | Bolus: 1mcgs/ kg over 10 mins followed by infusion of 0.3–1 mcg/kg/hr. | Vasodilatation with heart rate control.<br>Analgesic properties | Post op sedation. |
| Magnesium sulphate | Bolus: 20-60 mg/kg | Vasodilatation with heart rate control.<br>Analgesic properties | Prolonged neuromuscular block |

## Appendix III: Handover Form Used for Inter Hospital Transfer

***Patient details***

| Name: | Age: | Sex: M/F | MRN No: |
|---|---|---|---|
| Diagnosis: | | | |

| Brief clinical history: |
|---|
| Clinical summary written by: |

| Reason for transfer: | |
|---|---|
| Transfer out hospital: | Referring doctor: |
| Transfer in hospital: | Accepting doctor: |
| Inter -hospital transfer consent taken: Y/N | |

***Vitals before transfer:***

| HR: /min | BP: mm Hg | RR: |
|---|---|---|
| SpO2: % | O2: l/min | AVPU score: |
| Airway: Intubated and assisted / Intubated and spontaneous / Not intubated<br>Patent IV access:<br>Fluid on flow:<br>Medications on flow:<br>Monitors connected: ECG / Pulse oximetry / NIBP / Others | | |

***Transfer details:***

| Departure time: | Arrival time : |
|---|---|

| Duration of Transfer: |
|---|
| Accompanied by: |
| Critical events during transfer: |

***Vitals on arrival/admission:***

| HR: /min | BP: mm Hg | RR: |
|---|---|---|
| SpO2: % | O2: l/min | AVPU score: |
| Airway: Intubated and assisted / Intubated and spontaneous / Not intubated<br>Patent IV access:<br>Fluid on flow:<br>Medications on flow:<br>Monitors connected: ECG / Pulse oximetry / NIBP / Others | | |

***Handover details:***

Clinical summary: Y / N

Patient records: Y / N

Investigations: Y / N

| Handing Over Doctor | Taking over doctor: |
|---|---|
| Name:<br>Sign:<br>Date & time: | Name:<br>Sign:<br>Date & time: |

## Appendix IV: Inter-Hospital Transfer Guidelines

The transfer of the patient to a Centre where intensive care is available may sometimes be required if the facilities at the current hospital are inadequate. Most of these patients are critically ill and need the utmost care and planning to ensure safety during transfer. It is the responsibility of the referring team (surgeon as well as anaesthesiologist) to ensure a safe handover to the new treating team of doctors.

The following guidelines may be used to develop local protocols for inter-hospital transfer.

- The decision to transfer should be done by the treating team of doctors.
- Choose the appropriate hospital.
- The patient's family should be counselled by the treating doctor for the reason of transfer.
- Obtain consent from the patient's family after explaining the need as well as the risks involved in transfer.
- The administrative coordination between the two hospitals, e.g. checking the availability of beds, required doctors, equipment, etc. should be performed telephonically. The verbal consent to accept the patient by the destination hospital authorities should be done and documented.
- A short summary of the patient's clinical condition and handover document should be prepared.
- The transfer team should be identified. It should comprise at least 2 members who are adequately trained in handling sick patients, e.g. while transferring an intubated patient, the team should be trained in managing intubated patients. At least one doctor (preferably an anaesthetist) should accompany/supervise the patient during transfer especially sick patients.
- The departure checklist should include confirming the following:
  - Ambulance services.
  - Sufficient oxygen supply.
  - Shifting trolley.
  - Battery backup for equipment.
  - Mode of ventilation (for intubated patients).
  - Adequate monitoring (ECG, pulse oximetry, blood pressure).
  - Resuscitative medications (prefilled syringes).
  - Required paperwork—clinical summary, patient records and investigations.
  - Knowledge of destination hospital location and contact numbers.
  - Clinical stability of the patient should be confirmed before shifting.
- Patient should be stabilised before transfer. The following should be confirmed just before transfer—a patent IV line, a patent airway access, a functioning monitor with adequate battery backup. In case of an intubated patient –DO NOT EXTUBATE just prior to transfer.
- Note and record vital signs just before transfer.
- During transfer the vitals should be monitored continuously and documented frequently.
- Anticipation of problems during transfer and preparedness will help ensure safe transfer.
- Upon reaching the destination hospital, the transferring team should ensure that the patient is safely shifted to the desired critical care area and the hand-over formalities completed.

## References


1. Allman K, Wilson I. Oxford handbook of Anaesthesia. 3rd ed. Oxford, UK: Oxford University Press; 2011.
2. Shaw I, Kumar C, Dodds C, editors. Oxford textbook of Anaesthesia for Oral and maxillofacial surgery. Oxford, UK: Oxford University Press; 2010.
3. Sherwood MW, Douketis JD, Patel MR, Piccini JP, Hellkamp AS, Lokhnygina Y, et al. Outcomes of temporary interruption of rivaroxaban compared with warfarin in patients with nonvalvular atrial fibrillation: results from the rivaroxaban once daily, oral, direct factor Xa inhibition compared with vitamin K antagonism for prevention of stroke and embolism trial in atrial fibrillation (ROCKET AF). Circulation. 2014;129(18):1850–9.
4. Popat M. Difficult airway management. Oxford, UK: Oxford University Press; 2009.
5. American College of Surgeons Committee on Trauma. Advanced trauma life support for doctors. 6th ed. Chicago: American College of Surgeons; 1997.
6. Jacob R. Recognition and management of the difficult paediatric airway. In: Jacob R, editor. Understanding paediatric anaesthesia. 3rd ed. India: Wolters Kluwer (India); 2015. p. 184–94.
7. Kheterpal S, Martin L, Shanks AM, Tremper KK. Prediction and outcomes of impossible mask ventilation: a review of 50,000 anesthetics. Anesthesiology. 2009;110:891–7.
8. Reed MJ, et al. Can an airway assessment score predict difficulty at intubation in the emergency department? Emerg Med J. 2005 Feb;22:99–102.
9. Teasdale G, Jennett B. Assessment of coma and impaired consciousness. A practical scale. Lancet. 1974;2:81–4.
10. Mackay CA, Burke DP, Burke JA, Porter KM, Bowden D, Gorman D. Association between the assessment of conscious level using the AVPU system and the Glasgow coma scale. Pre-Hospital Immediate Care. 2000;4:17–9.
11. Chopra P, Dixit MB, Dang A, Gupta V. Dexmedetomidine provides optimum conditions during awake fiberoptic intubation in simulated cervical spine injury patients. J Anaesthesiol Clin Pharmacol. 2016;32:54–8.
12. Ramkumar V. Preparation of the patient and the airway for awake intubation. Indian J Anaesth. 2011;55(5):442–7.
13. Pavlakovic L, Lee G. Anaesthesia for maxillofacial surgery. Anaesthesia and intensive care medicine. 2014;15(8):379–84.
14. De Oliveira GS Jr, Castro-Alves LJ, Ahmas S, Kendall MA, RJ MC. Dexamethasone to prevent postoperative nausea and vomiting: an updated meta-analysis of randomized controlled trials. Anesth Analg. 2013 Jan;116(1):58–74.
15. WHO model list of essential drugs 17th list; March, 2011. http://www.who.int/medicines/publications/essentialmedicines/en/index.html

16. Rossaint R, Bouillon B, Cerny V, Coats TJ, Duranteau J, Fernández-Mondéjar E, et al. The European guideline on management of major bleeding and coagulopathy following trauma: fourth edition. 2016;20(1):100.
17. Rodrigo C. Induced hypotension during anesthesia with special reference to orthognathic surgery. Anesth Prog. 1995;42(2):41–58.
18. Bajwa S, Kaur J, Kulshrestha A, Haldar R, Sethi R, Singh A. Nitroglycerine, esmolol and dexmedetomidine for induced hypotension during functional endoscopic sinus surgery: A comparative evaluation. 2016;32(2):192–197.
19. Sajedi P, Rahimian A, Khalili G. Comparative evaluation between two methods of induced hypotension with infusion of Remifentanil and labetalol during sinus endoscopy. J Res Pharm Pract. 2016;5(4):264–71.
20. Morosan M, Parbhoo A, Curry N. Anaesthesia and common oral maxillo-facial emergencies. Continuing education in anaesthesia. Critical Care and Pain. 2012;12:5.
21. McDermott PJC. Reflex bradycardia in facial surgery. J Oral Maxillofac Surg. 1990;48(9):1015–6.
22. Kundra P, Garg R, Patwa A, Ahmed SM, Ramkumar V, Shah A, Divatia JV, Shetty SR, Raveendra US, Doctor JR, Pawar DK, Singaravelu R, Das S, Myatra SN. All India difficult airway association 2016 guidelines for the management of anticipated difficult extubation. Indian J Anaesth. 2016;60(12):915–21. https://doi.org/10.4103/0019-5049.195484.
23. Patel PK, Morris DE, Gassman A. Complications of orthognathic surgery. J Craniofac Surg. 2007;18(4):975–85.
24. Beck JI, Johnston KD. Anaesthesia for cosmetic and functional maxillofacial surgery. Continuing Education in Anaesthesia Critical Care & Pain. 2014;14(1):38–42.
25. Lupori JP, Van Sickels JE, Holmgreen WC. Outpatient orthognathic surgery: review of 205 cases. J Oral Maxillofac Surg. 1997;55:558–63.

# Part IV

# OMS and Medical Imaging

# 8

# Fundamentals of Radiology in Maxillofacial Surgery

Shyamsundar K. Joshi and Annie I. Kochuveettil

**Learning Objectives**

- To identify the strategies in building an effective working relationship with the imaging department and help plan appropriate imaging investigations.
- To understand the principles of various imaging techniques; the advantages and disadvantages of these techniques in varying clinical scenarios.
- To gain awareness about the benefits and risks of using ionizing radiation and understand the basic principles of radiation protection.
- To establish the role of imaging as a treatment guide following different maxillofacial surgeries.

## 8.1 Introduction

Accurate diagnosis is the mainstay of proper surgical management in a maxillofacial surgical patient. Definitive diagnosis may be possible in a few patients based on clinical evaluation in the outpatient department or emergency setup. Other cases may require the use of supplementary investigations, including radiological imaging.

Like other medical specialties, the scope of Radiology is vast, playing a significant role in disease management. Penning a chapter on Radiology for a clinical branch-like Maxillofacial surgery is an uphill task. As a clinician, the maxillofacial surgeon, after having made the diagnosis, has the desire to visualize and gain in-depth knowledge of the ongoing disease process within the patient. Radiology plays an important supporting role in helping the clinician visualize within the patient's body. It is hence necessary for clinicians to have basic knowledge of the key concepts of Radiology, helping them understand its applications in the diagnosis of a patient's clinical condition.

The scope of practice of a practicing MFS includes both surgical and nonsurgical problems that affect the orofacial region, and hence they need to be well versed with the imaging concepts of the head and neck region.

**Head and Neck Imaging**

Anatomy of the head and neck is complex and imaging in this region poses several challenges and an MFS needs to be cognizant of them.

Modern imaging has the unique advantage of being able to:

- Demonstrate intricate and critical anatomical structures packed in small compact space pockets.
- Define the anatomy pertinent to the region of clinical interest.
- Define the critical relation to vital structures like the brain and cerebral vessels.
- Define the related adjacent critical areas like the airway, orbital contents, and both intra- and extracranial neurovascular elements.
- Define the underlying pathological process.

Conventional Radiography is one of the modalities that have been available from early days, ever since X-rays were discovered by Wilhelm Conrad Roentgen in 1895. However, it is regarded as a poor choice for anatomical evaluation due to overlapping of anatomical structures especially in the head and neck region. Yet it still has a popular role in its own humble way. It is universally available, the least time-consuming imaging investigation, and gives a 'bird's eye view' of the region of interest. It provides instant practical

S. K. Joshi (✉) · A. I. Kochuveettil
Department of Radiology, SDM College of Medical Sciences and Hospital, Shri Dharmasthala Manjunatheshwara University, Dharwad, India

information on the status of the airway and osseous elements, helps inferring the underlying pathological process based on the presence of air pockets or bony destruction, and at times may even reflect systemic pathology. It guides the clinician as to the further steps to be taken for patient management or to the need for further imaging. Despite it being the era of advanced technology, conventional radiography should invariably be the first choice among imaging investigations. In cases of complex maxillofacial injuries and polytrauma, when the patient's clinical status demands the next level of investigation, CT may be performed first, bypassing conventional radiography.

Pioneers in the field of imaging had a yearning to develop modalities that could demonstrate finer anatomical details in the region of interest.

This, coupled with the technological evolution, has paved the way for the development of various radiological imaging technologies that include:

- Ultrasonography (USG)
- Color Doppler
- Computerized Tomographic (CT) scan
- Dentascan
- Cone beam CT
- PET scans
- Radioisotope scanning
- Magnetic Resonance Imaging (MRI)
- Functional imaging, etc.

These advances in imaging techniques have enabled the MFS to diagnose with greater confidence and refine their approach to surgical treatment. This has also led to a reduction in unexpected surprises springing up on the surgical table.

Considering that a range of imaging modalities are available, it is imperative that the MFS has basic knowledge about their functionality, being familiar with the advantages and disadvantages of each so that the appropriate imaging investigation that gives the most optimal information in a given clinical setup can be selected. The rationale behind choosing the right investigation is that it should be easily available, least time consuming, cause least possible discomfort to the patient and be economical. Appropriate use of the concerned imaging modality should provide the maximum possible anatomical and functional information. This is possible if a genuine effort is made by an MFS to understand the basic principles and other related components of specific diagnostic imaging relevant to his field of interest and establish a close rapport with the imaging department.

## 8.2 Requesting an Imaging Investigation

Prior to requesting a radiological investigation, the MFS needs to have a clear idea about the usefulness of an investigation, its limitations, and whether it will help to improve the patient outcome. A radiological imaging requisition must specify the choice of investigation and the surgeon's expectations from it, so that the information received strengthens his approach in treating the patient.

It must provide mandatory demographic and relevant clinical data, including the patient's symptoms, which primarily brought him to the MFS, their duration, clinical signs, and the clinician's differential diagnosis of the same. In addition to concentrating on the clinical data, entries made available through the Hospital Information system (HIS) and the Radiology Information system (RIS), accurate patient identification by the MFS is essential prior to referral to the imaging department.

## 8.3 Role of the Maxillofacial Surgeon (MFS) Vs. the Radiologist's expectation from the MFS

An MFS deals with patients suffering from maxillofacial disease processes, but being a clinician primarily he is expected to have basic knowledge of various systemic clinical problems as well. Systemic disease may manifest as disease in the maxillofacial region or vice versa. For instance, a cystic lesion in the jaw could be the primary radiographic finding in a patient suffering from hyperparathyroidism. Similarly, patients suffering from systemic diseases like osteopetrosis, fluorosis, fibrous dysplasia, and other marrow infiltrative disorders could also present with a disease in the maxillofacial region. Further, detection of congenital anomalies in the maxillofacial region is an indication for a more detailed survey to rule out associated anomalies elsewhere.

The surgeon should be able to identify radiological images, correlate the same with the report and the patient's clinical status, and focus on timely decision making and patient management, thus optimizing the patient's outcome. However, in a dire emergency when a radiologist's opinion is not available, or a delay is expected in obtaining the same, an MFS should be able to interpret radiographs that suggest life-threatening conditions like tension pneumothorax, aspiration bronchopneumonia, foreign body aspiration, or pulmonary edema among others. Imaging can help the MFS in narrowing down on the clinical diagnosis, in staging and evaluating the prognosis of a disease process, or in surgical planning by depicting the exact extent of a lesion after diagnosis is confirmed.

MFS' need to communicate with their radiology counterparts the expectations they have from imaging of a case so that the radiologist can provide the relevant anatomical and functional information from the region of interest. Each imaging modality has its own reporting language and the surgeon needs to be well versed with the language used and have a clear concept of principles of image formation, specific to the energy source used in the particular investigation.

## 8.4 Role of the Department of Imaging and the Radiologist

The responsibility of the imaging department is conducting the specified diagnostic imaging investigation, interpretation of the tests or procedures by the radiologist and providing the clinician with accurate reports of the performed investigation as early as possible. Clinical radiologists function as key members of multidisciplinary teams, being an integral part of patient care.

## 8.5 Energy Forms Used in Diagnostic Medical Imaging: Understanding the Basics

Different types of energies are used in diagnostic imaging. These energies are imperceptible to the human eye and when they are passed to the desired location in the body, they interact with the body tissues in different ways. The tissue interactions can reveal information about the tissue, but they need to be interpreted. Access to this information is possible only if it is converted into a visible form on a display system. In essence, the requirements for an imaging investigation are; a reliable and reproducible energy form, a subject (the patient) into whom the energy can be sent, and a format that can convert the invisible image into a visible display.

X-rays and gamma rays are photon energies and members of the electromagnetic spectrum having a wide range of wavelengths and frequencies. X-rays have very small wavelengths being lesser than 1 Å unit and greater than 0.1 Å units. This range of specific frequencies and wavelengths of X-rays give them special properties, gaining popularity in diagnostic imaging.

Gamma rays have shorter wavelengths and higher frequencies than X rays. They are used in nuclear medicine both for diagnostic and therapeutic purposes.

Conventional radiography, including mammography, fluoroscopy, computed tomography (CT), is a modality that generates images of the ionizing radiation. It works on the same basic principle, which essentially involves passing of an X-ray beam through the body followed by absorption and scattering of a portion of the X-ray energy by the body tissues and transmission of the resultant radiographic pattern formed by differential tissue absorption to a detector for recording or further computer processing.

The popularity of X-rays as an imaging modality is due to its optimum penetration power and photochemical and fluorescent properties. Its fluorescent property is useful in converting invisible images into visible light images, while the photochemical property is responsible for conversion of the visible light image into a permanent visible record called radiograph.

*Conventional radiography* includes plain radiographs of different body parts like chest, skull, PNS, etc., contrast studies of the gastrointestinal tract like Barium studies, contrast studies of the genitourinary tract like Intravenous urography (IVU), and contrast studies of the vascular system like Arteriography, Phlebography, etc.

*Fluoroscopy* involves a continuous display of real-time movements of moving structures as radiographic images on the monitor, e.g., act of swallowing, movement of the soft palate, movement of the temporomandibular joint, cardiac pulsations, diaphragmatic movements, etc.

*Computed Tomography* includes cross-sectional imaging with its modifications like 3D, Volume rendering, Multiplanar reconstruction images, C.T. angiography, etc.

*Ultrasound* imaging or sonography makes use of high-frequency sound waves that are transmitted from the transducer into the body. The reflection of these waves off the body structures forms the basis of ultrasound image formation. The information necessary for image production is provided by the amplitude of the reflected sound signal and the time taken for it to travel through the body. Commonly ultrasound is used in the imaging of the abdomen, fetus, breast, eye, heart, vessels, and the musculoskeletal system. In recent years, there has been much research into ultrasound of the maxillofacial region, and it has been found to have a range of unique applications, including the evaluation of cervical lymph nodes and the detection of space infections and cystic and solid lesions of the head and neck. In early cases of peripherally located carcinoma of the tongue, ultrasonography may be an initial mode of imaging for evaluation.

Ultrasound imaging is not associated with the same risks as ionizing radiation and is considered to be generally safe if used appropriately. Ultrasound energy does have the potential to produce biological effects on the body and can cause minimal heating of tissues and in certain cases produce tiny gas pockets in the tissues and body fluids known as cavitation.

*Magnetic resonance* imaging makes use of strong magnetic fields and radiofrequency energy to create images. The signals that produce an MR image originate from the protons present in water and fat molecules in the body. Application of a strong magnetic field by the MRI scanner causes the protons within the body to align themselves. Radiofrequency current is then passed into the patient's body creating a varying magnetic field that causes the protons to flip their spins. Turning off the radiofrequency pulse causes the protons to return to their normal spins, producing radio signals that are measured by receivers in the scanner and used to make digital images of the scanned area of the body.

Many forms of MRI exist, diffusion and functional MRI being the most common. Diffusion MRI helps in diagnosing disease processes like stroke that restricts diffusion of water molecules across body tissues, while functional MRI is used to visualize the functional activity of the brain. MRI does not use ionizing radiation but since it uses strong magnets, any form of metal implants like artificial joints and heart valves, pacemakers, cochlear implants, metal plates, screws, and rods do pose a hazard.

*Thermography* makes use of specialized cameras that can detect electromagnetic light energy in infrared wavelengths. Medical thermography produces a topographic heat map, displayed in the form of various color shades, based on the differential skin temperature at various dermatomes bearing resemblance to the visible image of the body. It is not a structural imaging technology providing information on structural changes like other modalities and does not provide a diagnosis, rather only aids in reaching a diagnosis. It is completely safe and painless, does not make use of any form of radiation, and is a unique form of imaging in that it can document pain, thus helping to differentiate malingering from an organic cause for the pain.

## 8.6 Basic Radiology for the Nonradiologist: What the MFS should know?

Plain radiographic film interpretation is an essential skill. The current implementation of electronic health records and digitization of the health care system has made radiographic images available throughout the hospital and an MFS may often have to interpret medical images. So, it is important that they know the basics of medical image interpretation, and this knowledge may prove to be crucial in an acute clinical setting. They should be aware of tissue appearances on radiographs and be capable of making a basic distinction between normal and abnormal.

Understanding the concept of density and contrast is fundamental to interpreting an X-ray image (radiographic image). Different body tissues, including bone, soft tissues, fat, and air, all attenuate the X-ray beam differently. Differential absorption of X-ray photons by the body tissues results in variable energy values of emerging photons producing an invisible image, which is converted into visible form as areas of different gray scales. The contrast on the image is the difference between adjacent densities. These densities range from white to black with varying gray shades in between them. If the densities of two tissues adjacent to each other are greatly different (say a white and a black density tissue), then they are said to have high contrast. If the densities of two tissues adjacent to each other are similar, then they are said to have low contrast. They appear similar in color, differing in their shades of gray. When two body structures of identical density are exactly side by side, the line of demarcation cannot be made out and whole of it appears as one structure.

Consider a chest radiograph. What do you think is the whitest component seen on the radiograph? Most commonly the answers given are heart, bones, below the diaphragm, and so on. Rarely does anyone mention that the "R" marker is the whitest. Similarly, if asked which the darkest component is, the popular answer given is, the lung surrounding the heart, very rarely does one mention that the air surrounding the chest is the darkest. Analyzing as to why the "R" marker is white and the air surrounding is dark, the reasoning is that the chest radiograph is nothing but a representation of the tissues in that region in various gray scales between extreme white and extreme dark, depending upon the variable absorption of X-ray photons in their path through the tissues.

The opacity produced on a radiograph by a specific body tissue is a representation of the actual penetrative ability of X-rays to pass through that tissue and then be incident on the film. Air and fat absorb less radiation, allowing more X-rays to pass through and be incident on the radiograph making their images appear black and pale gray, respectively. Bone and metal as is the "R" marker made of lead absorbs more radiation and so fewer X-rays are incident on the film making them appear white.

Continuing with the example of chest radiograph, what are branching structures that are seen in the lung fields? Are they arteries, veins, bronchi, lymphatics, or a combination of all these? The common answer given is bronchovascular. The correct answer is arteries and their branches, but not the bronchial tree. The explanation is simple. Air in the bronchi is surrounded by air in the alveoli and so no contrast exists between them and they are hence not seen. On the other hand, blood in the arteries is surrounded by air in the alveoli and hence they stand out. Veins do contain blood but are too less in number and do not significantly contribute to the branching structures. Lymphatics are too small to be detected.

If this basis of X-ray image formation is understood, you can easily interpret any radiographic image provided you have sound knowledge of the relevant anatomy, pathology, and pathophysiology.

## 8.7 Imaging Investigations

### 8.7.1 Imaging Investigations Using Ionizing Radiation (Photon Energies)

Electromagnetic radiation has a wide range of wavelengths ranging from being smaller than angstrom units to as large as many miles. Smaller wavelengths have greater energy and penetration power and are called photon energy meaning packets of energy and not particle energy. The two energies that are of concern in the present context are X-rays and Gamma rays. Passage of these energies through body tissues either for diagnostic or therapeutic purposes results in a series of events beginning with an incidence of the X-ray photon into tissue followed by sequential changes at molecular and atomic levels. The transformation of energy from the photon results in ionization, namely, in the discharge of an electron and a free radical. Hence, such energies are called ionizing radiation and the process involves breakage of enzyme bonds and formation of new molecules manifesting in the form of various repairable and irreparable biological effects.

The concept of photon energy and its effect on body tissues can be explained using the following example. Consider a hot iron ball being passed through a pile of corn (Fig. 8.1). The temperature of the ball after exiting the corn pile is grossly reduced. It is because the ball, during its transit through the pile, shares the energy with the corn in contact with it. The corn in very close contact to the ball is burnt to ashes, the corn a little farther away, is burnt to charcoal, corn still further away is converted to popcorn, while corn far away from the ball remains unaffected. The effect on the corn is directly proportional to the energy transferred from the hot iron ball to the corn. The same thing happens when photon energy passes through the body tissues with changes occurring at atomic level.

#### 8.7.1.1 X-Rays

X-rays are a form of electromagnetic radiation. Man-made X-rays are produced when fast-moving electrons undergo sudden deceleration on collision and interaction with the target anode in an X-ray tube. The electrons are emitted by the cathode, on being heated up by the electric current flowing through it.

Though conventional X-ray imaging has evolved over the past 100 years, the basic principle remains the same. On passage of an X-ray beam through the body, the beam is attenuated by the body's internal structures, being partly absorbed and partly scattered. The remnant of the X-ray energy is transmitted to a detector that records the image for later evaluation. The recording of the radiographic pattern may be on film or other electronic devices. The image created is due to weakening of the X-rays by tissues of varying density encountered along the beam's travel path. Bone being dense tissue, absorbs or attenuates a great deal of the X-rays, while soft tissue being much less dense attenuates or absorbs far less X-ray energy. These differences in absorption help in creating images that can clearly show normal tissue appearance as well as different forms of pathology.

Conventional radiography, fluoroscopy, and CT all work on the same basic principle differing only in their purpose. In radiography, a single image is recorded for later evaluation, in fluoroscopy X-ray images are displayed on a monitor in a continuous flow, thus allowing monitoring of a procedure or contrast passage in real time and in CT imaging a multitude of images are recorded as the detector rotates around the patient's body followed by reconstruction of the individual images as cross-sectional images of internal organs and tissues.

#### 8.7.1.2 Computerized Tomography (CT/Spiral CT)

Computerized axial tomography is a computer-controlled radiological study that produces a reconstructed image of a cross-sectional slice of the desired section of the body. Its features include the absence of superimposition, less scatter and better tissue differentiation of the anatomical slice, thinner slices producing a better reconstructed image. The major drawback of conventional radiography is the overlapping of anatomical structures resulting in difficulty in evaluation of desired structures in a particular plane. The imaging method 'Tomography' was introduced to overcome this drawback and involves imaging of anatomical structures at the desired plane with the blurring of overlapping structures. Classical conventional tomography had its own inherent drawbacks, which included poor-quality blurred images, high radiation dosage, and use of complicated techniques which led to it being replaced by tomography assisted by computer technol-

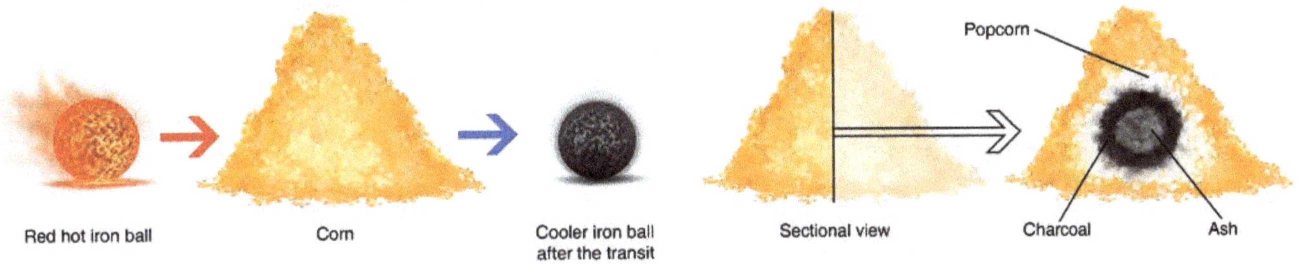


**Fig. 8.1** Illustration of passing a hot iron ball through a pile of corn and its effect on the corn

ogy called 'Computer assisted Tomography' (CAT). With a rise in popularity, CAT has been replaced by the word C.T. and technological advances have resulted in the development of better equipment capable of scanning the entire body within a few seconds. This provides fine anatomical details of submillimetric structures, allows tracing of blood flow in all its phases, and also permits clear depiction of information related to moving structures like the heart in real time as well as their external and internal morphology. Two types of CT have been described based on the shape of the X-ray beam, the traditional fan beam CT and cone beam CT.

**CT Unit Components** (Fig. 8.2a, b)

The essential components of a CT unit include:

- **The X-ray tube**—a specialized tube of high heat loading and dissipating capacity with a very small focal spot, as a source of X-ray energy
- **Detectors** that receive and quantify the attenuated X-ray photons
- **A computer** of high capacity that evaluates attenuated photon energy from detectors, stores the values, and converts these values to sectional images
- **A console** that manipulates all data stored in the computer, helping in reconstructing the image at desired planes with volumetric imaging or multiplanar reconstruction, 3D and volume rendering, followed by projection of the desired structures based on their density values, etc.
- **A gantry** that houses X-ray tubes, detectors, and related cables with a central aperture for the patient's body to enter for sectional imaging
- **A moving table** or a couch that facilitates the movement of the body with extreme accuracy at even submillimetric increment

CT scans have many benefits that far outweigh their risk. It is quick and easy, widely available, and provides superior anatomic and bone details. It has Volume Rendering Technique (VRT), Maximum Intensity Projection (MIP), 3D and Shaded Surface Display (SSD) capabilities, provides multiplanar reconstruction images in desired planes, and is the modality of choice for follow-up studies. (Figs. 8.3a, b, 8.4a, b, 8.5a,b, 8.6a, b, 8.7a, b, 8.8a, b, 8.9a, b, 8.10, 8.11, and 8.12).

The possible risks of using CT imaging include exposure to ionizing radiation and the predicament of suffering an allergic reaction due to use of contrast media. One drawback of CT when compared to MRI is the lesser resolution of soft-tissue detail. Other disadvantages are the associated cost and the limitations of its use in the pediatric age group due to the need of sedation.

**CT Limitations**

Motion and beam-hardening artifacts used to be considered as major drawbacks, but they have been markedly minimized with advances in technology. A physical limitation is that the patient needs to weigh less than 300 to 400 lbs. For

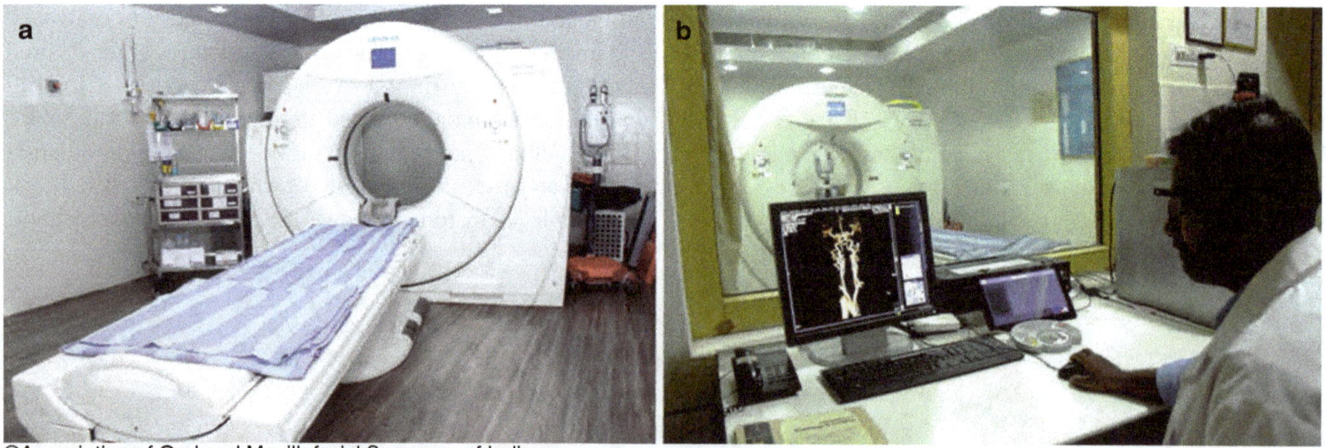




**Fig. 8.2** (**a**) CT room shows Gantry, Patient couch, Emergency crash trolley, Central suction, and Oxygen and Pressure Injector. (**b**) Control room showing a CT technician working with various controls and the image acquisition system

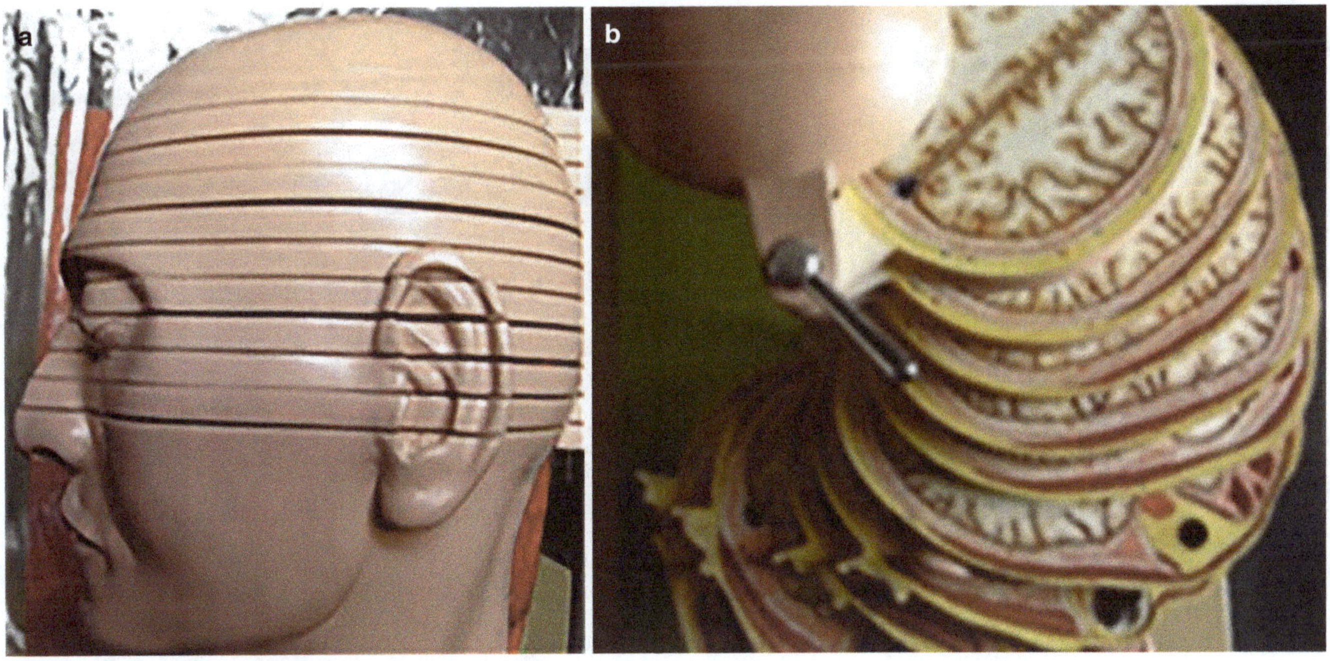




**Fig. 8.3** (**a**) Museum Model of head showing how axial slices are planned. The slice thickness varies from submillimeter to 10 mm, depending on the ROI (region of interest) and anatomical structure to be seen. (**b**) Stacked CT slices showing specific anatomy at a specific slice

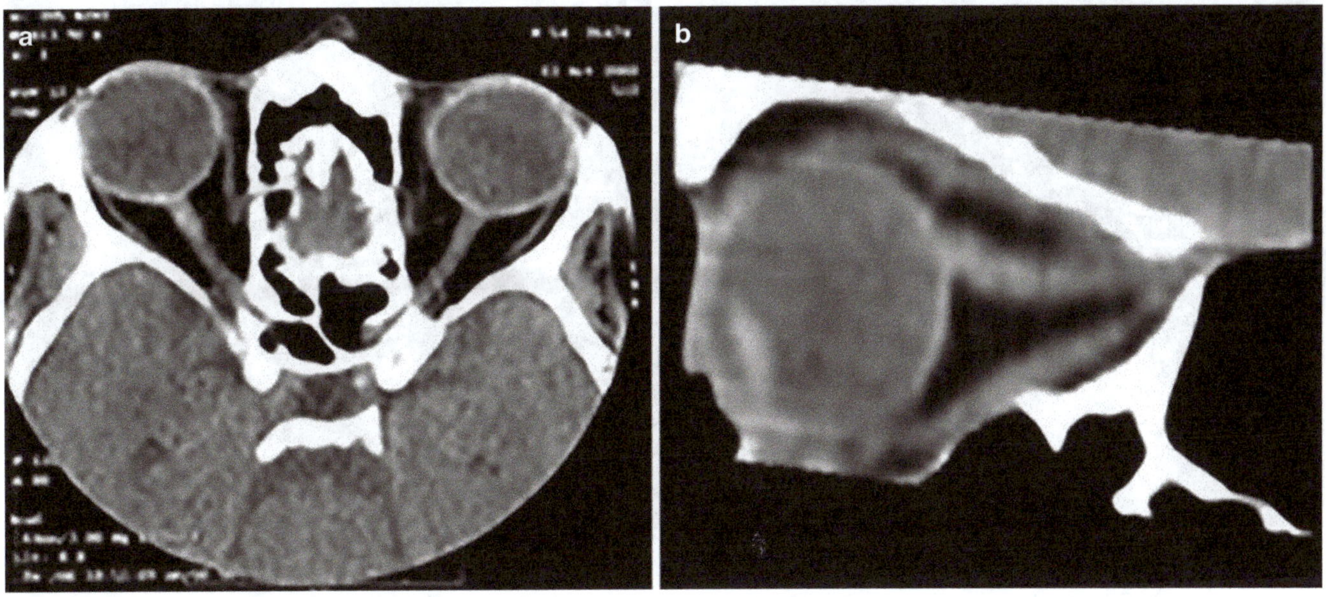




**Fig. 8.4** (**a**) CT axial primary slice soft-tissue window at the level of optic nerves showing mediolateral and anteroposterior relations and not supero inferior relations. (**b**) CT sagittal reconstructed image of the same patient at the level of optic nerve showing anterior, posterior, superior, and inferior relations

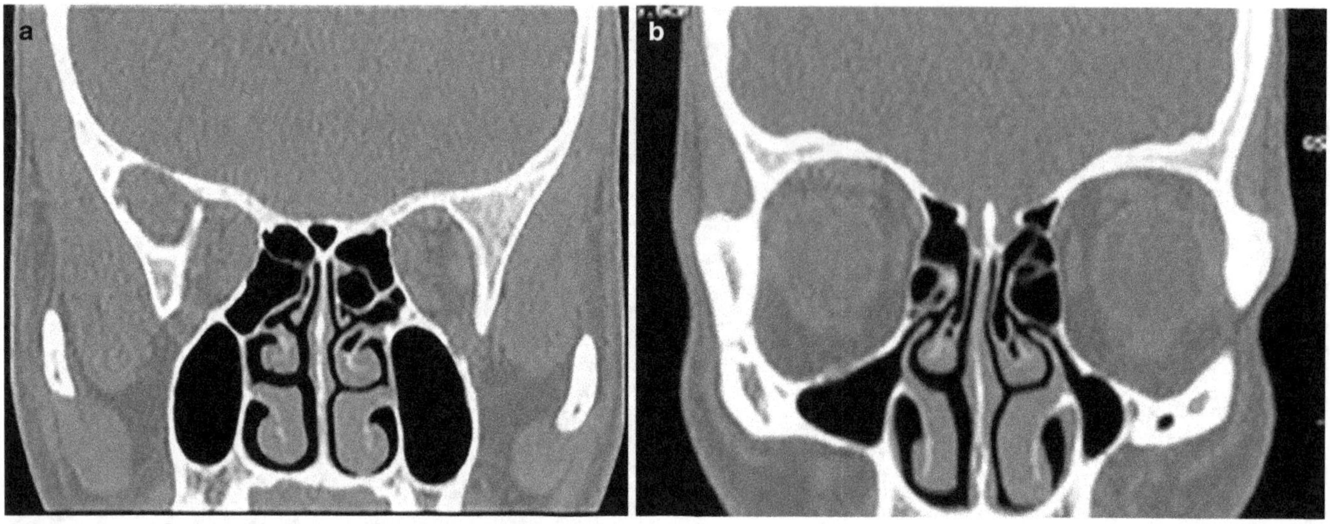




**Fig. 8.5** (**a**) and (**b**).CT coronal bone window primary images at different levels of paranasal sinuses

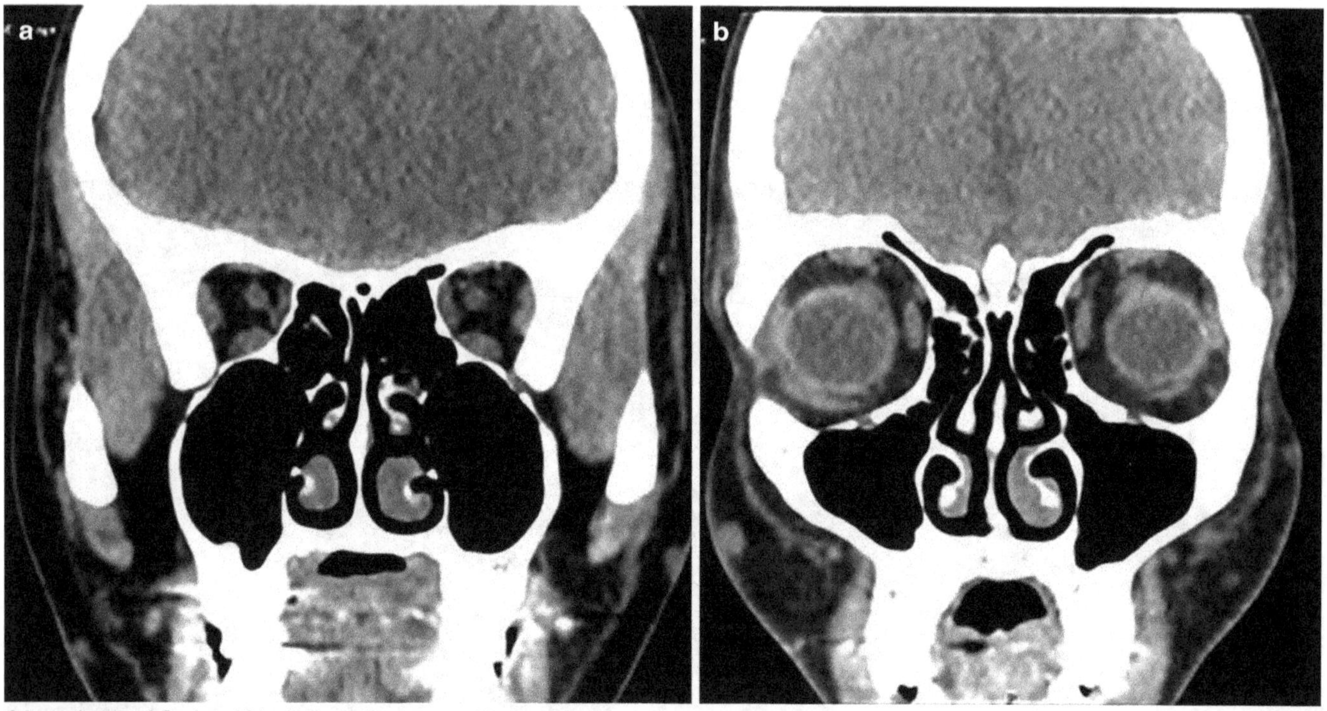




**Fig. 8.6** (**a**) and (**b**).CT coronal soft-tissue window primary images at different levels of Paranasal sinuses

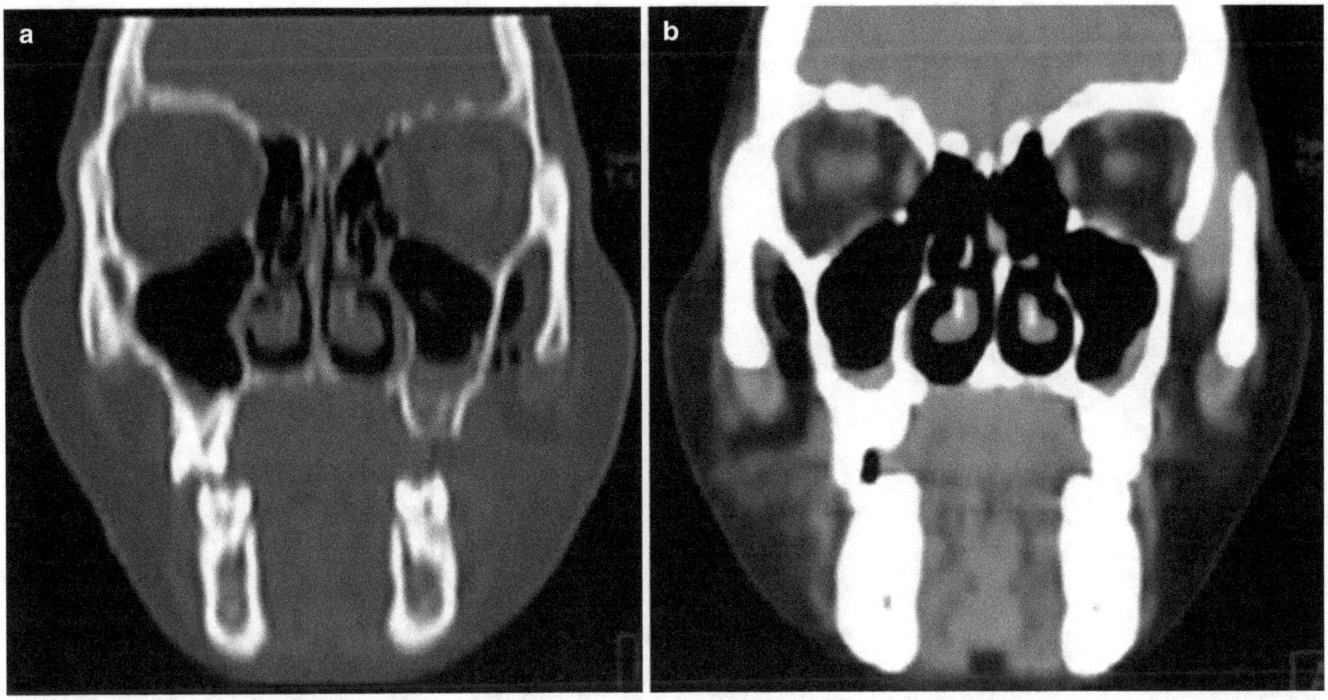




**Fig. 8.7** (**a**) and (**b**). CT reconstructed coronal images from thicker slices of paranasal sinuses at different levels. (**a**) bone window. (**b**) soft-tissue window. Note: coarse appearance

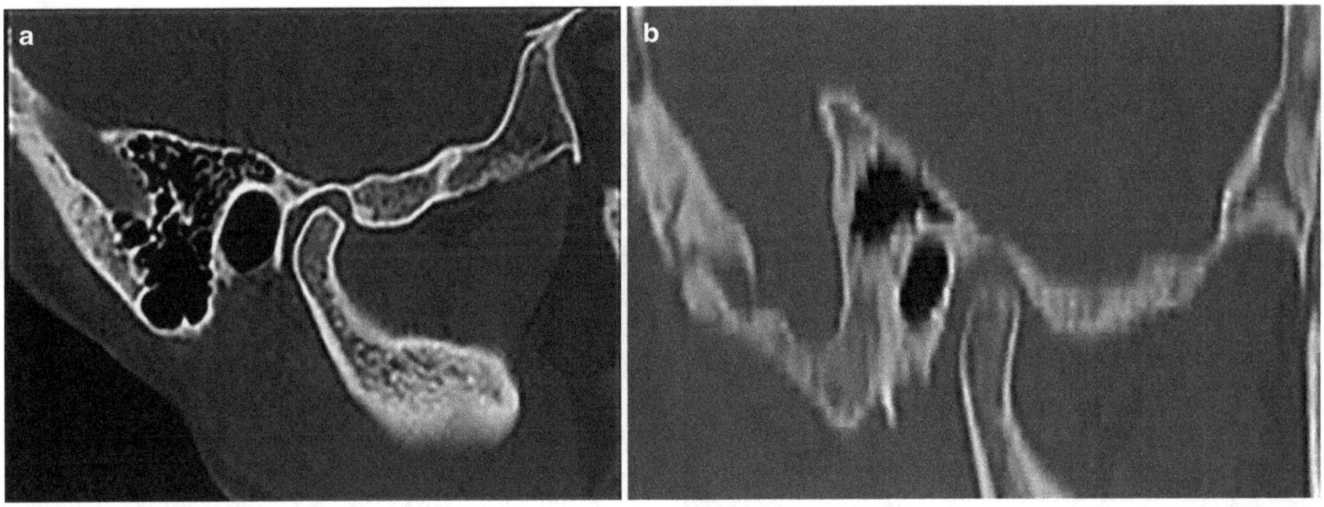




**Fig. 8.8** (**a**) CT direct slice of T.M. joint in its sagittal plane. Bone window. (**b**) CT reconstructed image from primary axial thick slices of T.M. joint in its sagittal plane. Note: coarse appearance

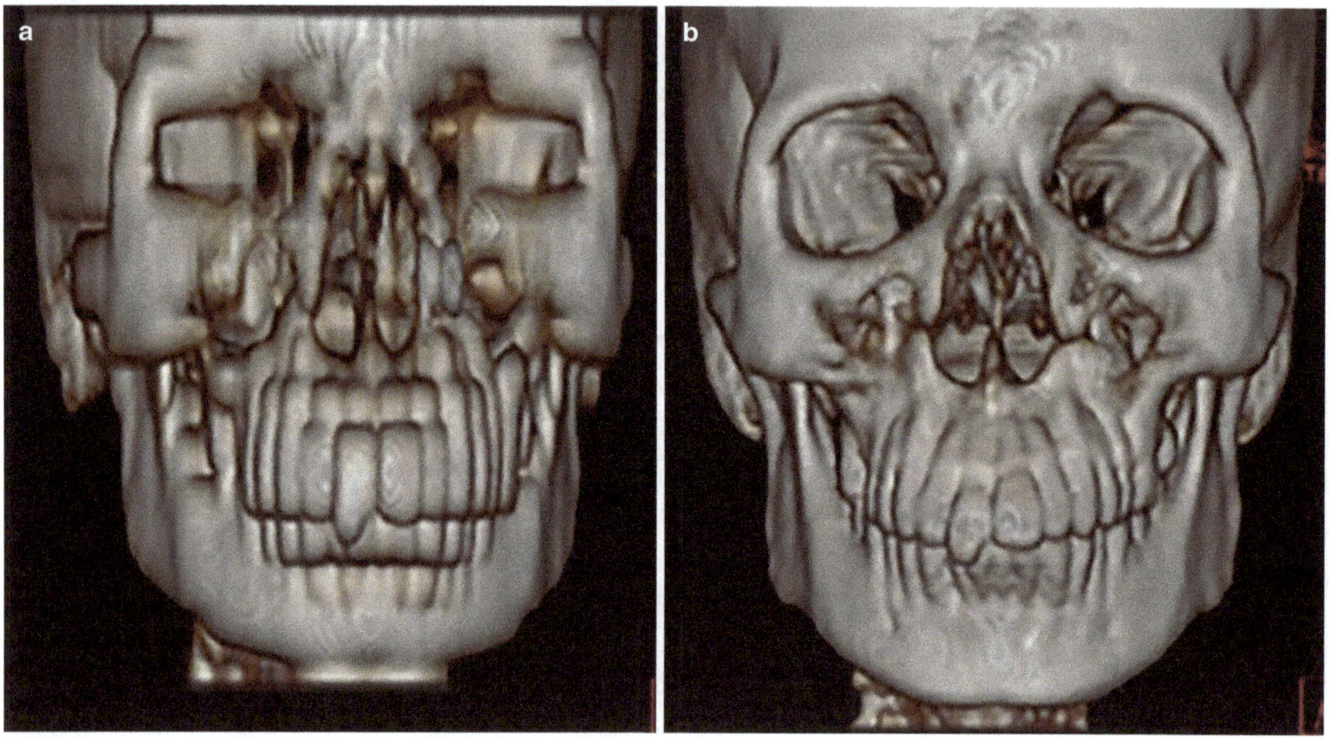



**Fig. 8.9** (**a**) CT 3D reconstructed image for surface bony details from thicker slices. Note: coarse appearance. (**b**) CT 3D reconstructed image from thin slices. Note: better and smoother image

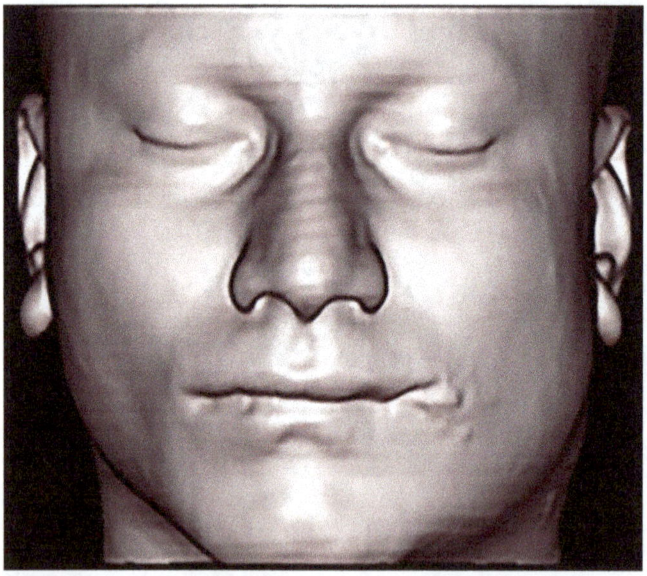



**Fig. 8.10** CT 3D surface rendering reconstructed image for surface soft-tissue details from thinner slices

CT imaging of the head region, axial and direct coronal slices are primarily possible, for the neck region, only axial slices are possible and in the temporomandibular joint region axial and direct sagittal slices are possible. It is through the raw data thus available that images are reconstructed in any desired plane.

**Dentascan**

*Basic principles of CT Orthopantomography (OPG) and Dentascan*

Conventional OPG is a first-level diagnostic exam that provides a gross panoramic view and just enough information about alignment of the teeth and any other related gross pathology. Unavoidable overlapping of some of the anatomical structures hinders accurate evaluation. To overcome these drawbacks, Dentascans and CT OPGs are used. They are extended applications of CT scan and involve the acquisition of thin axial submillimeter slices of the region covering the upper and lower jaws (Fig. 8.13). Reconstructed images obtained using these raw data image slices form the CT OPG or Dentascan image (Fig. 8.14a, b).

Coronal reconstructed images form the C.T. OPG (Fig. 8.15a, b, c). It is a second-level imaging technique wherein evaluation of the osseous elements of the maxilla and mandible is far better in comparison to conventional OPG. It provides the MFS with a better understanding of the morphology of the roots and the degree of contiguity between the roots and the mandibular canal. The information acquired is then used in planning and performing minimally invasive surgical procedures [1].

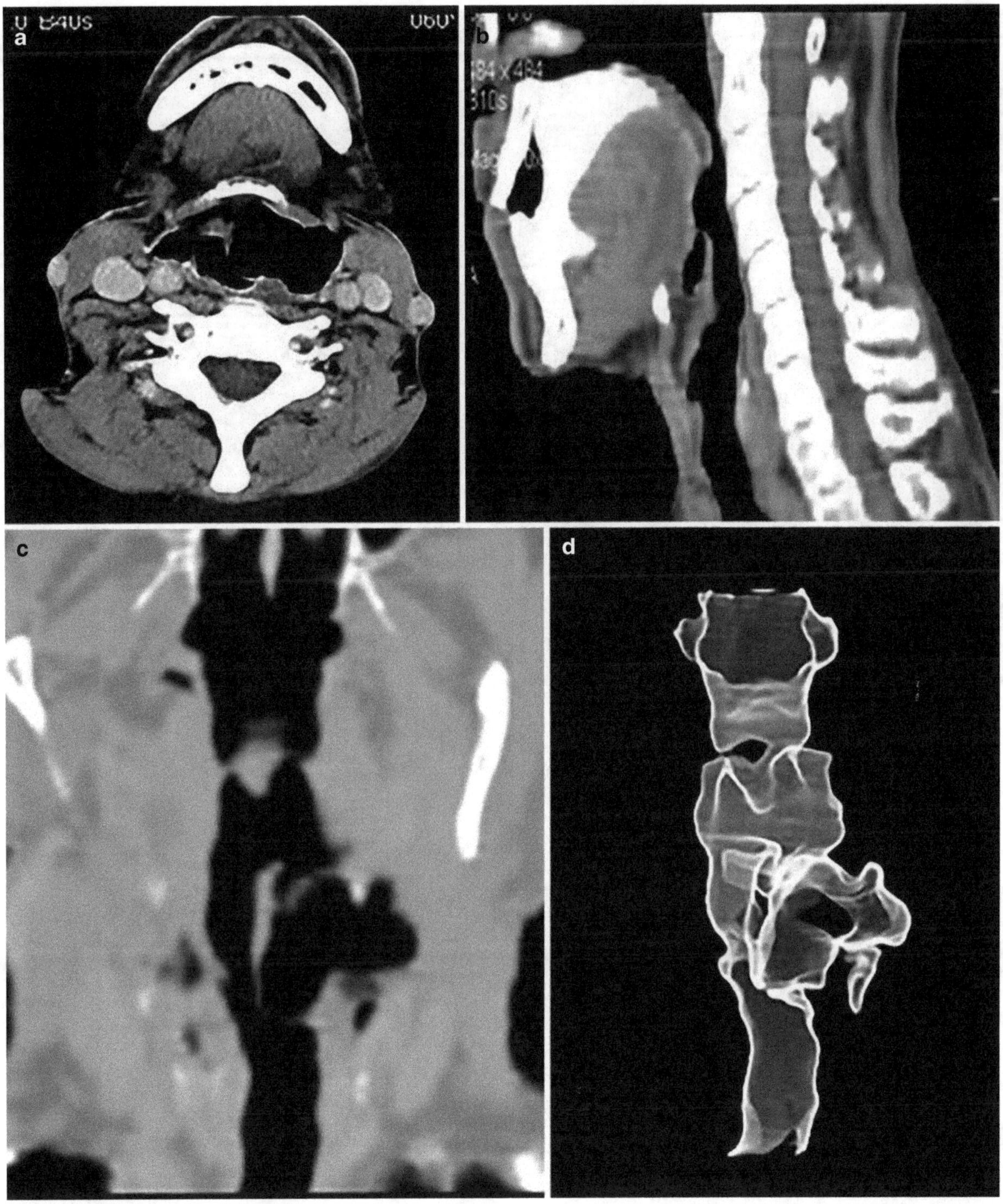




**Fig. 8.11** (**a**) CT Primary axial slice of neck at midlaryngeal level. (**b**) and (**c**) Sagittal and coronal reconstructed images from sequential CT primary axial slices. (**d**) CT Volume rendering technique (VRT) image of air column in the pharynx, larynx, and tracheal region as minimum density projection from primary axial slices (**a**). Note: Better visualization of laryngocele

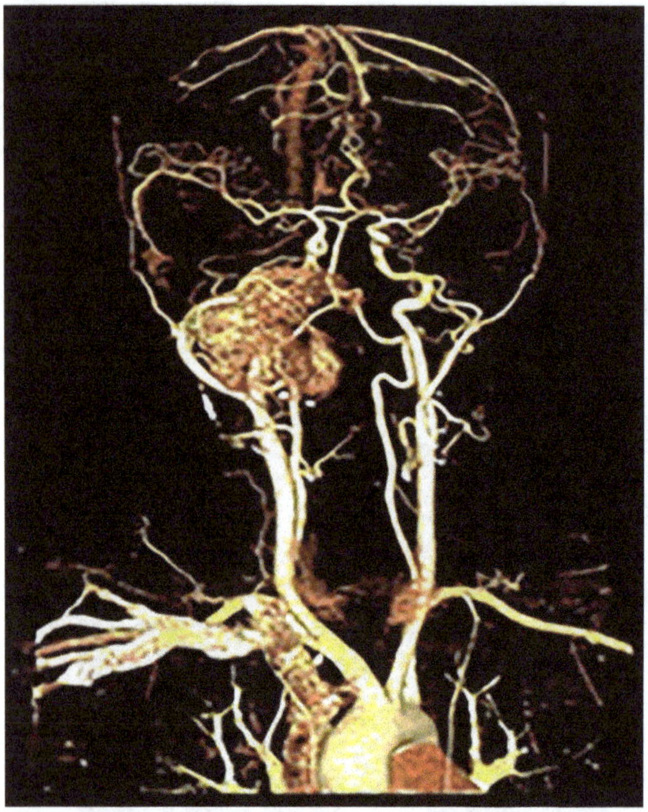



**Fig. 8.12** CT angiogram: 3D VRT (Volume Rendering Technique) displaying carotid arteries and its branches along with carotid body tumor. It is a reconstructed image from primary thin axial CT slices

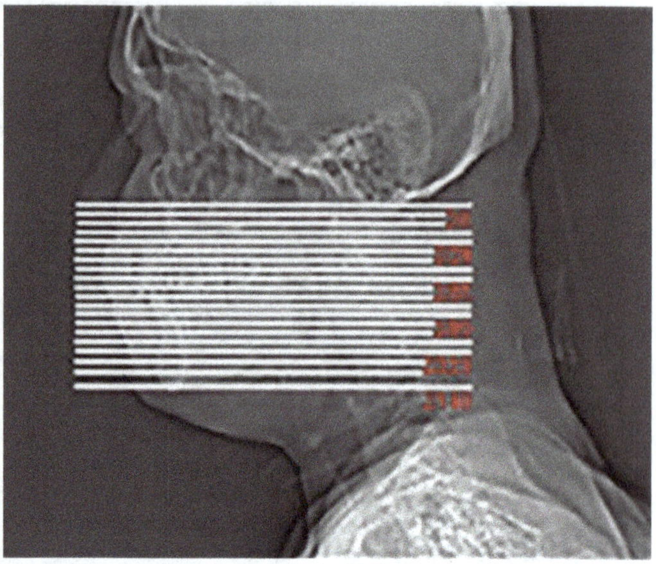



**Fig. 8.13** CT Scanogram for dentascan showing submillimeter axial slices planning in the region of maxilla and mandible

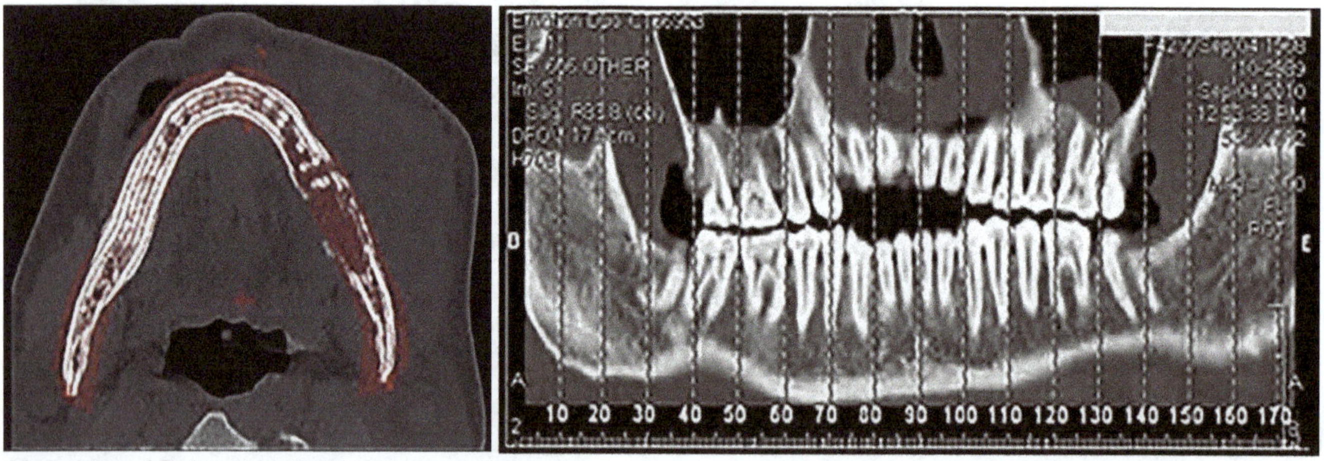




**Fig. 8.14** (**a**) and (**b**) .Reformatted panoramic CT images (**b**) are procured at desired plane of the jaw by curvilinear graphic lines drawn on the primary axial slice (**a**) selected

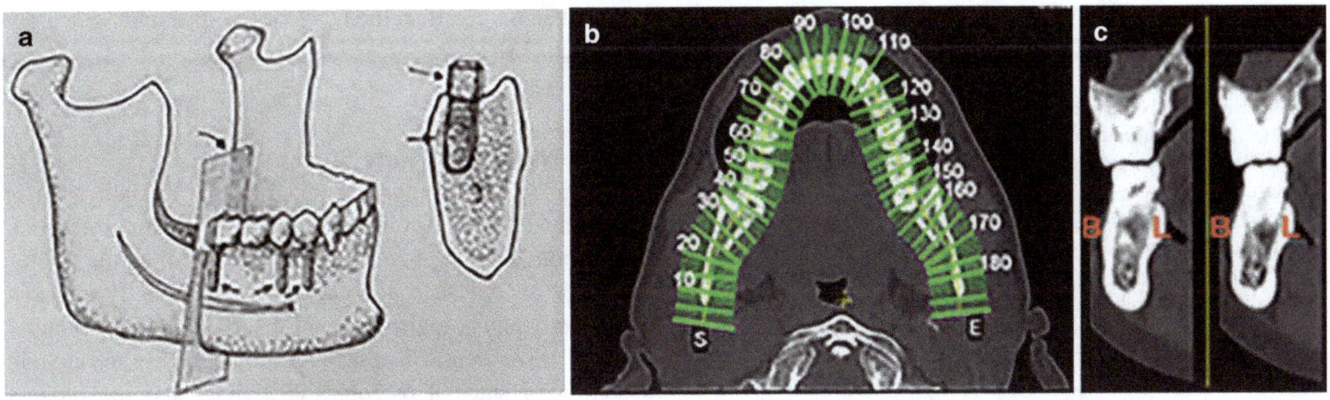




**Fig. 8.15** (**a**), (**b**), and (**c**). a and b show coronal plain image planning of individual tooth. c shows the coronal reformatted image of tooth

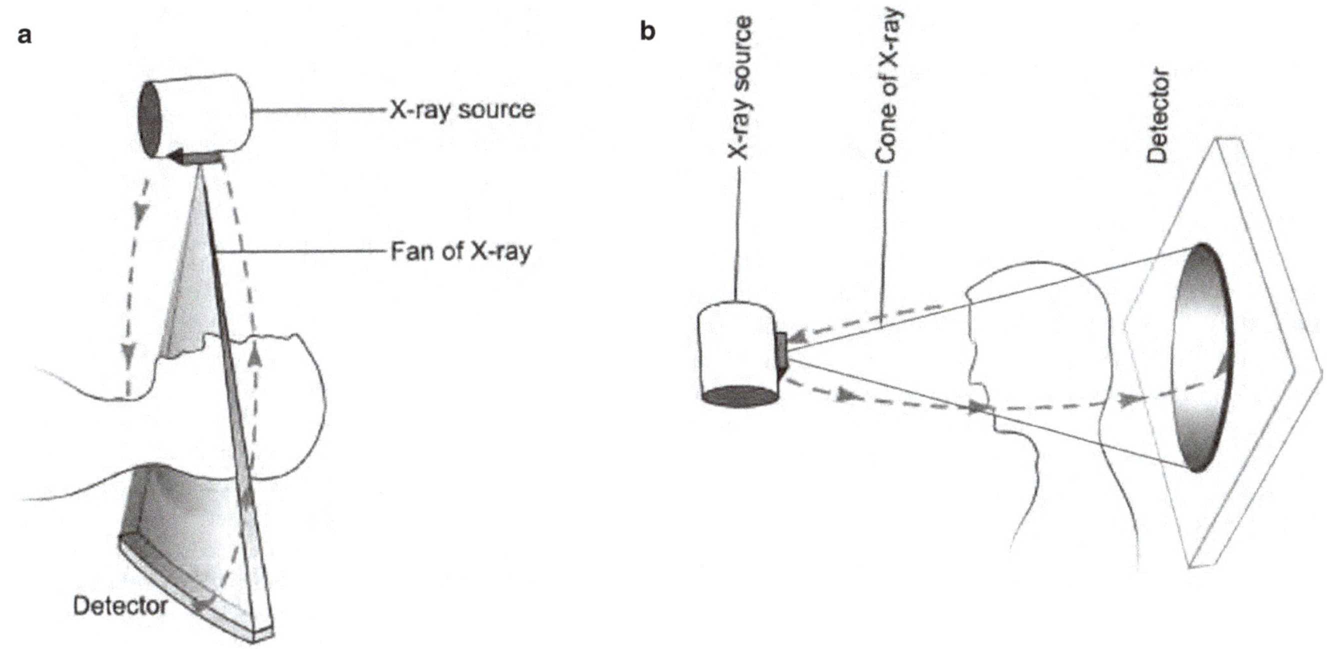




**Fig. 8.16** (**a**) and (**b**). Schematic diagram. (**a**) shows fan beam of X-rays from X-ray tube with curvilinear row of detectors. (**b**) shows cone beam of X-rays from X-ray tube with flat detector

## Cone Beam CT (CBCT)

*Indications for CBCT*

CBCT applications have proved helpful in a multitude of dental disciplines and the MFS needs to be aware of it. Its indications include periodontal and endodontic assessment, placement and evaluation of implants, evaluation of jaw bones, temporomandibular joints, bony and soft-tissue lesions, and alveolar ridge resorption and orthodontic evaluation.

### Working Principle and System Composition of CBCT System

As the name suggests, it is a form of computed tomography (CT). The basic process involved in CBCT is the scanning of the region of interest using a cone-shaped X-ray beam, making a single rotation around the vertical axis of the patient's head. The information obtained, from various angles about the structures in the region of interest, is in a digitized format relating to shape and density, which is then processed using

**Table 8.1** Comparison between CBCT and Fan Beam CT

| Fan Beam CT | CBCT |
|---|---|
| Conventional CT scanners make use of a fan beam and provide a set of consecutive slices of image. | CBCT makes use of a cone beam, which radiates from the x-ray source in a cone shape, encompassing a large volume with a single rotation. |
| Makes use of a lie-down machine with a large gantry | Makes use of a sitting up machine of smaller dimensions |
| Greater contrast and resolution | Ease of operation |
| Better differentiation between tissue types (bone, teeth, and soft tissue) | Commonly used for hard tissues Especially dental tissues |
| Higher radiation dose | Lesser radiation dose |
| Detector type X-axis only | Detector type X- and Y-axes |
| Volume acquisition requirements are sequential multiple gantry rotations | Volume acquisition requirements are single gantry rotations |
| Speed of examination is fast | Speed of examination is faster |

special software and a three-dimensional (3D) image is reconstructed [2].

CBCT occupies a special place in imaging of the Head and Neck region. It offers a number of advantages over traditional CT technology. It has a multitude of uses in the dental discipline, including dentoalveolar disease and anomalies, jaw tumors, vertical root and dentin fractures, among others. It has also had a positive impact on teaching students about oral and maxillofacial imaging making them adept at operating equipment and related instruments, resulting in greater accuracy in evaluation and analysis of the pathological characteristics of the disease process leading to a proper final clinical diagnosis. Both the traditional fan beam CT and CBCT are third-generation CT scanners but are different in some ways (Fig. 8.16a, b) (Table 8.1).

#### 8.7.1.3 Gamma Rays

Gamma rays are a form of Electromagnetic radiation (EMR). They are similar to X-rays but can be differentiated by the fact that they originate from the nucleus. Gamma-ray photons have the highest energy with their waves having the shortest wavelength in the EMR spectrum. The difference between the two is that X-rays are produced by accelerating electrons when they strike a target, while gamma rays originate from the nucleus of a radionuclide after radioactive decay. Gamma rays damage the DNA of cells and it is this action that is used in the treatment of cancerous tumors, care being taken not to affect the DNA of the surrounding healthy tissue cells [3].

#### 8.7.1.4 Nuclear Isotope Studies

Scintigraphy or radionuclide imaging is a modality that is readily available and relatively inexpensive. One drawback is that though it can provide specific information, the resolution is poor. It is a functional imaging modality and can assess early physiological changes even before bone mineral changes are evident. Bone scintigraphy is highly sensitive in detection of skeletal osteoblastic activity and the process involves uptake of the radiopharmaceutical Technetium-99 m (Tc-99 m), by the mineral component of the bone due to its affinity for bone. It has proven to be greatly useful in the study of malignant lesions and also in the evaluation of vascularized bone grafts used in reconstruction surgeries of the maxillofacial region [4]. Another use of radionuclide imaging is in evaluating patients with condylar hyperplasia. In these patients, radionuclide imaging of the temporomandibular joint is performed to exclude active condylar growth and in planning the extent of orthognathic surgery. A progressive condition necessitates the removal of the entire condyle and neck while trimming of the enlarged condyle suffices otherwise [5].

#### 8.7.1.5 Positron Emission Tomography (PET)

PET also is a functional imaging technique. It is unique in that it produces images reflecting in vivo changes in tissue metabolism, linking the changes to malignancy. Body images are produced when radiation is emitted from radioactive tracer substances like Carbon-11, Fluorine-18, Oxygen-15, or Nitrogen-13. When a positron emitted from the radioactive substance collides with an electron in the tissue, gamma rays are given off at the site, which are detected by a gamma detector. FDG-PET/CT fusion scans of the head and neck are not primarily for infection identification but for categorizing a clinically questionable lesion as malignant or not.

CT scans detect changes in body structure and only confirms the presence of a mass. PET scan is different from CT in that it can reveal the presence of disease earlier allowing for quicker diagnosis, can detect the extent of disease and whether a detected mass is benign or malignant, helps monitoring treatment and its effectiveness, and can detect abnormalities even before there is any anatomical change. This is based on the fact that glucose consumption by malignant cells and hence tissue is far higher than that of normal tissue.

The scan involves intravenous injection of a radiolabeled compound like 2-deoxy-2-(18F) fluoro-D-glucose (FDG). After uptake of the compound, it undergoes further break down in the cells. Since tumor cells have a high metabolic rate, it is also metabolized by the tumor cells. FDG is metabolized to FDG-6-phosphate, but the tumor cells are incapable of metabolizing it further and in consequence the FDG-6-phosphate accumulates and concentrates within the tumor cells. It is this accumulation that is detected and quantified. As compared to normal tissue, the uptake of FDG by malignant tissue is very high, making it a sensitive method to pick up early malignant tissue [6].

## 8.8 Radiation: Hazard Awareness and Principles of Protection

**Hazardous Nature of X-Rays**

When an X-ray photon is incident on tissue, it results in a series of changes at the molecular and atomic level. The trans formed photon energy results in the discharge of an electron and a free radical, or ionization in other words. Ionization results in the production of a new molecule due to breakage of enzyme bonds manifesting in the form of different biological effects. These effects may be repairable when there is no appreciable damage, or irreparable when there is definite occurrence of damage, the adverse effect being cumulative in nature.

**Myths and Facts about radiation in the field of Diagnosis:** Many myths exist regarding radiation hazards associated with medical diagnostic imaging. Possible rea sons for this are the available historical data, exaggerated social media reports, results of experimental studies and the complex nature of radiation biology making it difficult to evaluate its mechanism of action. Historical data relates to the reports of visible radiation hazards from studies on vic tims of the Hiroshima/Nagasaki bomb explosion in 1945 who were followed up for 15-18years. Exaggerated report ing by social media about nuclear reactor accidents like that at Chernobyl add to the existing myths. The extremely short time for which radiation interacts with matter ($10^{-5}$Sec) after absorption, makes it difficult to study the complex nature of radiation biology. The biological process of cell death can take days to months, carcinogenesis can take years to occur while generations may pass before a mutational change is seen.

In reality, the dose of received radiation from man-made X-rays that exist today is minute, in comparison with the massive radiation exposure that occurred in the aforementioned examples. It is true that in the infant stage following discovery of X-rays and its use in diagnosis, visible radiation hazards did occur, which was due to ignorance in the understanding of its potential hazards and the use of crude equipment resulting in high amounts of radiation leak. With passage of time, we have learnt to put the benefits of X-rays to full use, concurrently taking proper precautions to protect ourselves from its hazardous effects. Over the years, improvements in diagnostic equipment using ionizing radiation have led to the production of newer equipment providing the best possible image quality with minimal radiation exposure and improved devices that are protective against radiation. Yet, the fact remains that the best method to reduce the effects of radiation is using it only when it is an utmost necessity [7].

## 8.9 Imaging Investigations Not Involving Ionizing Radiation

### 8.9.1 MRI (Magnetic Energy Coupled with Radiofrequency Energy)

This imaging modality does not involve the use of ionizing radiation but makes use of magnetic and radiofrequency energy to obtain information of the internal organs. Components of an MRI unit include the magnet, the console, and the computer.

**Image Procurement by MRI**

Exploiting the body's magnetic property forms the basis of imaging using magnetic resonance. The human body is abundant in atoms with odd number of protons, or in other words ionized particles or charged atoms. A charged particle spinning around its own axis creates a magnetic field around itself behaving like a tiny bar magnet. Hydrogen represents one such atom that is present in water molecules and therefore in all body tissues.

The random orientation of the hydrogen atoms cancels out their magnetic fields and so there is no net magnetization at rest. When these protons are placed in a strong magnetic field, a net magnetization is produced that aligns parallel with the main magnetic field. To influence the human body, the external magnetic strength needs to be about 6000 to 80,000 times the earth's magnetic strength. The resultant net magnetization acts as the source of the MR signal and is used to produce MR images. Application of a radiofrequency (RF) pulse results in absorption of energy from the RF pulse causing the net magnetization to rotate away from the direction of the main magnetic field, the amount of rotation or flip angle depending on the strength and duration of the RF pulse. The strength and duration of the RF pulse can be controlled such that the net magnetization can be rotated to any angle [8]. Withdrawal of the RF pulse results in the liberation of energy, with the emission of signals based on the density of protons or hydrogen atoms. These signals are captured by the external antennae, fed into the computer, and processed to produce the image.

### Types of Magnets: Their Advantages and Limitations

- External magnets are of two types, the permanent magnet and the electromagnet.
- Permanent magnets are cheaper with no significant recurring cost. However, its limitations include limited strength of less than 0.5 tesla, heavy nature making transportation difficult, production of weak signals, and slower performance with limited range resolution.
- Electromagnets work by the passage of high current around ferromagnetic substances creating the required magnetic field. They are faster, have better resolution, produce better reconstructions, and are lighter than permanent magnets. The drawback is the production of large amount of heat that needs cooling using Liquid Helium. Other disadvantages include the high cost of infrastructure, high consumption of electricity, and recurring expenses.

### Preparing a Patient for an MRI

- Detailed history and clinical examination are mandatory.
- Specific history relating to previous surgery with the use of aneurysmal clips or metallic prosthesis needs to be ascertained.
- Patient compatibility for the procedure needs to be evaluated in view of the requirement of lying motionless for a minimum of 30 to 40 min, e.g., Orthopneic patients, COAD patients. Anesthesia might be required for agitated patients and infants.
- A double check for any metallic objects on the patient's body using a metal detector device is necessary.
- Claustrophobic patients need to be reassured and put at ease before the examination begins.
- The procedure needs to be explained in detail prior to the patient entering the MRI magnet room.

CT & MRI are complementary to each other. As far as the MFS is concerned, thin-slice CT with reconstruction is required while evaluating bony lesions, especially in cases of trauma. MRI on the other hand is good for evaluation of soft-tissue tumors and is contraindicated in penetrating injuries of the eye (Table 8.2).

**Table 8.2** CT and MRI: A comparison

| | CT | MRI |
|---|---|---|
| Multiplanar Imaging | Only axial slices are possible. Images need to be reconstructed in multiple planes following acquisition of primary axial sections. Direct sagittal and coronal slices are possible except for TM joint. | Direct multiplanar images can be primarily acquired in any desired plane. Excellent sectional images are possible. |
| Soft-tissue characterization | | Best with MRI than CT |
| Compact bone/ calcified lesions | Best analyzed by CT than MRI | |
| Bone marrow | | Assessment best with MRI than CT |
| Radiation | Ionizing radiation involved | No ionizing radiation involved |
| Motion artifacts | Relatively well managed with CT | Very sensitive to any kind of motion. May require anesthesia. Noisy breathing too may affect images |
| Time required | Faster, with whole body scan from vertex to toe taking 8–10 seconds | Takes longer. Minimum time required for scan of any part is 40–60 min |
| Contrast media | Invariably required and so contrast-related problems are unavoidable. | Contrast is less frequently used and is relatively safer. |
| Trauma | Best modality | |
| Ferromagnetic artifacts | | MRI is contraindicated in patients with pacemakers or recently placed implants. MRI compatible supportive gadgets: Pulse Oxymeter, anesthesia equipment, I.V. stands, etc. |

### How Does CT/MRI Differ from Conventional Radiography?

CT and MRI are sectional imaging methods, in which the whole body or the region of interest is sectioned into serial slices and further into cubes (Fig. 8.3a, b). Each slice surface represents the corresponding sectional anatomy with each slice being made up of small units or cubes with each cube representing the basic nature of the tissue in the digital form (Figs. 8.17 and 8.18a, b). Different modalities produce varied imaging appearances of the same structure. For instance, if a coconut is imaged using different modalities, the fine structural details of the interior of the tender coconut, and its contents are better seen on CT and MRI (Fig. 8.19a-c). Similarly, imaging of a pineapple in axial (Fig. 8.20a-d) and coronal planes (Fig. 8.21a-c) and using the volume-rendering technique (Fig. 8.22) reveals varied appearances on CT and different MRI sequences.

To summarize, in sectional imaging, the region of interest or the whole body is divided into slices and cubes with each cube representing the basic tissue of that region with thinner slices and smaller-sized cubes offering better resolution.

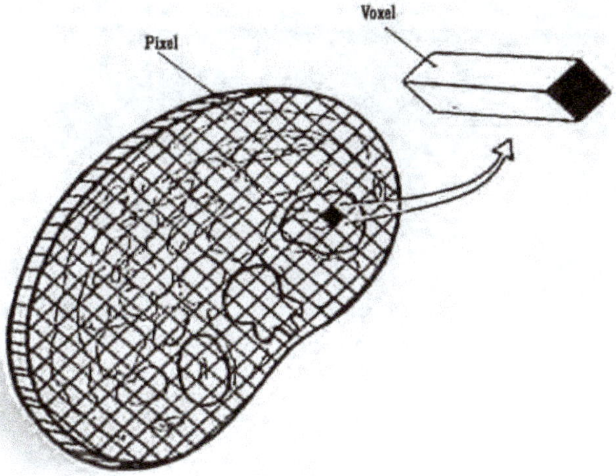




**Fig. 8.17** Each axial slice is divided into small cubes loaded with digitalized values representing corresponding tissue volume called voxel. Its surface represents a fraction of the grayscale image specific for that region called pixel. Thinner the slice and smaller the pixel, better is the resolution

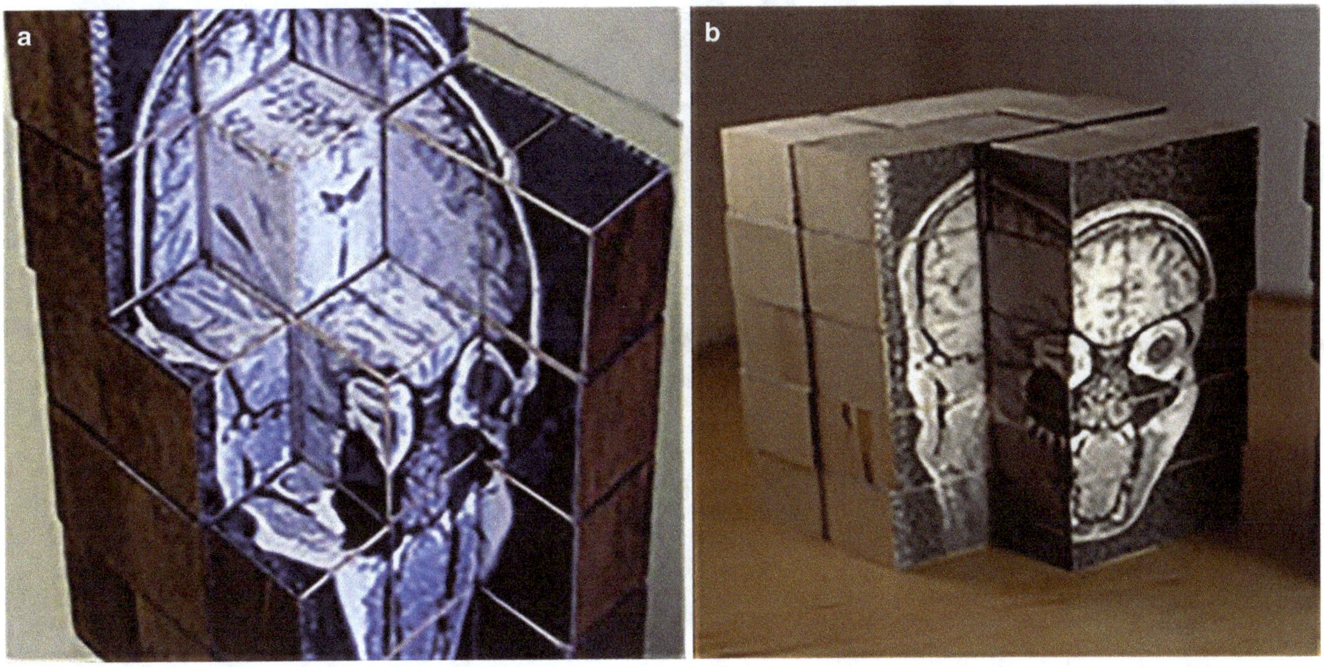




**Fig. 8.18** (**a**) and (**b**). Figures showing unit wise volumetric digitalized information of anatomical structures for retrieval and displayed as sectional anatomical slices

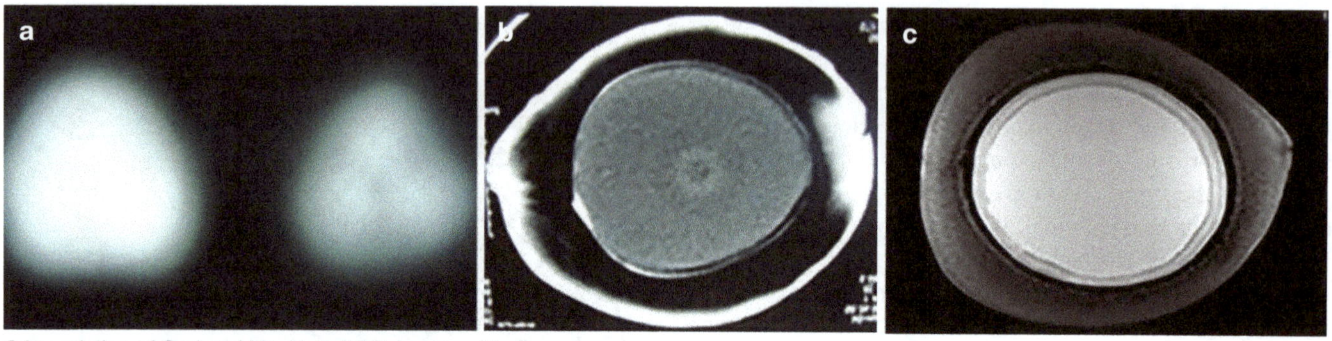


©Association of Oral and Maxillofacial Surgeons of India

**Fig. 8.19** (**a**), (**b**), and (**c**). Imaging of tender coconut. (**a**) Conventional plain Radiograph. (**b**) CT Axial sectional imaging. (**c**) MRI sectional imaging. Note: added information with each of these modalities

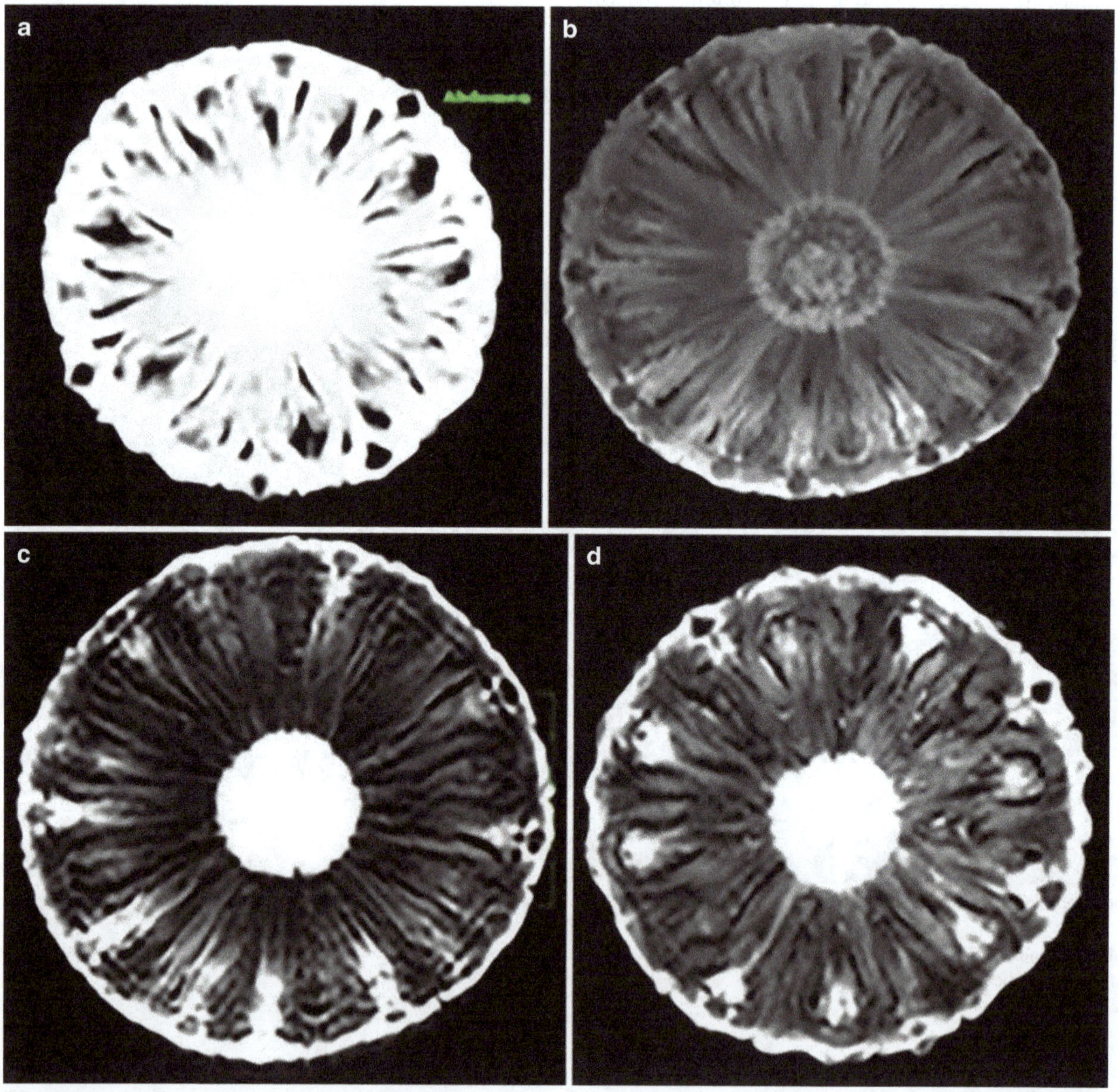


©Association of Oral and Maxillofacial Surgeons of India

**Fig. 8.20** (**a**), (**b**), (**c**), and (**d**). Axial sectional images of pineapple taken at the same level (**a**) CT. (**b, c, d**) MRI various sequences. Note: superior soft-tissue resolution in MRI, highlighting various components of soft tissue in various sequences

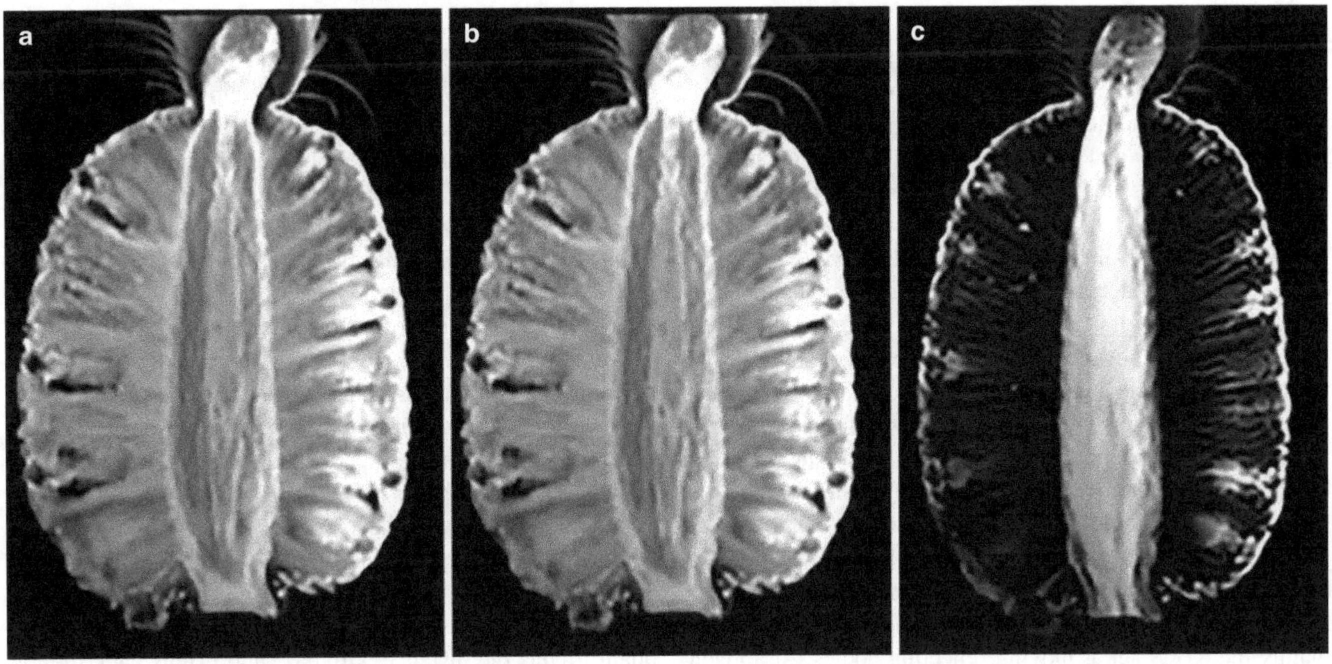



**Fig. 8.21** (**a**, **b** and **c**). Various sequences of MRI of a pineapple showing multiplanar capability to procure sections in any desired plane without reconstruction unlike CT

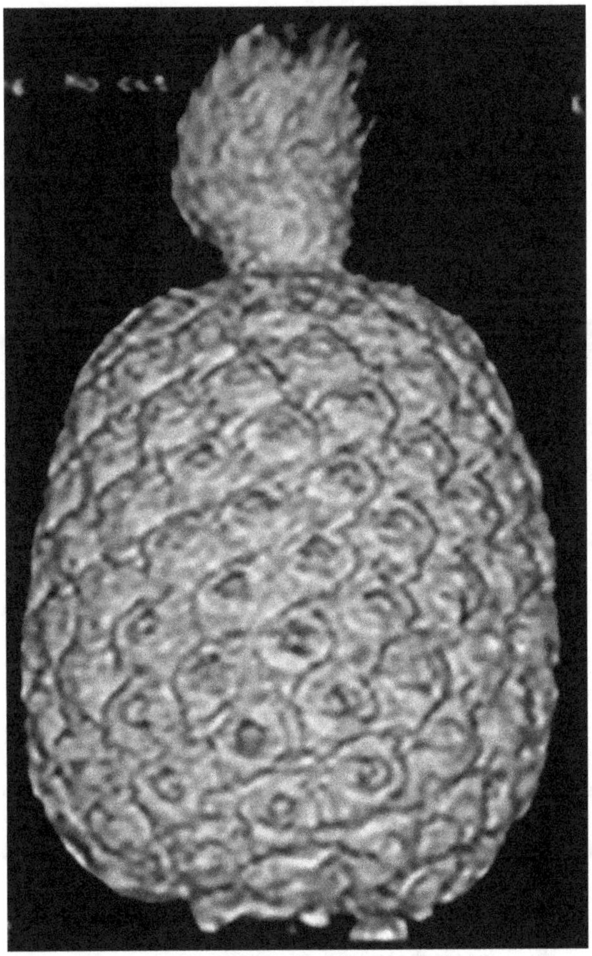



**Fig. 8.22** CT 3D surface rendering image of Pineapple

### 8.9.2 Ultrasound

It seems implausible that sound waves can produce informative images of internal organs of a human body. Yet it is true that technology has evolved so much over the years that it is now possible to obtain information of body structures using sound waves by making use of the echo and Doppler properties of sound waves.

Sound waves can be classified, based on their wavelength and frequency as audible sounds (20 to 2000 cycles/sec), infrasound (less than 20 cycles/sec), and ultrasound (>20,000 cycles/sec). Ultrasound in the range of 2 to 20 MHz is used in medical imaging [8]. The source of these ultrasound waves is piezoelectric crystals. These crystals have the special property of generating electrical pulses on being subjected to pressure. In addition, the passage of electricity through the crystals causes them to get compressed or deformed. Essentially, these crystals are unique in that they have the dual property of converting electrical energy into mechanical energy and mechanical energy into electrical energy. Intermittent passage of electrical current through the crystals makes them alternate between compression and relaxation, resulting in vibration of the crystal, in consequence producing sound energy of small wavelength in the ultrasound range.

Devices, equipped with piezoelectric crystals, having the capability to convert electrical energy to mechanical energy and finally to sound energy as well as having the reverse capabilities of converting sound energy to electrical energy, are termed as Transducers.

Sound waves are useful in imaging due to their property of echo/reflection and due to the Doppler effect. Echo property refers to the property of sound waves to get reflected at the interface of two media, the strength of the reflected sound echo depending on the density difference of the media through which they traverse. Reflected sound energy gets converted to mechanical energy and finally to electrical energy on striking the crystal, and this electrical energy is represented on a monitor as bright dots of variable gray scales.

Varying density interfaces throughout body tissues, produces variable image brightness with gray scales ranging between extreme bright dots to black dots, representing different organ or tissue sections. The Doppler effect of sound refers to the change in the apparent frequency of a wave when the observer and the source move toward or away from each other. Motion causes a change in pitch with a higher frequency being heard when the sound source approaches the observer, and a lower frequency being heard when the sound source moves away. This Doppler property is used in evaluating the direction and velocity of flow of blood in vessels. The transducer is considered as the fixed source of sound and the blood component, mainly the RBCs act as moving reflecting bodies. At a given point in the vessel by calculating the sudden change in the frequency of reflected sound, we can calculate the velocity of blood and also the direction of blood flow. This helps in the evaluation of percentage of stenosis in a vessel.

### B Mode

A grayscale sectional image has specific echo texture based on tissue content with the display mode being called as the 'B' mode (Brightness mode) or grayscale mode. Higher sound frequency provides better image resolution with delineation of finer tissue components, however, at the expense of depth of penetration. Higher-frequency transducers (7 MHz to 20 MHz) are hence used for imaging superficial structures like cheek, the maxillofacial region, neck spaces, breast, thyroid, testis, eye, musculoskeletal system and skin, regions where finer analysis of tissue structure is expected. Deeper structures are evaluated by using transducers with frequency in the range of 2 to 5 MHz.

The relation between frequency, resolution, and depth can be understood well, using the hypothetical example of two friends—an ant and an elephant (Fig. 8.23a, b). Both of them are commanded to perform the same tasks, the first being to pick up and bring back a crystal of sugar dropped at a distance of 100 cm from the start line and the second to pick up and bring back a log of wood placed 100 meters from the start line. Both of them proceed to perform the first task. The ant being small is able to easily identify the sugar crystal and get it back; however, the elephant keeps moving around unable to identify the crystal. As to the second task, the ant is able to travel only a short distance after which it dies of exhaustion, unable to reach the log of wood while the elephant travels the distance with ease and brings back the log of wood.

The ant is comparable to the high-frequency short-wavelength sound wave that is able to travel a short distance and bring back finer information about superficial tissues. If, on the other hand, it travels a long distance all its energy is absorbed by interaction with tissues. The elephant is comparable to the low-frequency sound wave with long wavelength that can travel deeper into the tissues and get information of deep structures, but limited tissue details. In a clinical setup, both the ant (high-frequency sound) and the elephant (low-frequency sound) are essential for evaluation, depending on the clinical situation and region of interest.

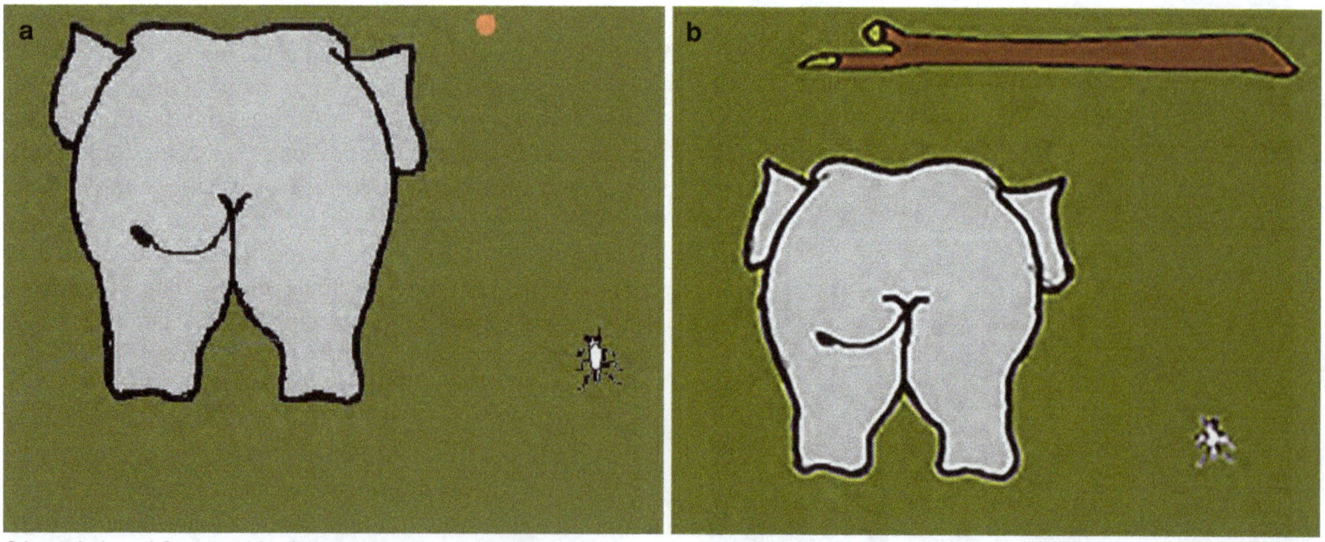




**Fig. 8.23** (**a**) and (**b**). Example of an elephant and an ant demonstrating their varying capability in picking up large and small objects from varying distances—a pictorial representation for understanding the difference in the penetration capacity of high- and low-frequency sound waves. (Explained in the text)

**Color Doppler**

The display of flow of blood in a vessel is color coded. The flow toward the probe is depicted as red and flow away from the probe is blue. Arterial and venous flow, in a given anatomical region, is in opposite directions. Red generally represents flow in arteries, while blue represents venous flow. Turbulent flow is depicted using a mixture of colors.

**Power Doppler**

This display mode of Doppler conveys information about the overall flow in a given tissue, for instance, assessment of blood flow in a tumor. It helps to determine whether the tumor is hyper- or hypovascular.

**Strengths of Ultrasound**

- Ultrasound imaging is inexpensive and is free from the risk of radiation.
- Excellent soft-tissue resolution is possible and dynamic studies too can be performed under ultrasound guidance.
- It is the first line of investigation for hepatic, biliary, and renal disease and is an excellent modality for cyst imaging,
- Gynecological and prostate disorders are imaged using endocavitary ultrasound, Doppler studies allow assessment of blood flow, and real-time ultrasound imaging helps in guiding interventional biopsies and drainages.

**Weaknesses of Ultrasound**

- A long learning curve exists for some areas of expertise and image resolution is dependent on the machine that is available. Ultrasound does not give information of structure behind a bone and also gas filled structures.

**Specific Role of High-Resolution Ultrasonography (HRUSG) in the Maxillofacial Region**

HRUSG is a grossly underutilized modality in evaluating lesions of the maxillofacial region. This is due to the lack of awareness of its application. The tissues in the maxillofacial region are ideal for sonographic evaluation and hence is widely applied to help diagnose a number of clinical conditions. It can serve as the best possible initial parallel imaging investigation for all the superficial soft-tissue structures of head and neck region.

It is noninvasive and does not involve use of radiation. There are no contraindications to the use of ultrasound, and it can even be performed as a bed side examination. No prior specific preparation is required except for shaving of the beard, which might hamper the study. The study results are immediately available, and it is an excellent modality for evaluating various soft-tissue planes of the cheek. Evaluation of various anatomical spaces such as superficial masticator space, parotid space, carotid space, superficial neck spaces, visceral space, floor of the mouth, and all the infrahyoid neck spaces like the submandibular and sublingual spaces are possible using HRUSG, as are also pathologies like pre- and paravertebral abscesses, cellulitis, Ludwig's angina, and ranula [9].

High-resolution ultrasound is also capable of evaluating the nature of lymph nodes, assessing fluid and solid components and also assessing tissue vitality. Procedures like drainage of abscesses and biopsies can be conveniently performed under ultrasound guidance. Being a highly economical imaging modality, it is excellent for follow-up studies, excellent as a screening method, and at most times proves to be the conclusive examination [9].

**Drawbacks of Ultrasound Examination of the Maxillofacial Region**

Drawbacks include difficulty in assessing structures behind bony elements and structures containing gas. In case of huge masses, only partial information may be obtained, while short-necked individuals and obese patients are difficult to evaluate. Structures at the base of the skull cannot be evaluated as are structures medial to ramus. Another limitation is that ultrasound cannot provide information about structures behind bone or any gas-filled structure. Scanning using a hockey stick probe might help overcoming this limitation. Scans need to be performed by individuals having vast experience and expertise.

There needs to be an increase in awareness regarding the developments in the application of HRUSG in the maxillofacial region and a close interaction between the surgeon and the sonologist for creating an atmosphere of better understanding among them.

### 8.9.3 Thermography

Medical thermography is used for early preclinical diagnosis and treatment of homeostatic imbalances. It is noninvasive and safe since it does not use any radiation. It makes use of body heat to diagnose a wide range of health conditions. By using high-speed computers and thermal imaging cameras, body heat is processed and recorded in the computer as an image map that can be analyzed. The analysis is based on determining the presence of abnormal hot and cold areas that can relate to different conditions.

**Applications in the Maxillofacial Region**

A variety of conditions related to blood flow in the head and neck vessels can be assessed by thermal imaging. Easy visualization of facial blood vessels by thermography is possible because of its superficial location. Common venues of thermographic use in the head and neck region include evaluation of pain related to differentiation of different types of headache, facial nerve injury following a blow to the face or an accident, and visualization of disorders of the temporomandibular joint.

## 8.10 Role of Chest Radiograph in the Practice of Maxillo Facial Surgery

One of the most frequently requested investigations by an MFS is the Chest radiograph. Hence, interpretation of chest radiographic findings is of prime importance in determining the patient's clinical status.

### 8.10.1 Chest Radiographic Evaluation for Optimum Diagnostic Quality

An ideal chest radiograph, in terms of quality, is one that fulfills the following criteria (Fig. 8.24)

(a) Well-positioned patient without rotation.
- *Purpose*—Avoiding problems related to improper positioning that can obscure certain lung regions like the hila and mediastinal lines, can prevent clarity of borders, or can result in distorted position of structures like the trachea, which can be misinterpreted as a paratracheal mass.
- *Ideal radiograph*—The vertebral spinous processes are equidistant from the medial ends of the clavicle

(b) Proper lateral location of both scapulae on the radiograph.
- *Purpose*—avoids superimposition of scapulae over the lung fields
- *Ideal radiograph*—Medial border of the scapulae should be out of the lung field

(c) Inclusion of anatomical structures.
- *Purpose*—inclusion of entire lung fields from apex to diaphragmatic domes
- *Ideal radiograph*—must include the lower neck, both shoulders, lateral chest walls, and both diaphragms, including upper abdomen

(d) Proper identification references
- *Purpose*—Proper patient and radiographic verification.
- *Ideal radiograph*—must include the patient name, medical record number, date of acquisition, and the side marker (the most important of all)

(e) Optimum technical factors.
- *Purpose*—Clear visualization of the normal anatomy or presence of any pathology
- *Ideal radiograph*—
  - Posterior third of ribs faintly visible through heart shadow
  - Intervertebral spaces faintly visible through the heart shadow
  - Obtained in deep inspiratory effort as revealed by position of diaphragms

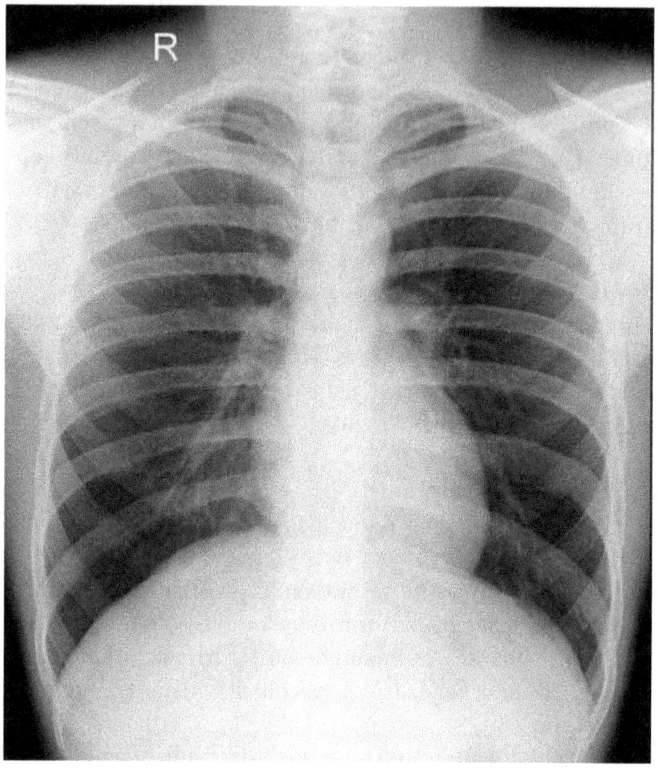




**Fig. 8.24** A Normal Chest Radiograph

### 8.10.2 Reading a Chest Radiograph: Interpretation Basics

The aim of reading a chest radiograph is to scan the whole image in a methodical way such that no anatomical part included in the radiograph is missed. While interpreting the radiograph, it is necessary for the interpreter to actually feel the structural component of the anatomical part being evaluated.

If, for example, a rib is being evaluated it needs to be traced, consciously keeping in mind, its component parts, the two cortical margins seen as white lines representing compact bone and the less dense central component representing marrow with fine normal trabeculae. This is in addition to evaluation of its number and shape. This meticulous evaluation will prevent missing of rib lesions and interpretation of the lesion is easier with prior knowledge of possible pathologies that affect ribs.

Many ways of methodical scanning have been documented in literature. The WHO-recommended method involves chest radiographic evaluation by beginning at one corner of the film, continuing to horizontally scan till the other corner, followed by sliding down and again continuing to scan toward the other edge, continuing till the whole of the radiograph has been scanned. As part of the examination, both sides of the chest must be compared.

It can be likened to the painting of a wall by a professional painter with a perfect finishing touch. Once the initial primary scan is complete, specific areas called the lawyer's zone or hidden areas of the lung need to be looked over a second time. These areas include both the hilar regions, both cardiophrenic regions, both apical and clavicular regions, and finally also through the heart and diaphragms.

### 8.10.3 Requesting a Chest Radiograph: Clinical indications

#### 8.10.3.1 Preoperative evaluation

i. Cleft lip and palate/any other congenital maxillofacial anomaly
ii. Infections of the maxillofacial region
iii. Known malignancy in maxillofacial region
iv. Trauma.

#### 8.10.3.2 Intra- / Postoperative recovery room

i. Sudden choking and breathlessness
ii. Sudden cyanosis
iii. Sudden cough
iv. Chest pain.
v. Fever
vi. Evaluation of chest tubes and catheters (suggested reference for further reading).

### 8.10.4 "The Chest Radiograph. A Mysterious Treasure"...the More you Search, the More you Find!!

#### 8.10.4.1 Consolidation

It is one of the most common terminologies used in Radiology. Clinicians and pathology textbooks, however, commonly use the term pneumonia. Any infection of the lung parenchyma is broadly referred to as pneumonia. Involvement of the alveolar components of the lung parenchyma by the infection is called parenchymal consolidation [10]. It is a disease process in which the air normally present within the small lung air sacs (alveoli) is replaced by liquids like pus, blood, or other fluids, or solids like tumor cells.

Radiologically, consolidation appears opaque [11]. Normally, the alveoli are filled with air and so the normal opaque pulmonary vasculature can be visualized against the dark background of air. However, as discussed earlier, the replacement of the air spaces by any form of fluid or solid material makes the normally visualized pulmonary vessels inapparent with the air containing bronchi being visualized against the opaque background, which is called the air bronchogram (Fig. 8.25a–c).

The consolidation process involving a single lobe and limited by a fissure is called as lobar pneumonia, while the involvement of the entire lung is known as whole-lung consolidation. At times, the process is not as uniform and is distributed in the form of patchy opacities with intervening nonopacified alveoli, an appearance referred to as the air alveologram, which is seen in Bronchopneumonia.

**Pulmonary Edema**

Maxillofacial surgeons are often faced with the problem of patients going into a state of sudden breathlessness in the postoperative recovery room for which the MFS asks for a portable chest radiograph. One of the most common causes of sudden breathlessness in the postoperative recovery room is pulmonary edema. The common confusion for which MFS postgraduates seek the radiologist's opinion is whether the cause of breathlessness is bronchopneumonia or aspiration bronchopneumonia.

In case of acute cardiogenic pulmonary edema caused either due to left ventricular failure or fluid overload, the characteristic radiographic abnormality would reveal bilateral symmetrical areas of consolidation predominantly in the

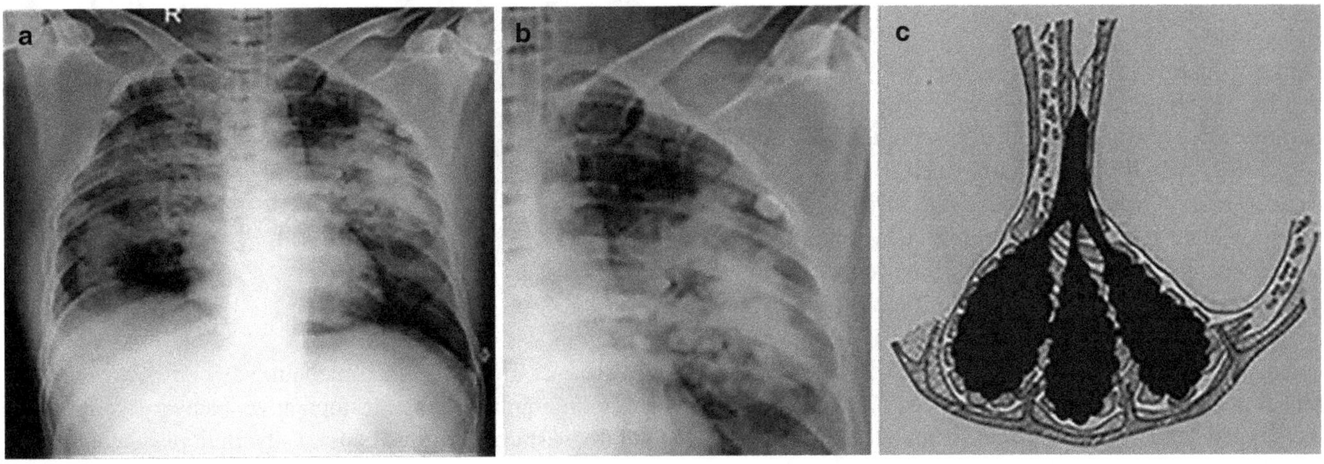




**Fig. 8.25** (**a**) and (**b**) Consolidation: Homogeneous opacities with "Air-bronchogram" sign. (**c**) Schematic diagram showing group of alveoli filled with fluid replacing normal air

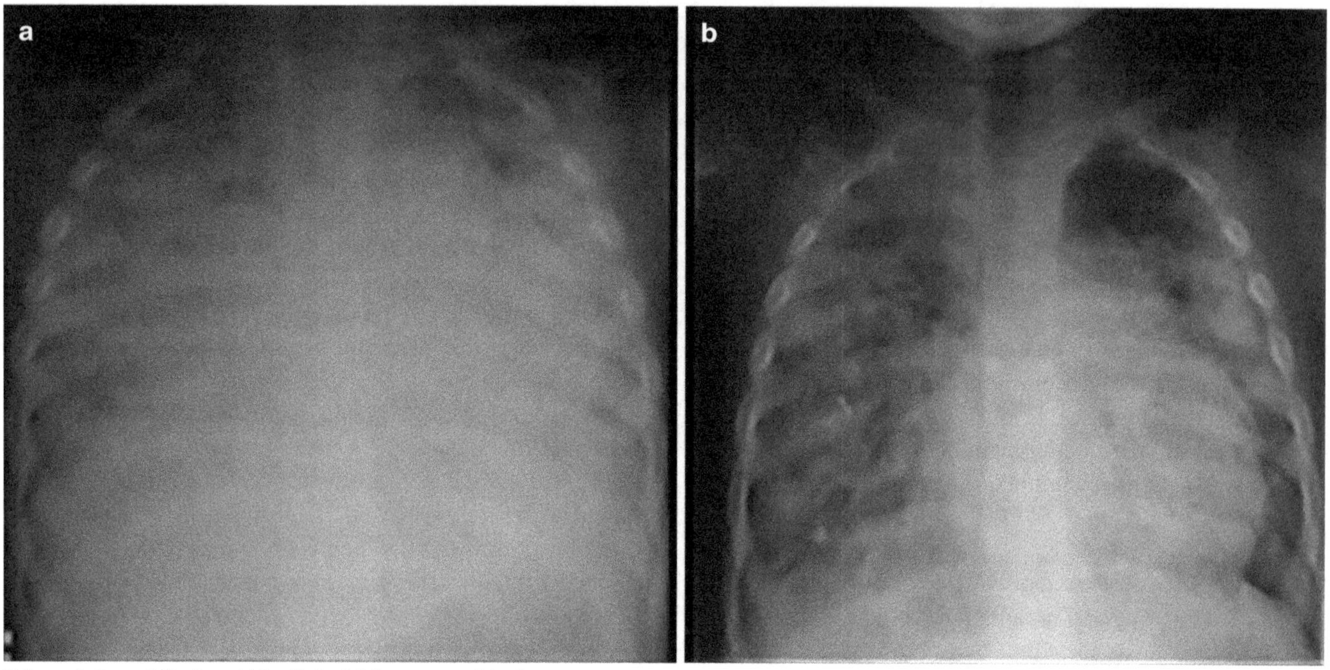




**Fig. 8.26** (**a**) Congestive cardiac failure with cardiomegaly and pulmonary edema. (**b**) Resolution of pulmonary edema after treatment

perihilar and lower lung zones [10] (Fig. 8.26a, b). Noncardiogenic pulmonary edema caused by different pathologies, including fluid overload, acute glomerulonephritis and adult respiratory distress syndrome among others, affects the permeability of the pulmonary capillary membrane (Fig. 8.27). The distribution can vary depending on the position of the patient. The opacities seen on the portable radiograph should not be confused with the appearance of pneumonia (Fig. 8.28).

Rare causes of unilateral pulmonary edema, including raised intracranial pressure and the administration of fluid through the central venous catheter inadvertently placed in the pulmonary artery, need to be kept in mind as well.

### Atelectasis

Diminished air within the lung associated with reduced lung volume is termed atelectasis manifesting radiologically as pulmonary opacity accompanied by volume loss. The causes are varied, including resorption, relaxation, adhesive and cicatrization atelectasis. Of these, the form of atelectasis a maxillofacial surgeon commonly deals with is resorption atelectasis, where there is an obstruction in the communication between the alveoli and trachea. The obstruction may be at any level from the common air way to the segmental bronchus; however, common air way obstruction resulting in bilateral atelectasis is a rare occurrence [11]. Radiologically, the appearance is that of a homogeneous opacity without an air bronchogram sign, with loss of lung volume and displacement of structures toward the opacity.

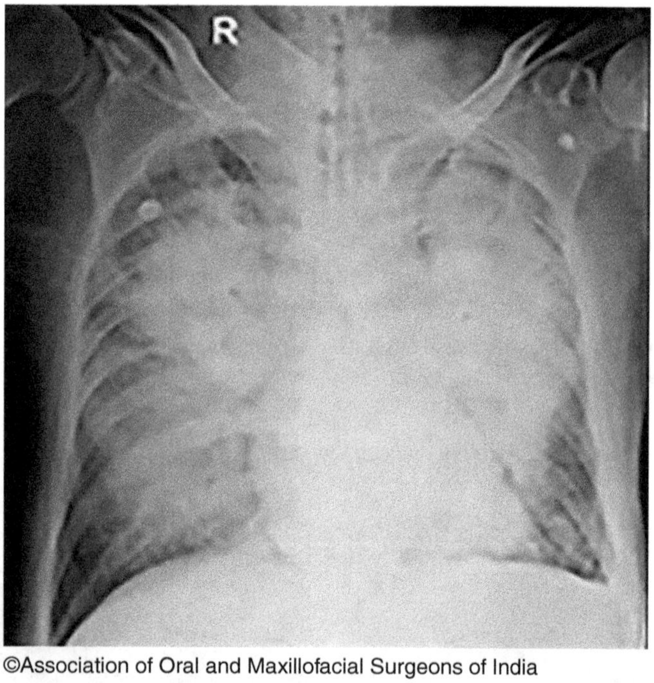




**Fig. 8.27** Noncardiac pulmonary edema in a patient with renal failure

The maxillofacial surgeon commonly comes across similar radiographs in the postoperative recovery room. The commonest cause of this is the inadvertent placement of the endotracheal tube into one bronchus, causing occlusion of the other bronchus, and resulting in atelectasis as a

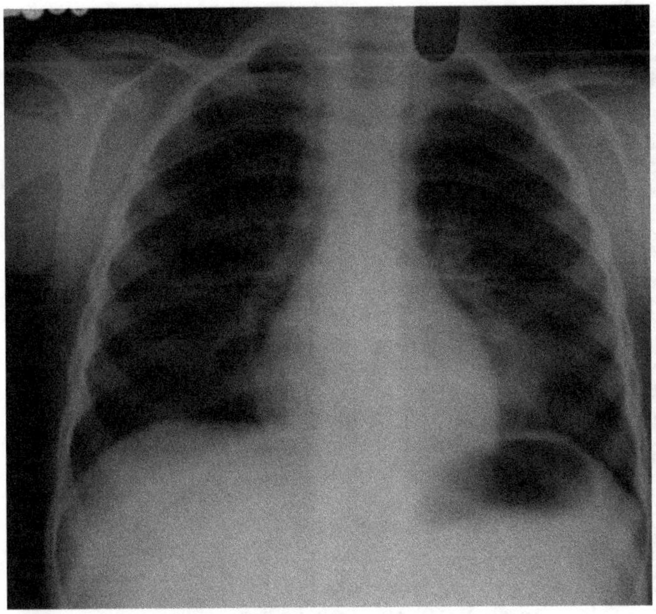



**Fig. 8.28** Aspiration Bronchopneumonia

consequence. Early detection and diagnosis with readjustment of the endotracheal tube is bound to be life saving, helping prevent long-term complications (Fig. 8.29a–c). Thick mucus plugs are other common occluding elements, seen in postoperative recovery rooms resulting in lobar or segmental opacities with loss of volume. Again, early detection and good respiratory physiotherapy are keys to improved lung compliance with a radiograph taken at a later date as follow-up.

**Relaxation Atelectasis**

Normally negative intrapleural pressure is caused by competing thoracic pressures. Lung elasticity and surface tension of the alveolar fluid create an inward tension, pulling the lung inward, which is countered by opposing forces from the pleural fluid and thoracic wall, the pleural cavity surface tension, and the parietal pleural attachment to the thoracic wall causing outward pull of the lungs. The outward pull is slightly higher than the inward pull with a negative intrapleural pressure of about -4 mm of Hg. When this intrapleural negative pressure is lost as occurs commonly in cases of pneumothorax or pleural effusion, the lung has a natural tendency to recoil, with the loss of lung volume being proportional to the amount of air or fluid collected in the pleural space [11].

**Pneumothorax**

The presence of air in the pleural space is called pneumothorax, the most common cause of which is trauma either accidental or iatrogenic. In the absence of such causes, it is called spontaneous pneumothorax. Radiological findings of pneumothorax include increased peripheral translucency, absence of lung markings within this area of translucency, and the identifiable visceral pleural margin of the collapsed lung (Figs. 8.30 and 8.31). The detection of a pneumothorax should prompt the search for an underlying cause like a fractured rib or a ruptured bulla or iatrogenic causes like a central venous catheter procedure. Associated lesions like pneumomediastinum and surgical emphysema should also be looked for.

A maxillofacial surgeon might have to read supine portable radiographs of patients presenting with clinical signs suggesting respiratory distress and the presence of pneumothorax might be missed. In such a scenario, the MFS should look for radiographic evidence of pneumothorax at sites adjacent to the diaphragmatic silhouettes on either side and the cardiophrenic and costophrenic angles and he should also be able to appreciate the appearance of an exceptionally sharp cardiac border [11]. The MFS needs to be aware that air trapped within the skin folds can mimic pneumothorax (Fig. 8.32).

Identification of an air fluid level would prompt the diagnosis of a hydropneumothorax. It is difficult to characterize the nature of the fluid as being transudate, exudate, blood, or chylous. An MFS may be unable to diagnose a hydropneumothorax, on an AP supine portable radiograph as the fluid level will not be identified. Here, the collapsed lung tends to float on the fluid, which is dependent posteriorly giving a veil effect (Fig. 8.33).

**Pneumomediastinum**

It is the collection of air within the pleural boundaries of the mediastinum and can arise secondary to barotrauma from mechanical trauma, intrathoracic, or iatrogenic trauma and infection or can occur spontaneously. A radiographic diagnosis of pneumomediastinum requires depiction of normal anatomic structures being outlined by air as they leave the mediastinum. The mediastinal air can cause elevation of the thymus, collect anterior or posterior to the pericardium, surround the pulmonary artery or its branches, or can collect adjacent to the major aortic branches or major bronchi (Fig. 8.34).

Most cases of pneumomediastinum described in maxillofacial surgery literature are as a result of dissection of air down the fascial planes of the neck. Chest radiographic findings need to be carefully examined to make the diagnosis of pneumomediastinum, which is crucial to the MFS in planning appropriate treatment of affected patients. On rare occasions, a significant amount of air in the mediastinum can cause vessel or tracheal obstruction and induce symptoms and signs of tamponade and decreased venous return.

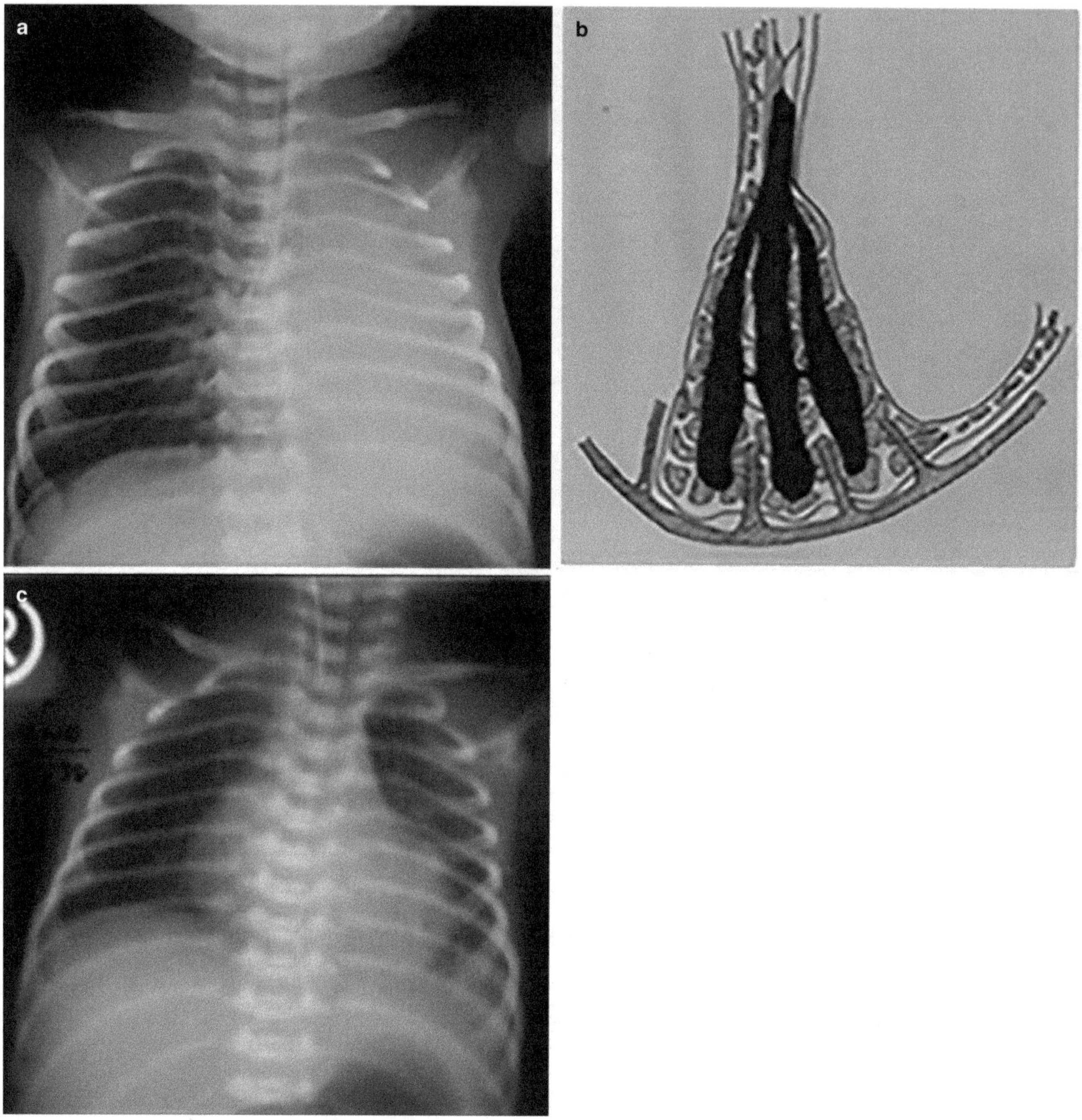




**Fig. 8.29** (**a**) Whole lung collapse: Left hemithorax is homogenously opaque with loss of volume of left lung with displacement of mediastinum to left. Note: Abnormal placement of endotracheal tube blocking the (Lt.) Bronchus. (**b**) Schematic diagram showing loss of volume of alveoli as seen in collapse with absence of air. (**c**) Reversion of normal left lung aeration after repositioning of endotracheal tube

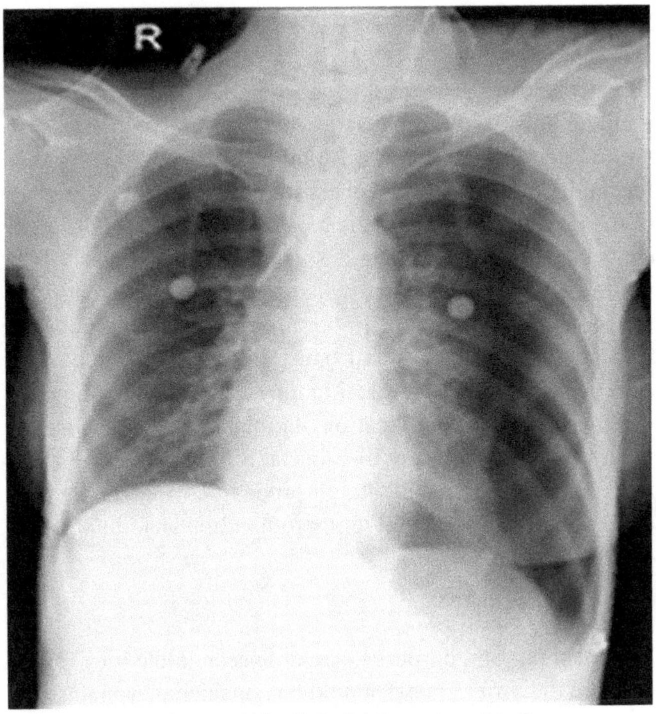




**Fig. 8.30** Left-sided pneumothorax

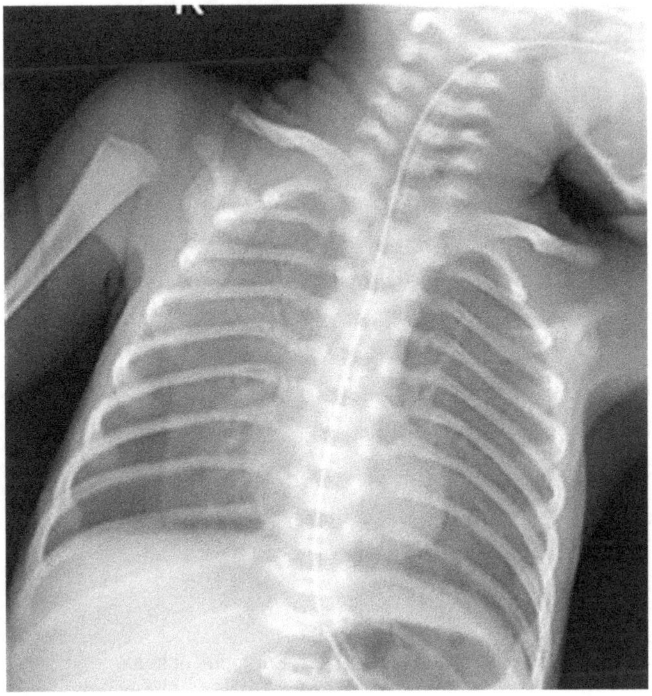



**Fig. 8.32** Right-sided pseudopneumothorax due to air trapped in skin fold

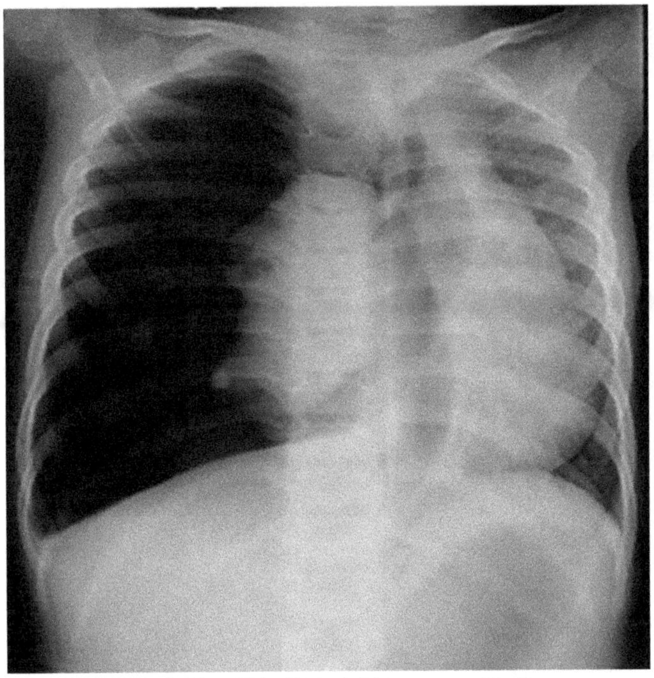



**Fig. 8.31** Right-sided tension pneumothorax

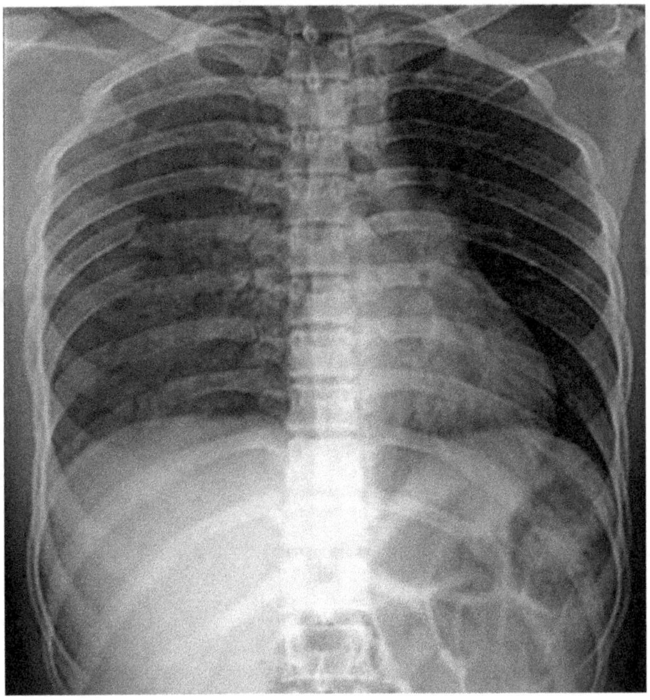



**Fig. 8.33** Right-sided hemopneumothorax with multiple rib fractures as seen in supine radiograph

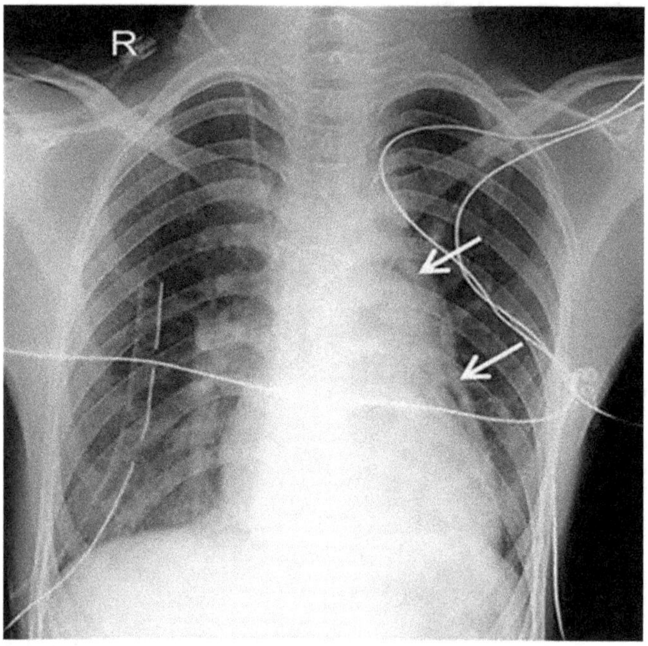




**Fig. 8.34** Pneumomediastinum. Air around the pulmonary artery and heart.

## Surgical Emphysema

Though subcutaneous emphysema or surgical emphysema actually means gas in the subcutaneous tissues, it also includes soft-tissue emphysema that dissects into the deeper soft tissues and musculature along fascial planes. The translucent air spreads over the chest wall and axilla into the root of the neck. Fascial planes clearly outline the pectoralis muscle and neurovascular bundles in neck (Fig. 8.35a, b). If trauma is the cause, the gas by itself may not need treatment, but its identification is of importance as it may be the only indication of the presence of other serious injuries requiring urgent management. Surgical emphysema can uncommonly occur as a serious complication of oral and maxillofacial surgical procedures. It may also occur following teeth extraction, endodontic treatment, or procedures like restorative dentistry, periodontal and temporomandibular joint surgery, or facial fracture repair.

## Pulmonary Nodules

For all intents and purposes, a nodule seen in the lung (especially in the lower zones) should be considered as metastasis unless proven otherwise, by a maxillofacial surgeon.

**Fig. 8.35** (**a**) and (**b**). Surgical emphysema with pneumothorax

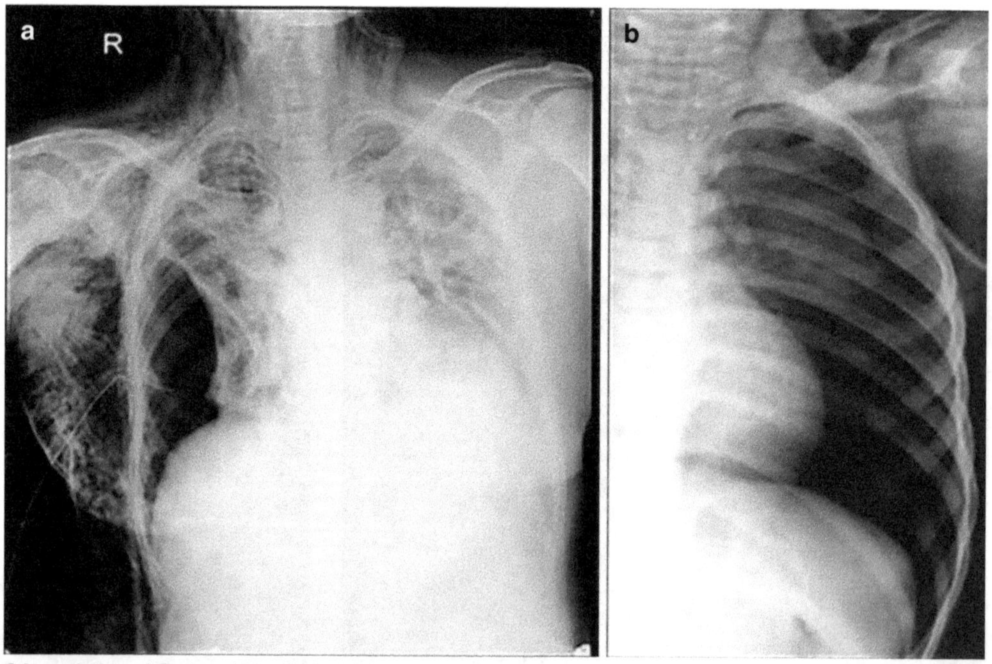

*Pulmonary nodules* can be characterized, based on some signature findings. In the absence of these findings, the nodule remains nonspecific. Common causes of pulmonary nodules are granulomas, bronchogenic cysts, hydatid cysts, hamartomas, pulmonary hematoma following laceration, rheumatoid nodules, fungal granulomas, and pulmonary metastasis.

*Tuberculomas* usually range in size from 1 to 3 cm in diameter, have central calcific lesions, and are surrounded by satellite scarred lesions. They are commonly seen in the upper zones, but they can occur anywhere in the lung (Fig. 8.36).

*Bronchogenic cysts* are well-defined nodules, around 3 to 4 cm in size, usually seen in the parahilar region, and are sometimes purely in the mediastinum (Fig. 8.37a–e).

*Hamartomas* are nodules that can occur anywhere in the lung having well-defined margins with central popcorn-like calcification (Fig. 8.38a, b).

*Hydatid cysts*, too, can occur anywhere in the lung. They have a stenciled outline and vary in size from 1 to 10 cms. The radiographic air crescentic sign is pathognomonic of a hydatid cyst, appearing like the arc of the moon caused by the separation of the endocyst from the exocyst. Continued separation of the endocyst from the exocyst results in an air fluid level typically called the 'water lily' appearance. Pulmonary hydatid cysts do not calcify.

Presence of a solitary nodule in the lower lung without any characteristic findings makes pulmonary metastasis a strong possibility, which should be further evaluated with imaging and HPR. Multiple nodules of varying sizes in the lower zones are very much suggestive of pulmonary metastasis.(Fig. 8.39a, b).

**Role of Chest Radiograph in Cases Developing Sudden Onset of Breathlessness in Postoperative Period**

1. Aspiration Bronchopneumonia
2. Pneumothorax
3. Foreign body (Fig. 8.40a–c)
4. Abnormal placement of Endotracheal Tube (Fig. 8.41)
5. Pleural effusion
6. Pulmonary edema and pulmonary embolism

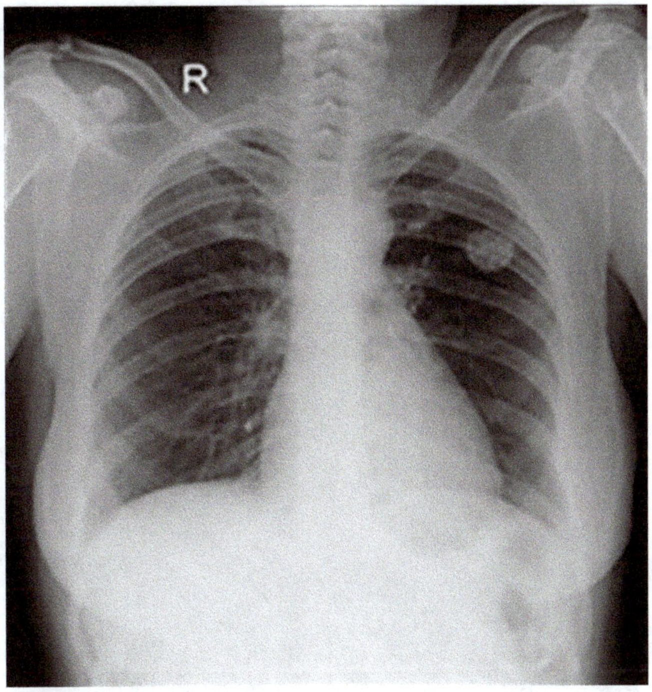




**Fig. 8.36** Pulmonary Nodule—Tuberculoma

A maxillofacial surgeon should be capable of identifying all of these causes of sudden onset of breathlessness in a postoperative patient in the event of the absence of availability of expert radiological opinion and act accordingly. They also need to be aware that patients on ventilators may develop ventilator-dependent complications.

**A glance into the future of imaging for Maxillofacial Surgeons**

1. Magnetization Transfer Imaging
   This is a modified MRI study that helps in
   - Prediction of whether the primary tumor is benign or malignant (possible in 80 to 90% cases).
   - Differentiation of reactive versus malignant adenopathy.
     This modality is still in the preliminary stage and needs further study.
2. MRI-guided biopsy procedures need MRI compatible equipment. The procedures are feasible and are usually done in cases that are not amenable to USG guidance.
3. Functional imaging of swallowing.

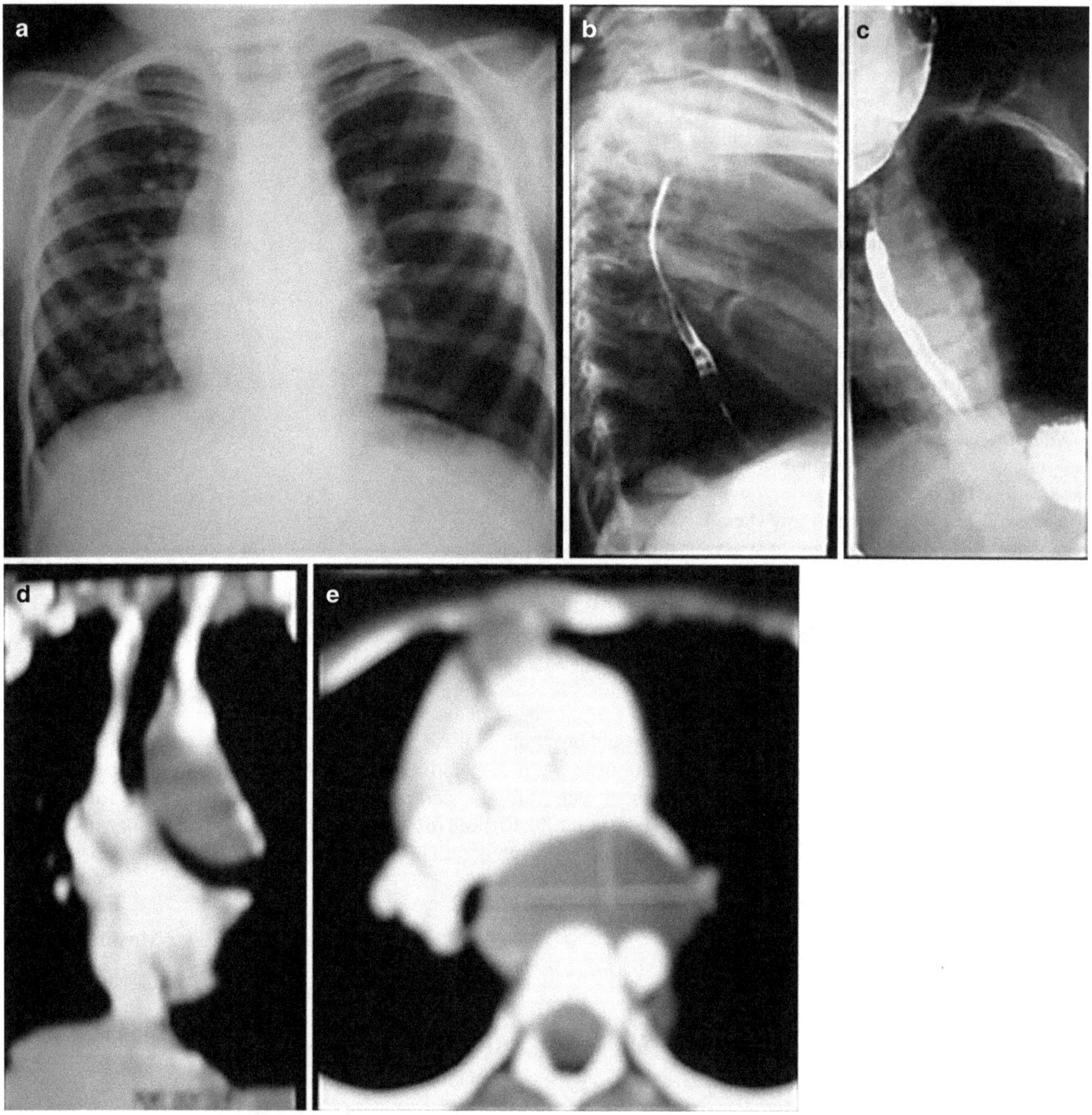




**Fig. 8.37** (**a**), (**b**), and (**c**). Preop chest radiographs of a patient with cleft lip presenting with dyspnea, more with changing position. (**d**) **and** (**e** Mediastinal mass—Bronchogenic Cyst confirmed on CT

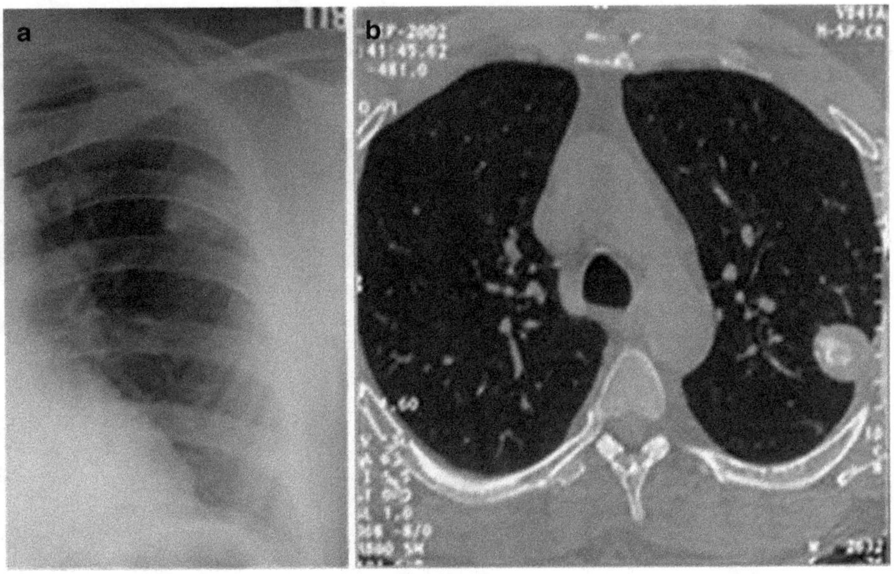




**Fig. 8.38** (**a**) Pulmonary Nodule-Hamartoma. (**b**) Confirmed on CT

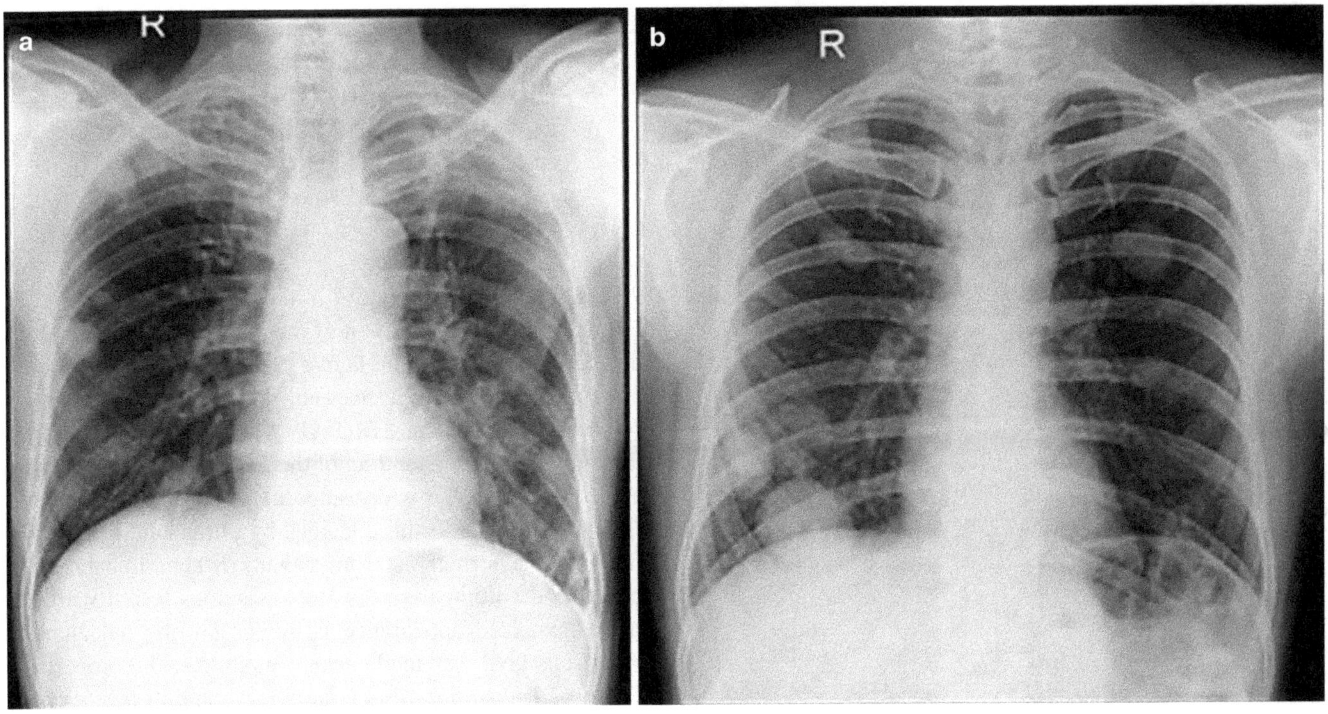




**Fig. 8.39** (**a**) and (**b**). Pulmonary metastasis

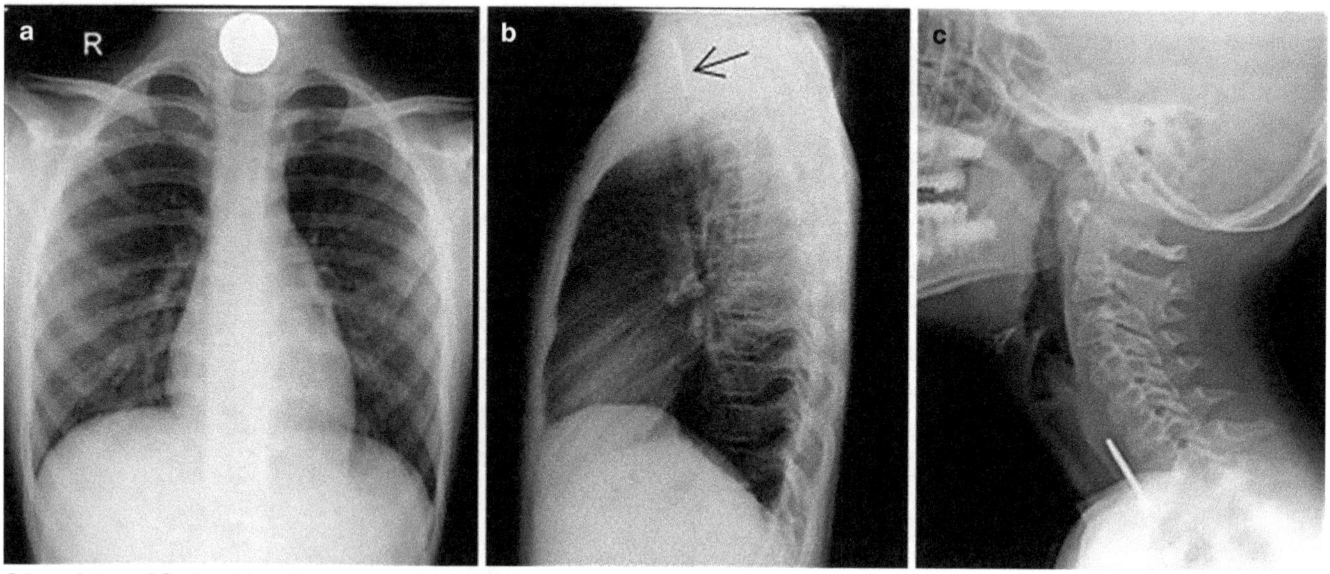




**Fig. 8.40** (**a**), (**b**), and (**c**). Foreign body, a coin in the cervical esophagus

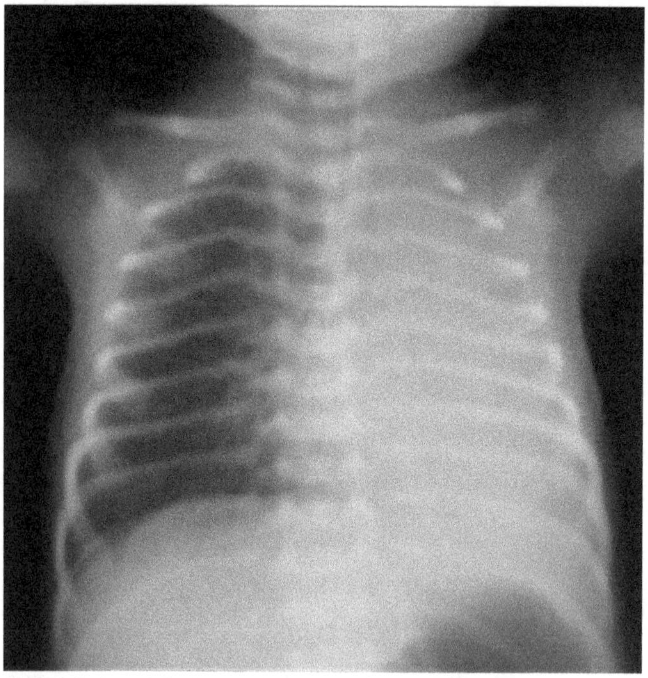



**Fig. 8.41** Abnormal placement of endotracheal tube with collapse of left lobe

## 8.11 Role of High Resolution Ultrasonography (HRUSG) as a Diagnostic Aid in the Practice of Maxillofacial Surgery

### 8.11.1 Preface

Primarily the use of HRUSG in the maxillofacial region is directed toward investigation of the cheek and the structures adjacent to it. Despite the layers of the cheek and the adjacent structures having a classical sonographic appearance, literature available on HRUSG of the cheek is limited. Having proper understanding of the relevant anatomy is critical in discerning the wide range of diseases affecting this region. Evaluation of these lesions by ultrasound is possible only once the normal ultrasound anatomy at various levels is defined and a comparison of the suspicious lesion with the normal expected appearance is made. An original attempt toward this goal was made at our institute with comparison of normal cadaveric sections at corresponding levels taken by HRUSG.

High-resolution ultrasonography has broad applications in the maxillofacial region especially in the cheek, which include evaluations of the unilateral or bilateral swollen cheek painful or pain less, restricted mouth opening, painful chewing without obvious clinical findings, and varied causes of facial swelling. Since early detection decisively influences patient prognosis in case of malignancy, it is one of the prime concerns in a presenting patient. Further, differentiation of lesions as being of benign, malignant, infective, or inflammatory etiology is important in deciding on a treatment plan. HRUSG should however be used to complement and not replace other imaging modalities as it does have its limitations.

Compared to other facial components, the cheek is predominantly composed of adipose tissue and is relatively small in size. Swelling of the cheek is easily visible and palpable in most patients presenting with cheek masses. Most lesions have nonspecific characteristics on computed tomography (CT) and magnetic resonance imaging (MRI). In contrast, HRUSG is ideal for evaluation of cheek lesions, because of its capability to differentiate between tissues like skin, fat, muscle, gland, ducts, and vessels especially since bony and gaseous interfaces are absent. Further, the superficial location of the cheek makes it easily accessible to ultrasound. Vestibule can be evaluated with fruit jelly technique obliterating the void space.

This short review attempts to aid the MFS in his understanding of HRUSG of the maxillofacial region, with special reference to the cheek.

## 8.11.2 Gross Cheek Anatomy

In simple terms, the cheek is the fleshy portion of the face, below the eye, extending from the angle of the mouth to the ear. Anatomically, it pertains to the buccomasseteric region comprising the buccal space and its contents, masseteric and buccinator muscles, the buccal fat pad, and Stenson's duct.

The region is continuous anteriorly with the lips. Its external anterior demarcation is formed by the nasolabial fold and groove extending from the side of the nose to the angle of the mouth. The mucosa lining the inner aspect of the cheek adheres to the buccinator muscle, while the gingival mucosa covers the mandibular and maxillary alveolar processes. The gingivobuccal sulcus is the junction formed between the gingival and buccal mucosae. The vestibule is the region of the mouth between the teeth, lips, and cheek, which is bound superiorly and inferiorly by buccal mucosal reflections onto the mandible and maxilla. Posteriorly the vestibule is continuous with the oral cavity proper (Fig. 8.42) [12, 13].

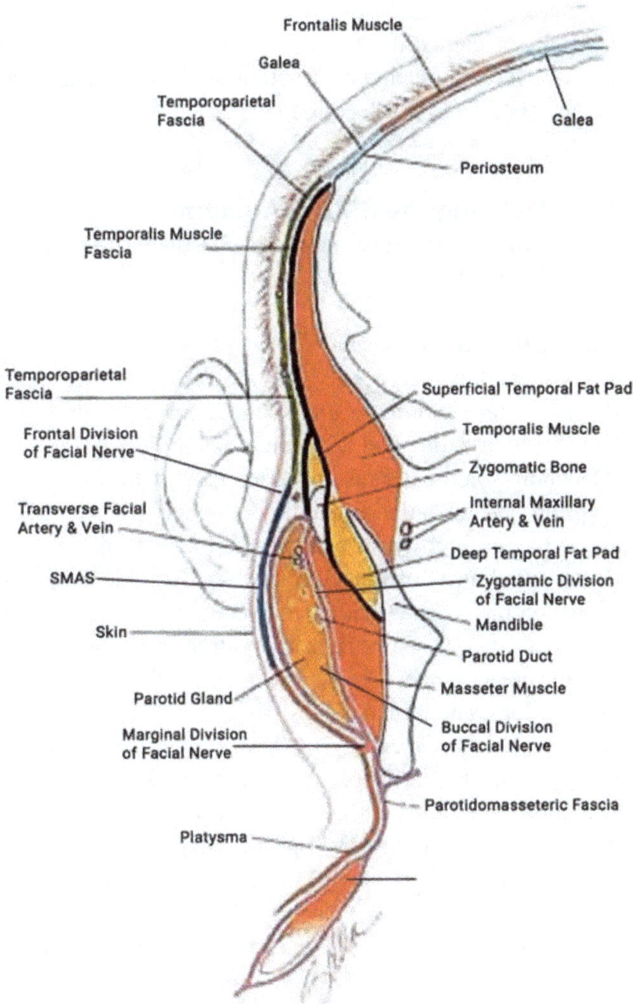




**Fig. 8.42** Anatomical layers of the cheek

## 8.11.3 Floor of Mouth, Anatomy (Relevant to HRUSG)

The part of the oral cavity located underneath the tongue is called the floor of the mouth and it can be involved by a myriad of pathological processes. Superficial lesions involving the mucosal surface are easily visualized and may not need imaging. Disease involving the deeper structures of the floor needs to be evaluated by imaging, and HRUSG is many times the first line of investigation because of its superior soft-tissue differentiation capability, thus allowing for clear depiction of contents of the floor [14].

Inflammatory processes, malignancies, and vascular abnormalities can affect the floor contents, while certain conditions like ranula and obstruction of the submandibular gland are specific to this location [14].

### 8.11.4 Defining the HRUSG Anatomy of Maxillofacial Region (Predominantly Cheek)

**Normal Ultrasound Cheek**
Various cheek layers have varying sonographic echogenicity and echotexture, and hence ultrasound is an invaluable tool in the characterization and localization of cheek lesions.

Depending on tissue density, the sound wave transmission, absorption, or reflection capability of each tissue varies. Tissues, having high water content like blood, appear black and are called anechoic because they conduct sound waves well. In contrast, tissues that are poor conductors reflect most of the sound wave energy back to the transducer appearing bright and are termed hyperechoic, examples of which include bones, tendons, and fascial planes. Tissues like muscle reflect less of the sound wave energy and have a hypoechoic appearance. In the cheek, the mucosal and submucosal layers appear hyperechoic, the mucosa more so. Muscle tissue appears hypoechoic, while fatty tissue appears echogenic (Fig. 8.43).

Compared to other imaging modalities, ultrasound has proven to be superior as regards identification of small lesions, detection of lesion plane, and lesion characterization (Fig. 8.44).

The cheek layers and neighboring structures that can be identified by HRUSG are.

**Cheek**
- Skin
- Subcutaneous plane
- Buccal pad of fat
- Buccinator muscle
- Submucosal layer
- Mucosal layer
- Masseter muscle and its lateral relations.
- Temporalis muscle
- Temporomandibular joint (TMJ)

**Neighboring Structures**
- Vestibule
- Gingiva
- Buccogingival Sulcus
- Periodontal tissue, etc.
- Tongue, lips
- Floor of mouth, Sublingual space
- Submandibular space
- Parotid gland / duct
- Retromandibular space
- Interdental space
- Alveolar margin
- Mental foramina
- Infraorbital foramina
- External nose
- Various other facial planes and spaces
- Arteries

### 8.11.5 Techniques of HRUSG of Cheek

For ultrasound examination, the cheek is considered to be a rectangular area bordered as follows (Fig. 8.45).

- by an imaginary line beginning at the angle of mandible and extending along its lower border to the level of angle of mouth inferiorly,
- by an imaginary line beginning at the angle of mandible and running along the posterior border of the mandibular ramus to include the temporomandibular joint posteriorly,
- by an imaginary line along the zygomatic arch superiorly and,
- by an imaginary vertical line at the level of angle of mouth that joins the superior and inferior lines anteriorly [15].

Various techniques, including the resting (neutral) and Puffed (Blow out) cheek technique, the tongue touch technique, and fruit jelly technique, were experimented with, each having their own advantages and limitations [15].

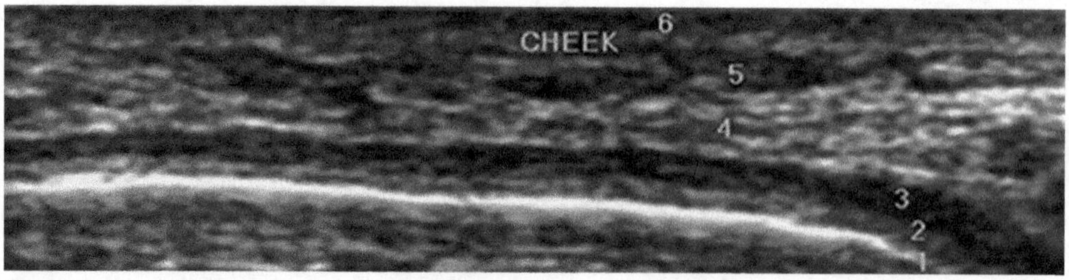




**Fig. 8.43** Normal Cheek/ Buccal layers on ultrasound

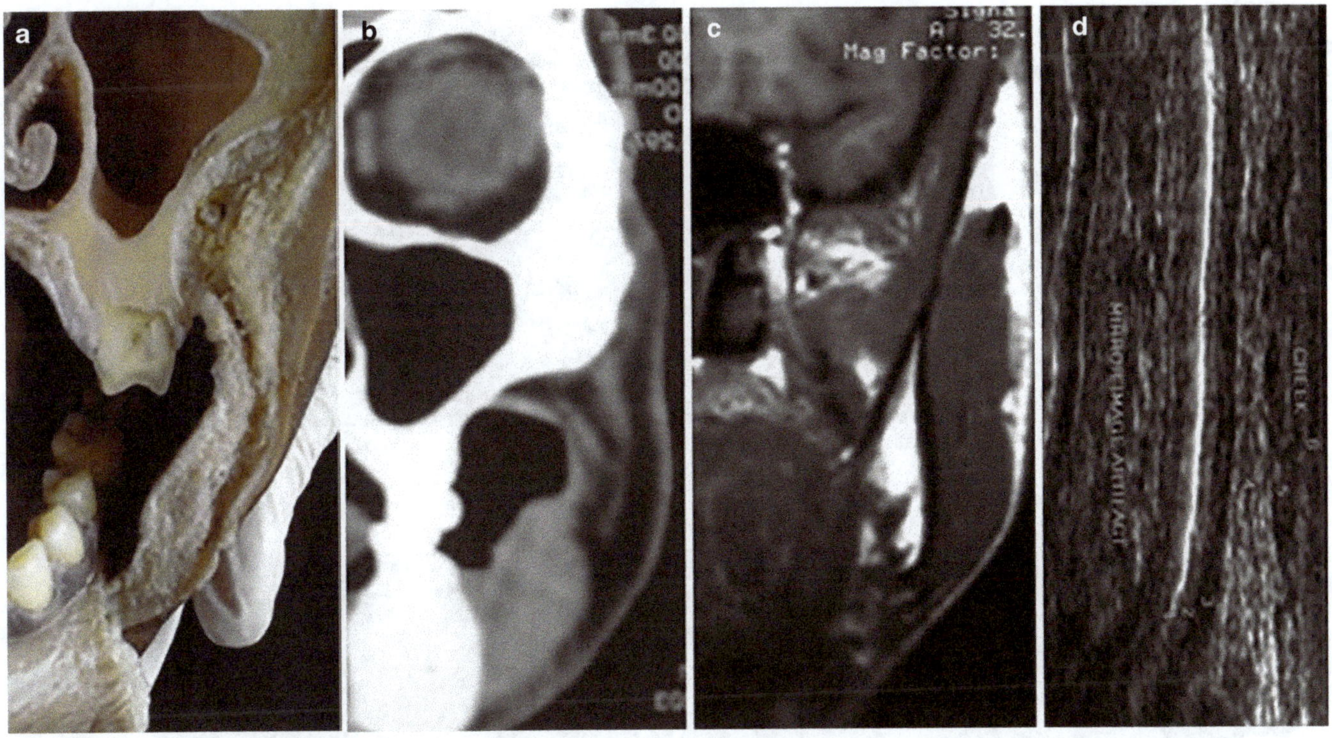




**Fig. 8.44** (**a-d**) Cheek anatomy—a comparison. Comparative cheek anatomy- (**a**) cadaveric specimen, (**b**) CT, (**c**) MRI, and (**d**) Ultrasound

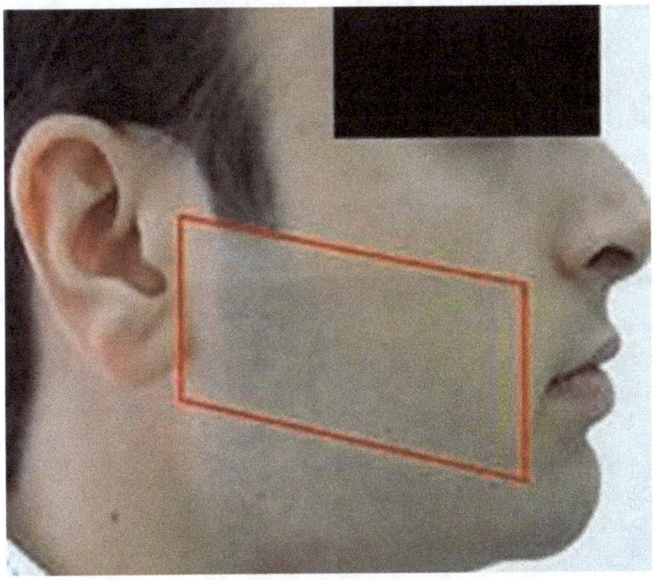



**Fig. 8.45** Area of Cheek ultrasound study

(a) *Resting (Neutral) and Puffed (Blow out) Cheek Technique* (Figs. 8.46 and 8.47).
   - Patient is instructed to blow, and ultrasound is performed in puffed cheek status.
   - Images obtained in axial and coronal planes.
     Advantage: Improved visibility of cheek layers and accurate definition of lesion size.
     Limitation: Occurrence of mirror image artifact.
     Less sensitivity in evaluation of lesions of the vestibule (gingivobuccal sulcus).

(b) *Tongue Touch Technique (*Fig. 8.48a–c).
   - Patient is instructed to feel the cheek lesion with the tongue.
   - Lesion is brought closer to the probe creating a better acoustic window.
   - Lesions of the superficial buccal mucosa and tongue lesions on its anterior half and corresponding lateral borders can be evaluated better.
     Advantage: Better visualization of lesion details.
     Limitation: Inaccessibility to tongue lesions along the posterior half and corresponding lateral borders.

(c) *Fruit Jelly Technique.*
   (Figs. 8.49a, b, and 8.50a–d)
   - Commercially available edible "Fruit jellies" are placed in the upper and lower gingivobuccal sulcus.
   - Patients are then instructed to close their mouth and ultrasound is performed.

Advantages:
- Useful in elderly and facial nerve palsy patients having difficulty holding puffed cheek for prolonged periods.
- Absence of artifacts due to vestibular air.
- Enhanced structural delineation and better evaluation of vestibular extension of lesion.

Limitation: Inability to evaluate lesions involving far posterior aspect of Vestibule.

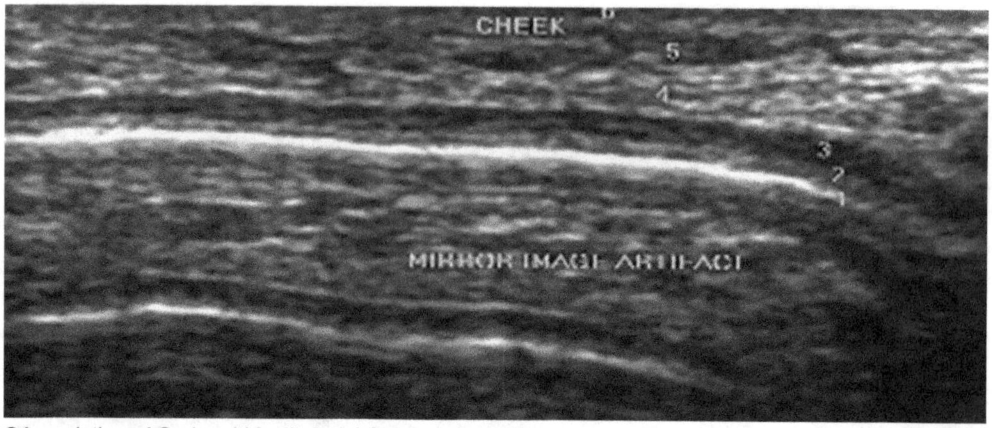




**Fig. 8.46** Cheek layers by "Puffed Cheek" Technique. (1) Mucosa. (2) Submucosa. (3) Buccinator. (4) Buccal fat. (5) Subcutaneous tissue. (6) Skin

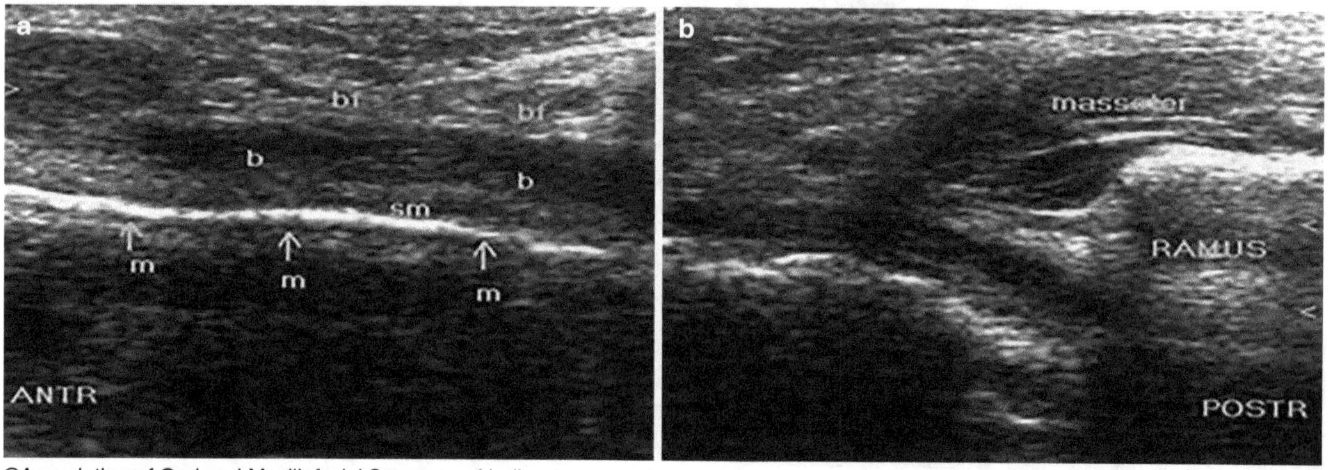




**Fig. 8.47** (**a**, **b**) Cheek layers by "Puffed Cheek" Technique. m-mucosa, sm-submucosa, b-buccinator, bf-buccal fat

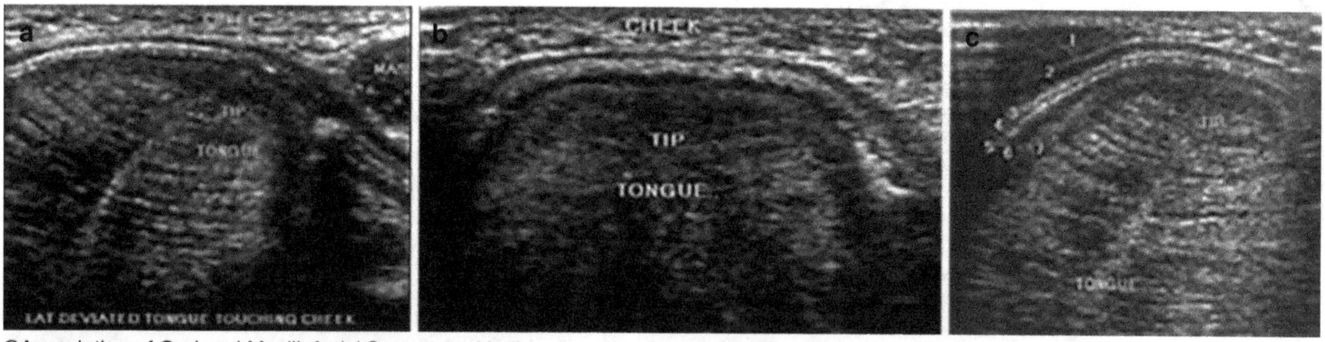




**Fig. 8.48** (**a**), (**b**), and (**c**). "Tongue Touch" Technique. Anterior tongue, its tip and lateral borders and cheek layers

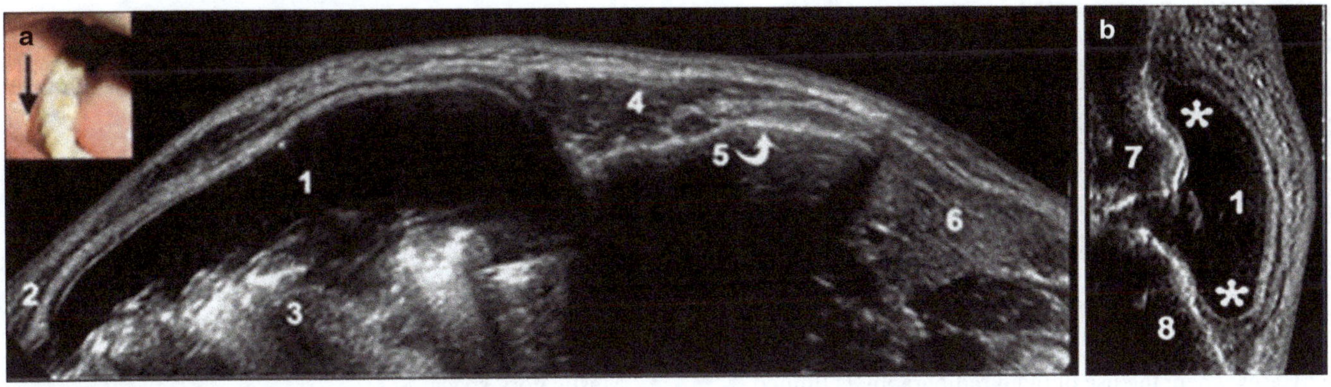




**Fig. 8.49** (**a**) Axial panoramic (**b**) Coronal Cheek layers by "Fruit Jelly" Technique. (1) Jelly (2) Angle of mouth (3) Alveolar process (4) Masseter (5) Mandible (6) Parotid (7) Maxilla (8) Mandible (Asterisk)- Upper and lower gingivobuccal sulcus

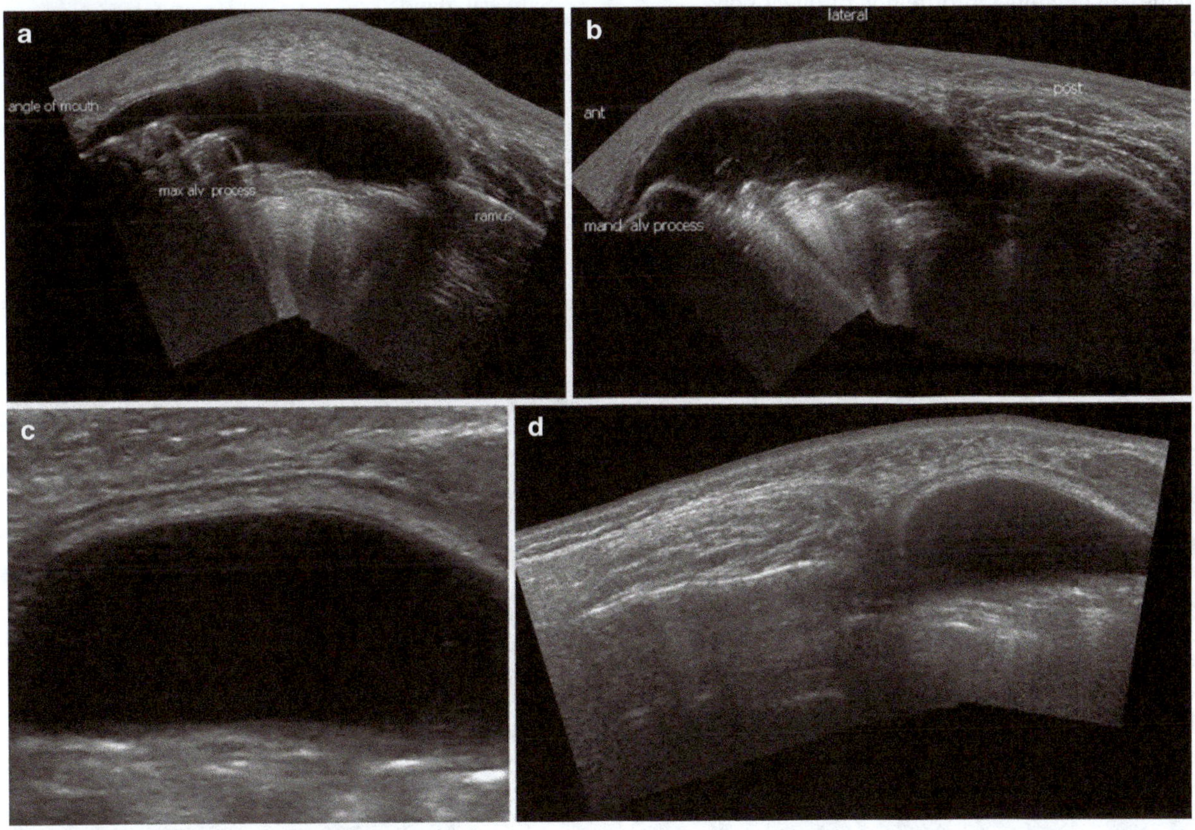




**Fig. 8.50** (**a, b, c,** and **d**).Cheek layers by "Fruit jelly" Technique. Panoramic axial slices. Coronal slices showing superior and inferior vestibules along with layers of cheek/alveolar surfaces

### 8.11.6 Case Presentation

**HRUSG Cheek: Scope of Use and Limitations**
Scope of practice of HRUSG cheek includes

- Cases where limitations are posed by the clinical presentation as in case of trismus or lesions that mimic others in their clinical presentation resulting in diagnostic difficulty
- Estimation of the extent of a lesion, thus helping in tumor staging
- Cases where the use of plain radiography is limited
- Inherent drawbacks of imaging modalities like CT and MRI and their high cost

**Limitations**
- Structures medial to the mandibular ramus
- Difficulty in obtaining information of intact bone
- Intra-articular structures of the temporomandibular joint
- Postoperative scar tissue or a large external wound
- Very thick patients, muscles, and nerves of the face

**Clinical Conditions that Can Be Evaluated**
- Swollen cheek: Painful, painless, unilateral, or bilateral.
- Limited mouth opening
- Painful chewing
- Swelling of the face involving the midline or parasagittal plane, floor of the mouth, TM joint region, submandibular region, nose, lip, gums, etc.
- Tongue lesions (Lateral margin).

**Notifiable Lesions**
- Cheek—Growth, hemangioma, lymphangioma, Oral submucous fibrosis, abscesses, discharging sinuses, etc.
- Masseter—evaluation of contraction, benign hypertrophy, trauma, Space infection, trauma, etc.
- Masticatory space.
- TMJ—swelling, click.
- Lytic lesions of jaws.
- Gum—evaluation. Lip lesions.
- Midline swellings.
- Tumor staging.
- Salivary gland.
- Space infections.
- Tongue.
- Lymph node evaluation.

1. **Inflammatory / Infective Pathology**
   (a) *Cheek cellulitis with evolving abscess (Fig. 8.51a–d).*

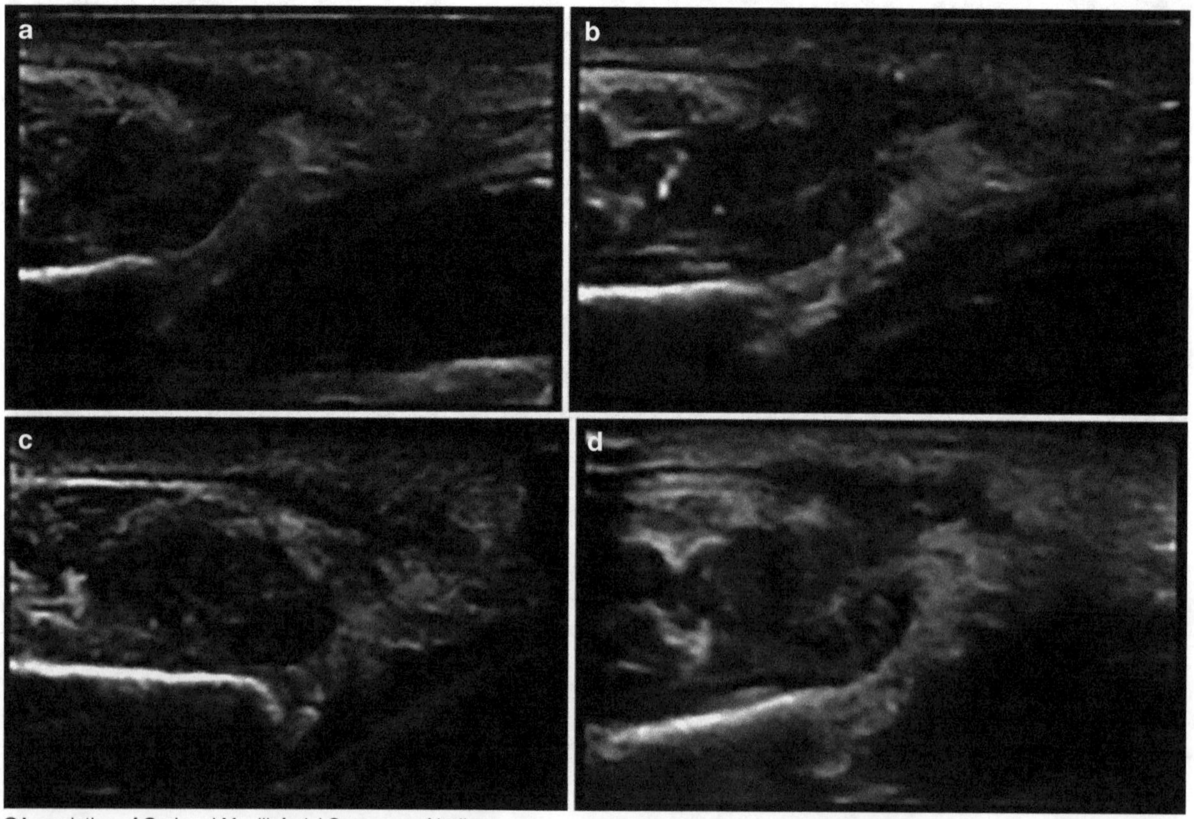




**Fig. 8.51** (**a**, **b**, **c**, and **d**).Cheek cellulitis with evolving abscess. Diffuse soft-tissue thickening, edema of deep subcutaneous fat plane, edematous buccinators and submucosal plane with mild echogenic tracking collection within the fascial planes

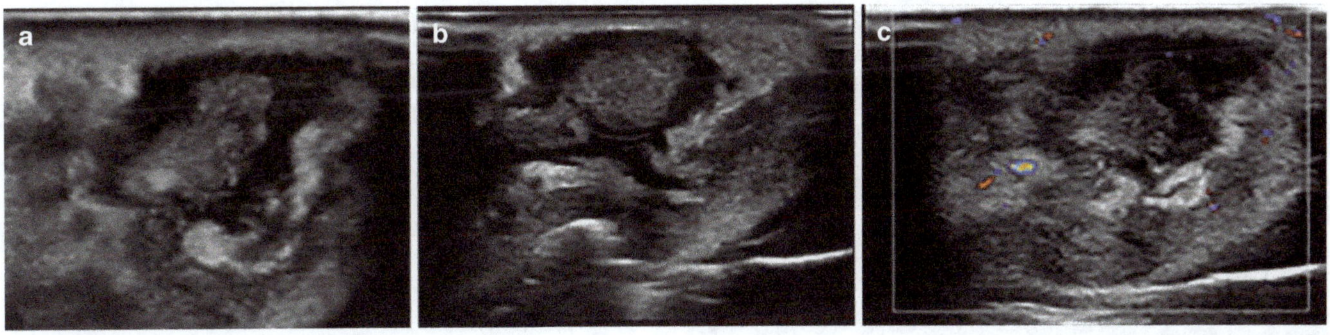



**Fig. 8.52** (**a, b** and **c**). Cheek abscess. Focal organized thick echogenic collection in the deep subcutaneous plane with minimal extension into buccinator muscle (45 year old male, with habit of chewing betel nut)

**Fig. 8.53** (**a–d**) Chronic osteomyelitis mandible. HRUSG showing hyperechoic lesion with hypoechoic halofungal granuloma

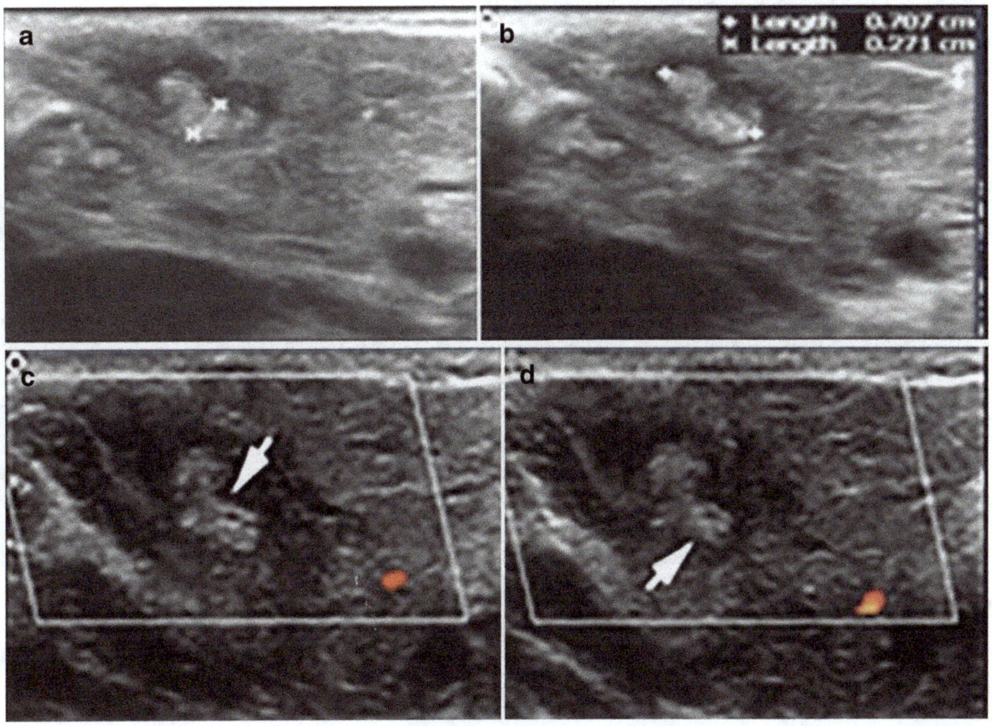



(b) *Cheek abscess (Fig. 8.52a–c).*
(c) *Chronic osteomyelitis mandible (Fig. 8.53a, b).*
(d) *Cysticercosis parotid (Fig. 8.54).*

2. **Benign Pathology.**
   (a) *Oral submucosal fibrosis (OSMF) (Fig. 8.55a–c).*
   (b) *Lesion at opening of Stenson's Duct (Fig. 8.56a, b).*
   (c) *Intraoral Mucocele (Fig. 8.57a, b).*
   (d) *Cheek lymphangioma (Fig. 8.58a–d).*
   (e) *Epidermoid cyst of cheek (Fig. 8.59a, b).*
   (f) *Painless unilateral swollen cheek (Intramasseteric lipoma) (Fig. 8.60).*
   (g) *Stenson's Duct calculus (Fig. 8.61a, b).*
   (h) *Polycystic disease of parotid (Fig. 8.62a, b).*

3. **Malignant Pathology.**
   (a) *Buccal mucosal malignancy with intact submucosa and buccinator (Fig. 8.63).*
   (b) *Buccal mucosal squamous cell carcinoma (Fig. 8.64 a-c).*

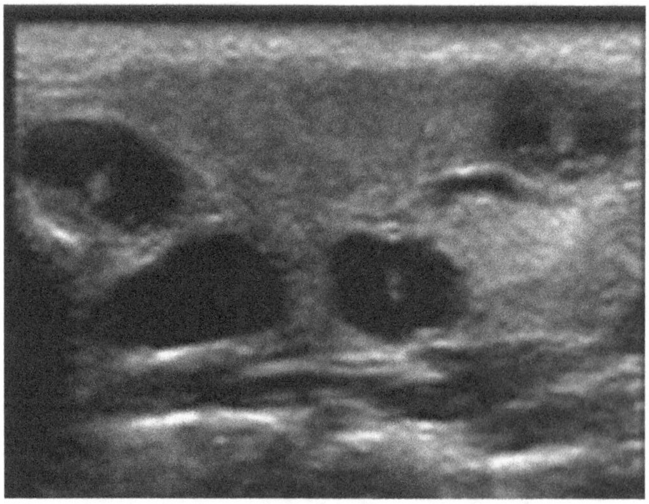



**Fig. 8.54** Cysticercosis parotid

(c) *Buccal mucosal carcinoma with mucosal and submucosal involvement, mandibular destruction and sparing of buccinator (Fig. 8.65).*
(d) *Buccal mucosal carcinoma comparative evaluation. (Fig. 8.66a, b).*
(e) *Superior vestibular malignant mass (Fig. 8.67a–c).*
(f) *Tongue malignancy-Tongue touch technique (Fig. 8.68a, b).*
(g) *Buccal malignancy with mandibular infiltration (Fig. 8.69a–d).*

4. **Vascular malformations**
   (a) *Arteriovenous malformation cheek (Fig. 8.70a–d).*
   (b) *Cheek hemangioma (Fig. 8.71).*

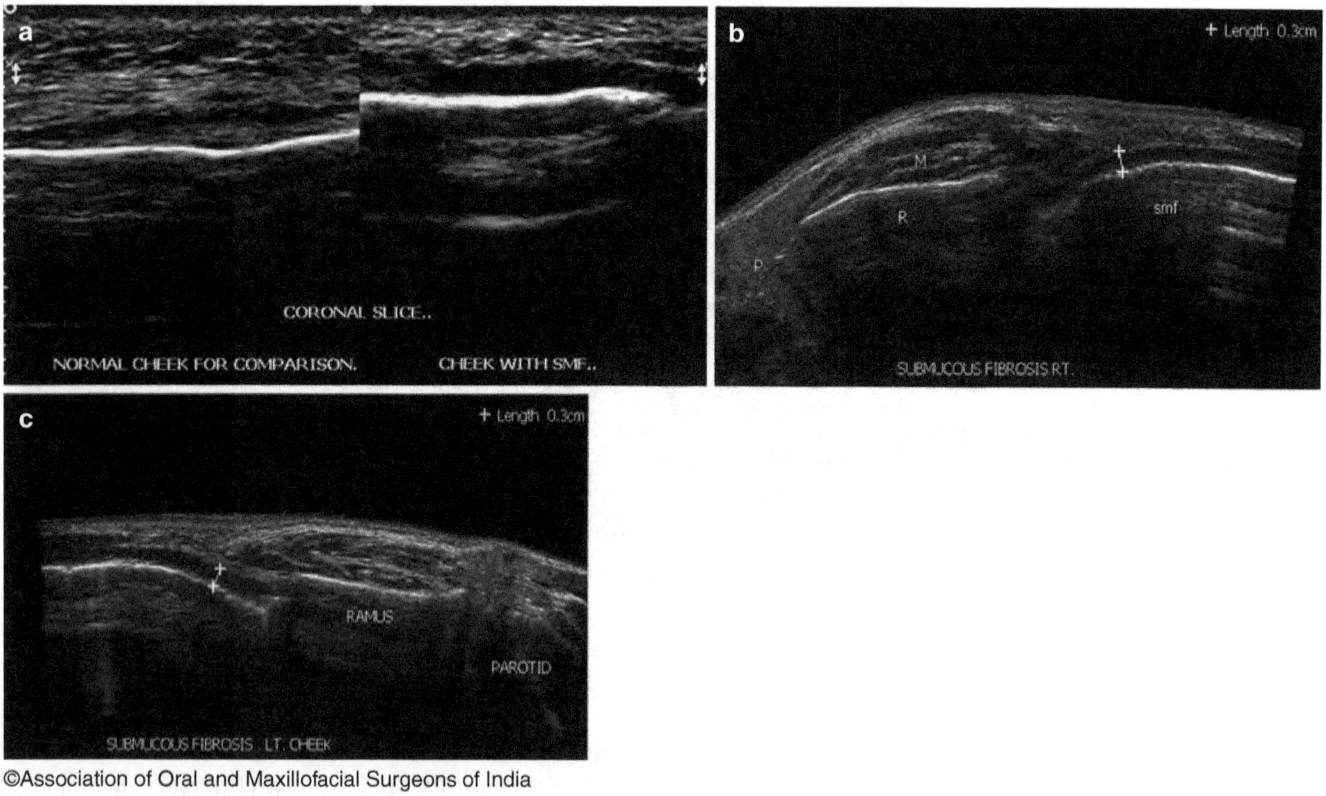




**Fig. 8.55** (**a, b** and **c**) Oral submucosal fibrosis. Axial slice showing thickening of the submucosal layer in OSMF in comparison to the normal thickness of the submucosal layer

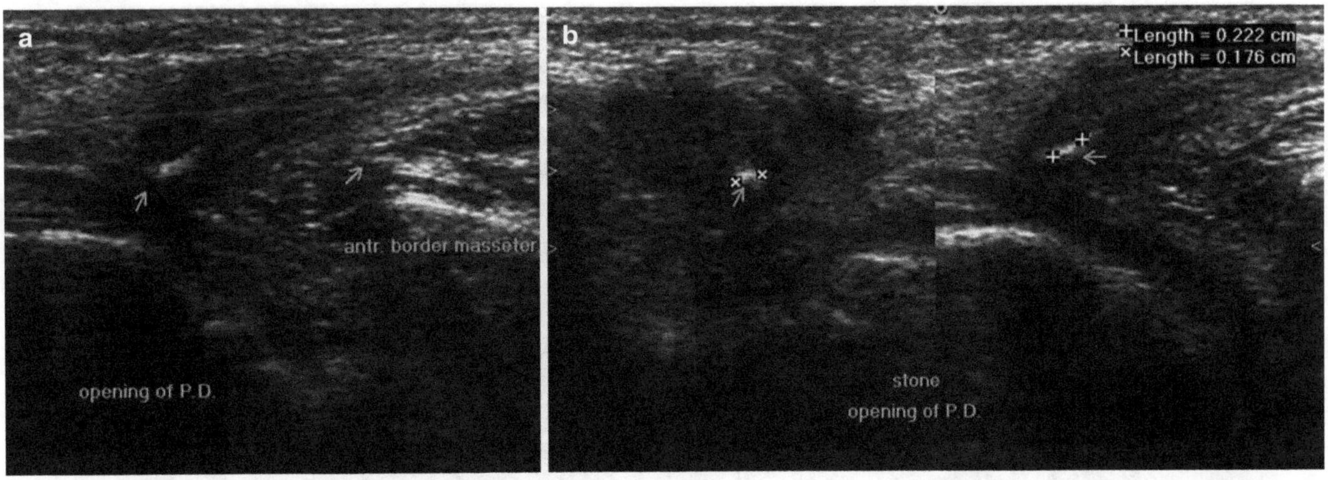




**Fig. 8.56** (**a**) and (**b**). Tiny calculus of about 1.2 mm revealed by HRUSG at Stenson's duct opening. (Pain while chewing food. No swelling)

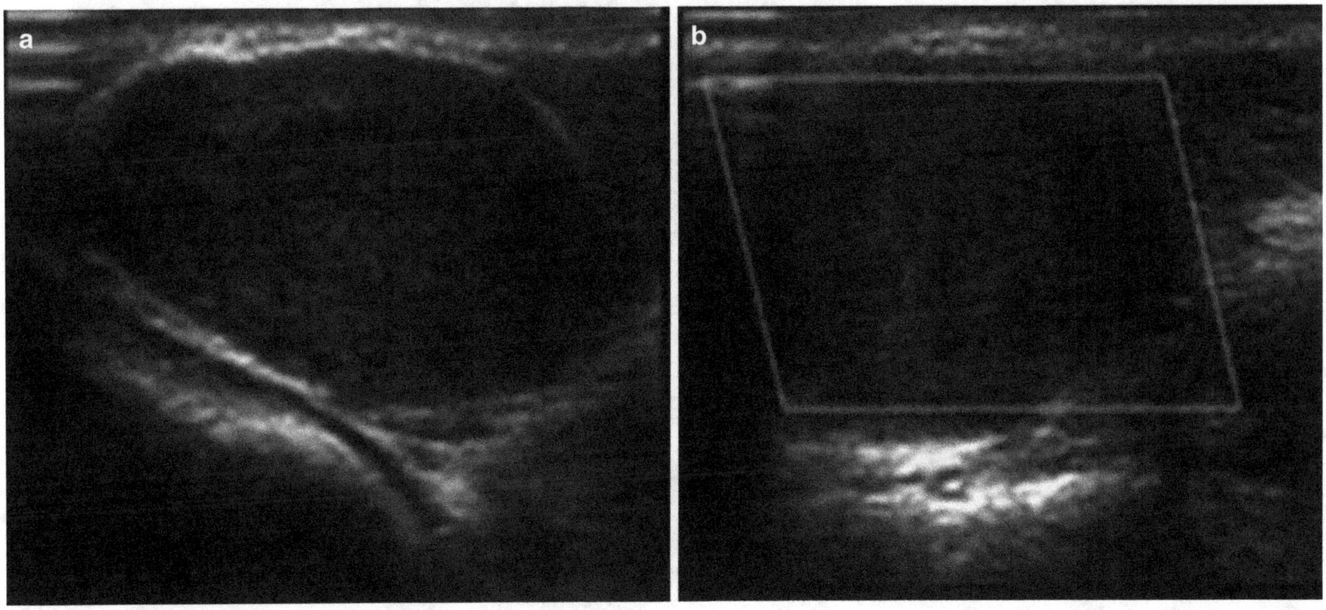




**Fig. 8.57** (**a**) and (**b**). Intraoral Mucocele. Well-defined cystic lesion in the submucosal layer with internal minimal echogenic contents. Possible diagnosis of mucocele given, later confirmed by HPR. (35 year old female, presenting with right-sided cheek swelling and mild pain)

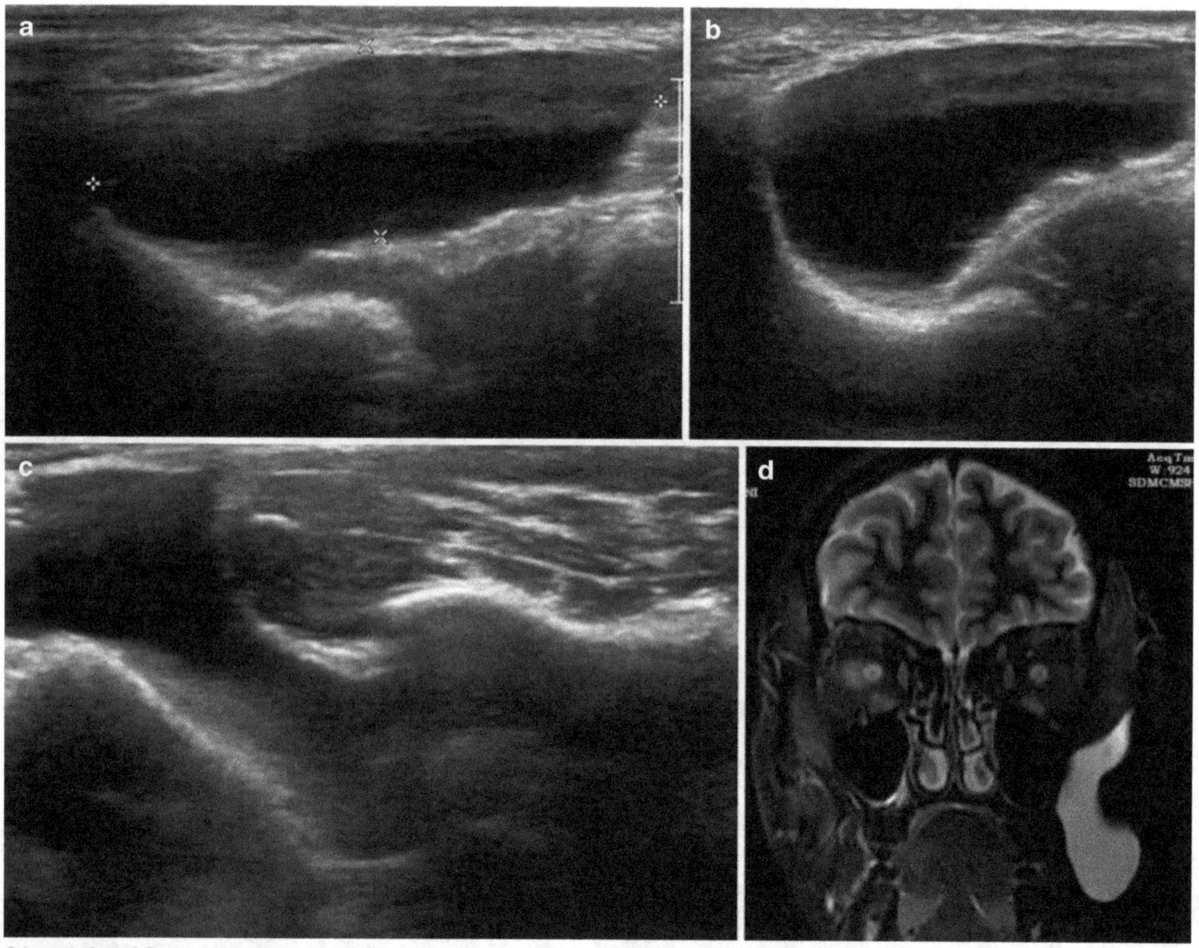



**Fig. 8.58** (**a**, **b**, **c**, and **d**). Cheek lymphangioma. Fluid-filled cystic lesion deep to submucosal layer with deep space extension adjacent to the masseter medial to mandibular ramus MRI coronal T2W imaging confirms hyperintense fluid along left side of cheek extending into infratemporal fossa (25 year old male, presenting with soft, painless swelling of left cheek)

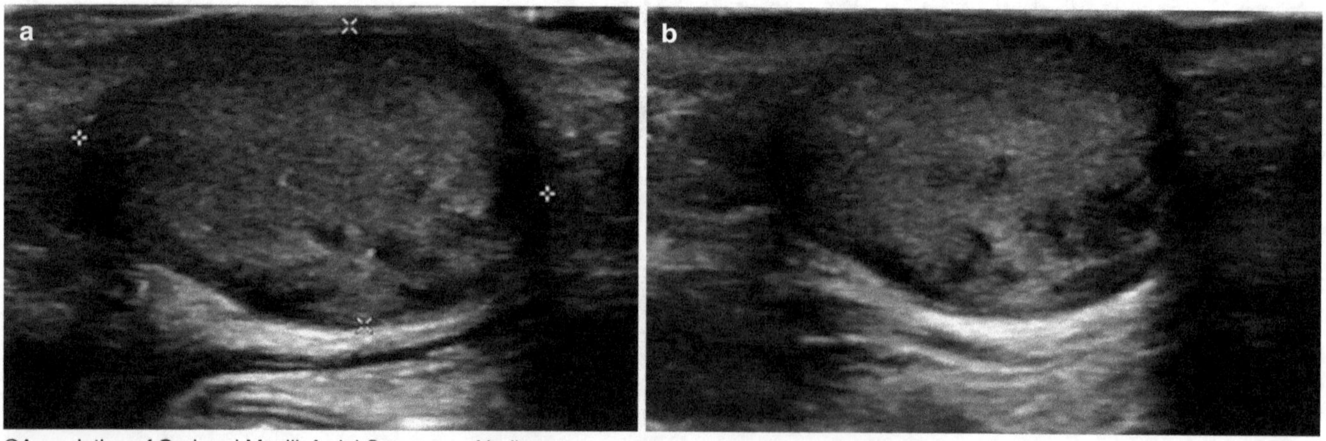



**Fig. 8.59** (**a**) and (**b**). Epidermoid cyst of cheek. Well-defined complex cystic lesion in the subcutaneous plane with internal echogenic contents causing displacement of underlying cheek layers (28 year old male presenting with painless left cheek swelling)

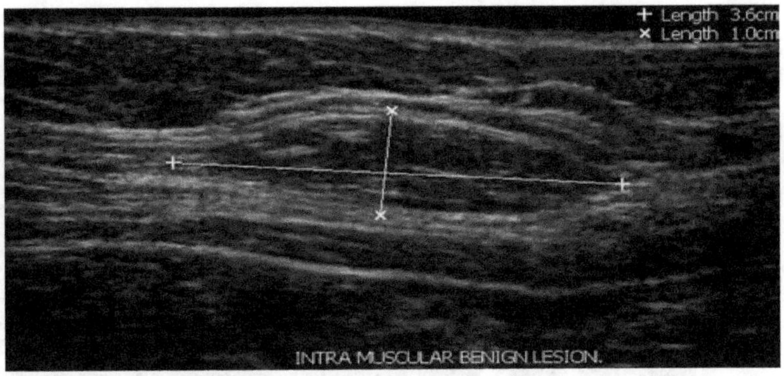


Association of Oral and Maxillofacial Surgeons of India

**Fig. 8.60** Intramasseteric Lipoma. Elongated intramuscular lesion isoechoic to the subcutaneous fat with internal echogenic strands representing intramasseteric lipoma. (30 year old female, presenting with painless swelling of cheek)

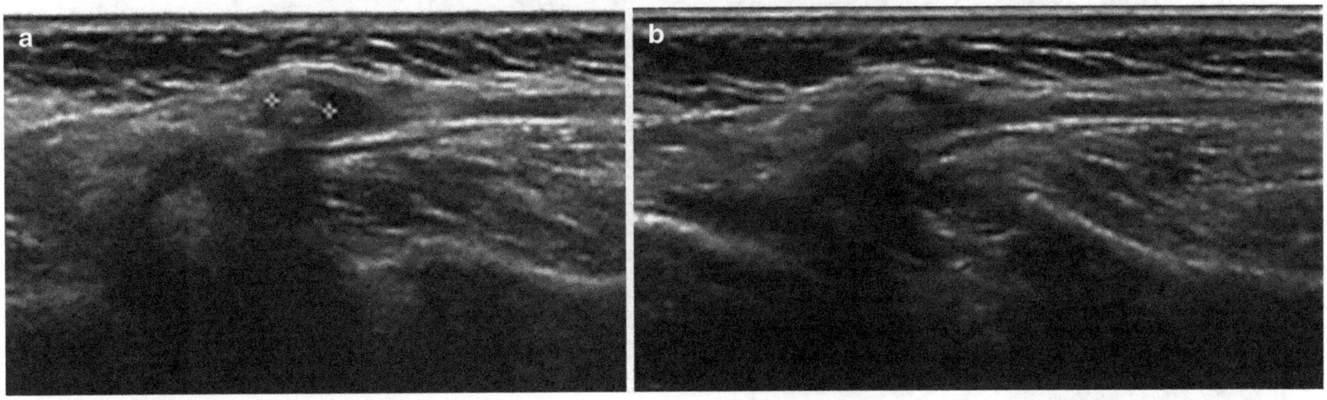


Association of Oral and Maxillofacial Surgeons of India

**Fig. 8.61** (**a**) and (**b**). Stenson's duct calculus. Hyperechoic calculus in the Stenson's duct with nondilated duct proximal to the calculus (23 year old male, with history of intermittent pain on right side of the cheek)

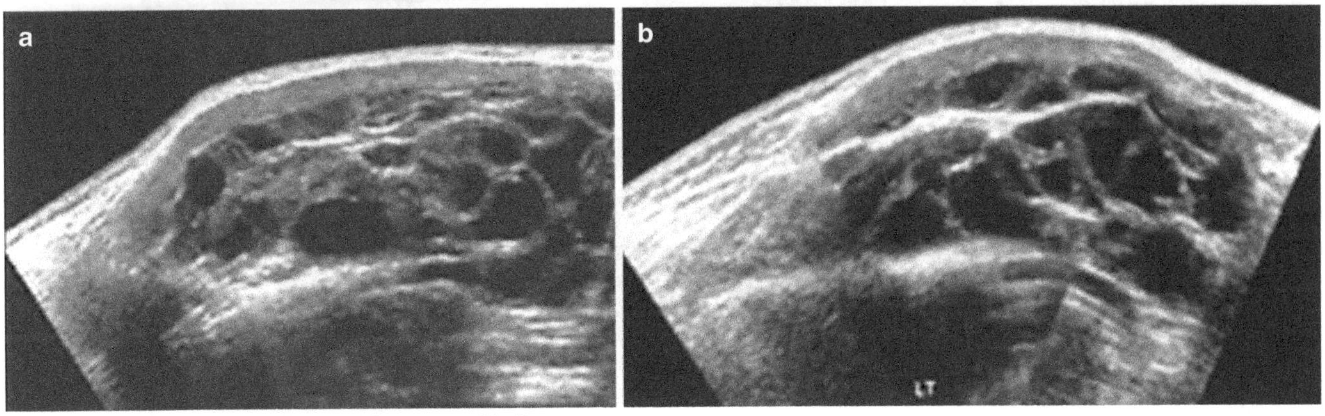


©Association of Oral and Maxillofacial Surgeons of India

**Fig. 8.62** (**a**) and (**b**). Polycystic disease of parotid. (22 year old male Bilateral painless swollen cheek 7–8 yrs duration)

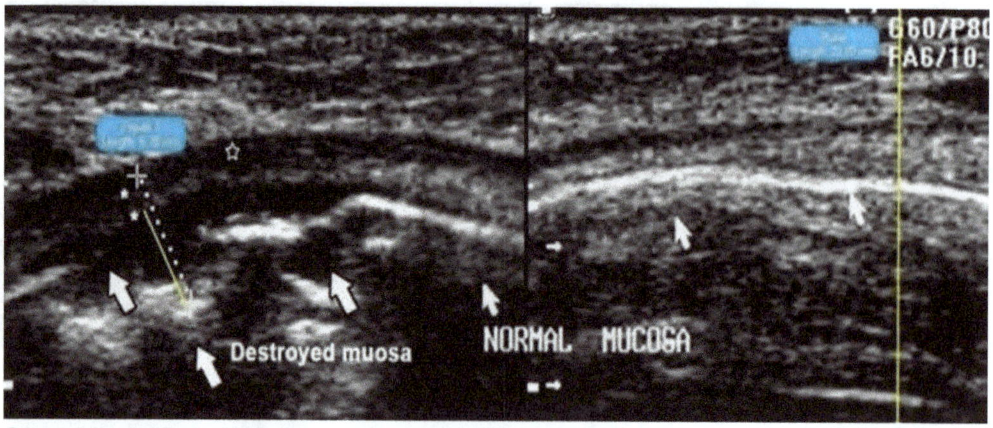




**Fig. 8.63** Buccal mucosal malignancy with intact submucosa and buccinator. Growth predominantly involving the mucosa, distinct from submucosa (between asterisk) buccinator (star) appears normal. (55 year old male with irritating nonhealing ulcer left cheek)

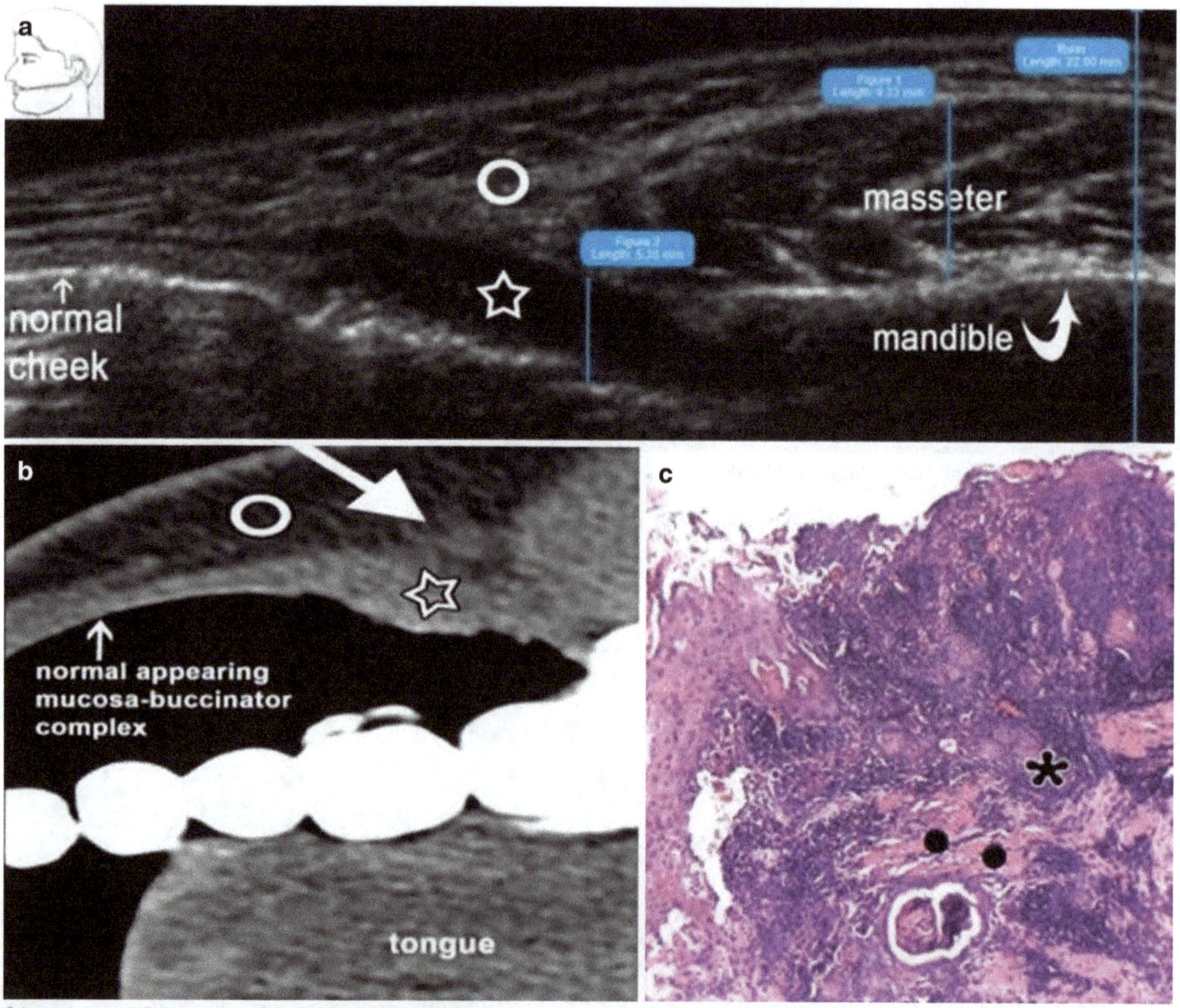




**Fig. 8.64** (**a, b,** and **c**). Early Carcinoma of the cheek better seen on HRUSG than by CT slice at the same level. Proved by Histopathology (52 year old male with squamous cell carcinoma of the buccal mucosa)

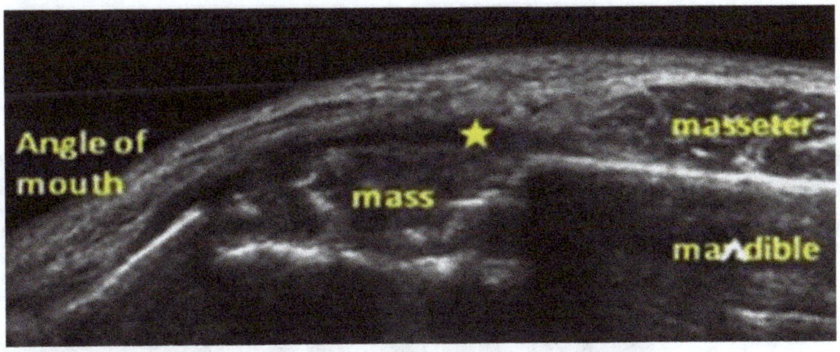




**Fig. 8.65** Buccal mucosal carcinoma

**Fig. 8.66** (**a**) Buccal mucosal carcinoma (Resting phase). (**b**) Buccal mucosal carcinoma (Fruit jelly technique). Patient was unable to perform the puffed cheek technique. Mass involving the mucosa, submucosa, buccinator, and fat

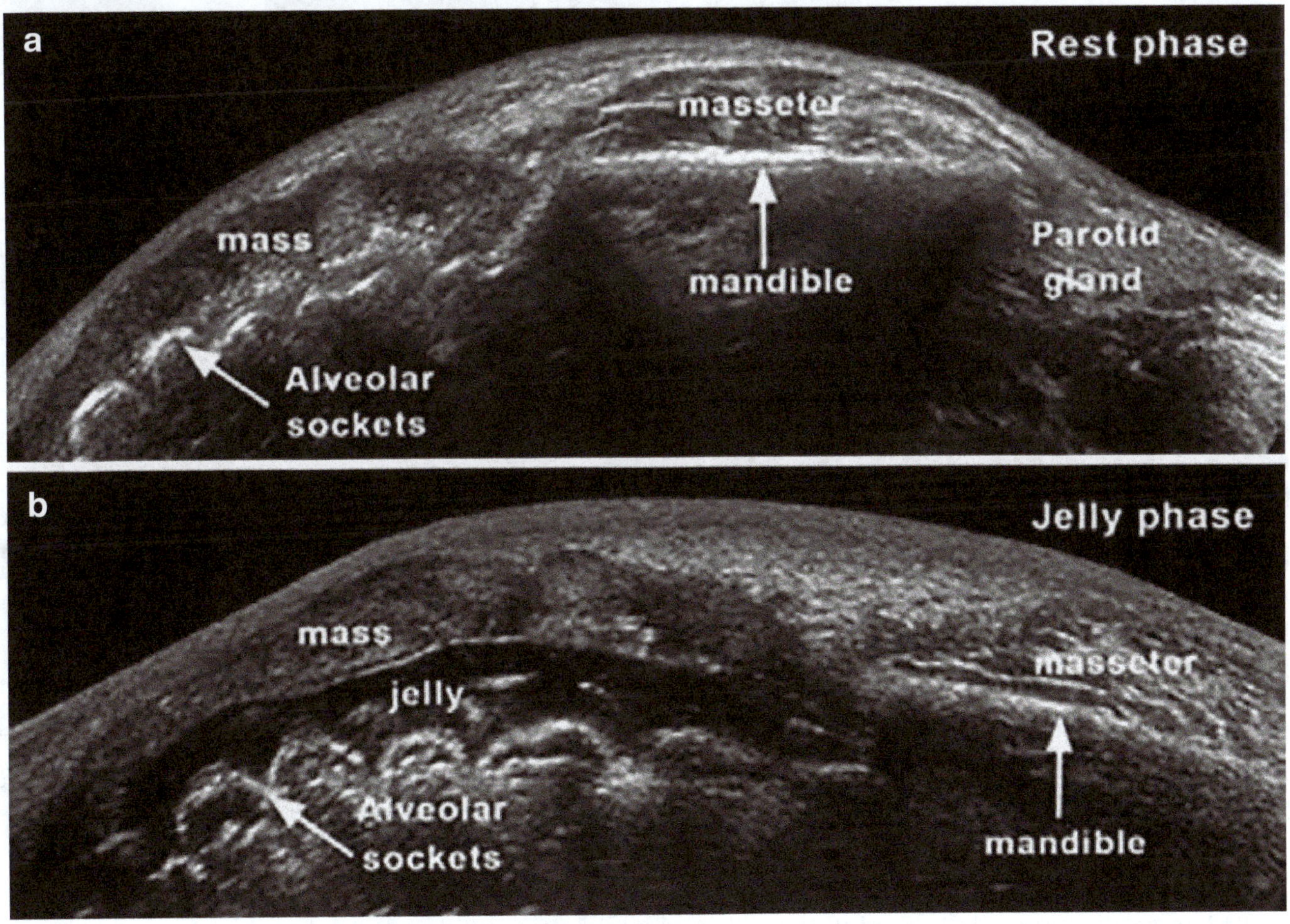

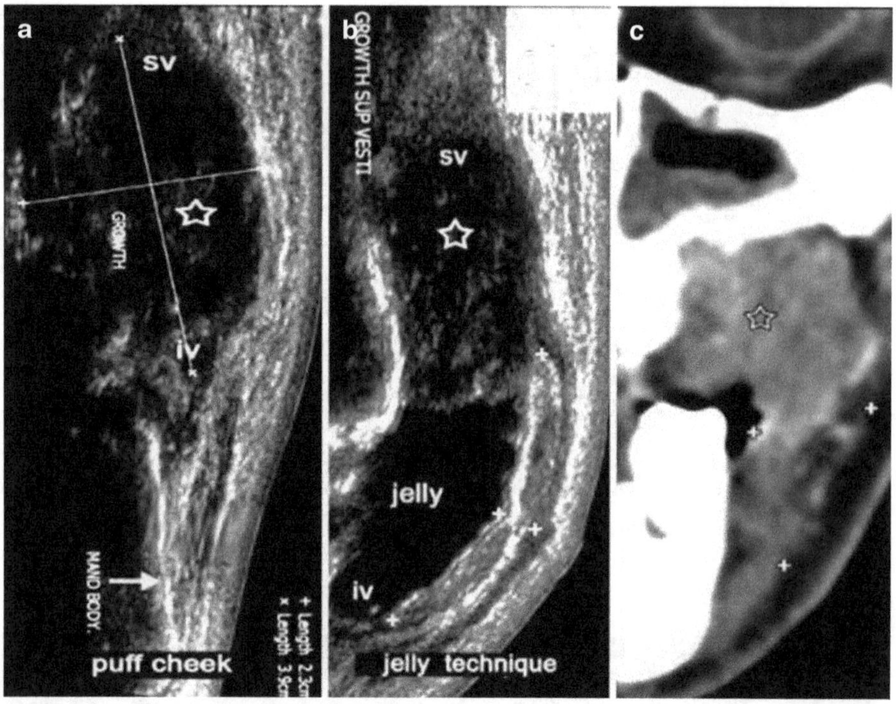




**Fig. 8.67** (**a, b** and **c**). Superior vestibular malignant mass. Coronal sections revealing predominantly hypoechoic, superior vestibular mass with irregular margins extending into cheek layers and causing underlying bony destruction. Comparison between (**a**) neutral cheek, (**b**) fruit jelly Technique and (**c**) CT

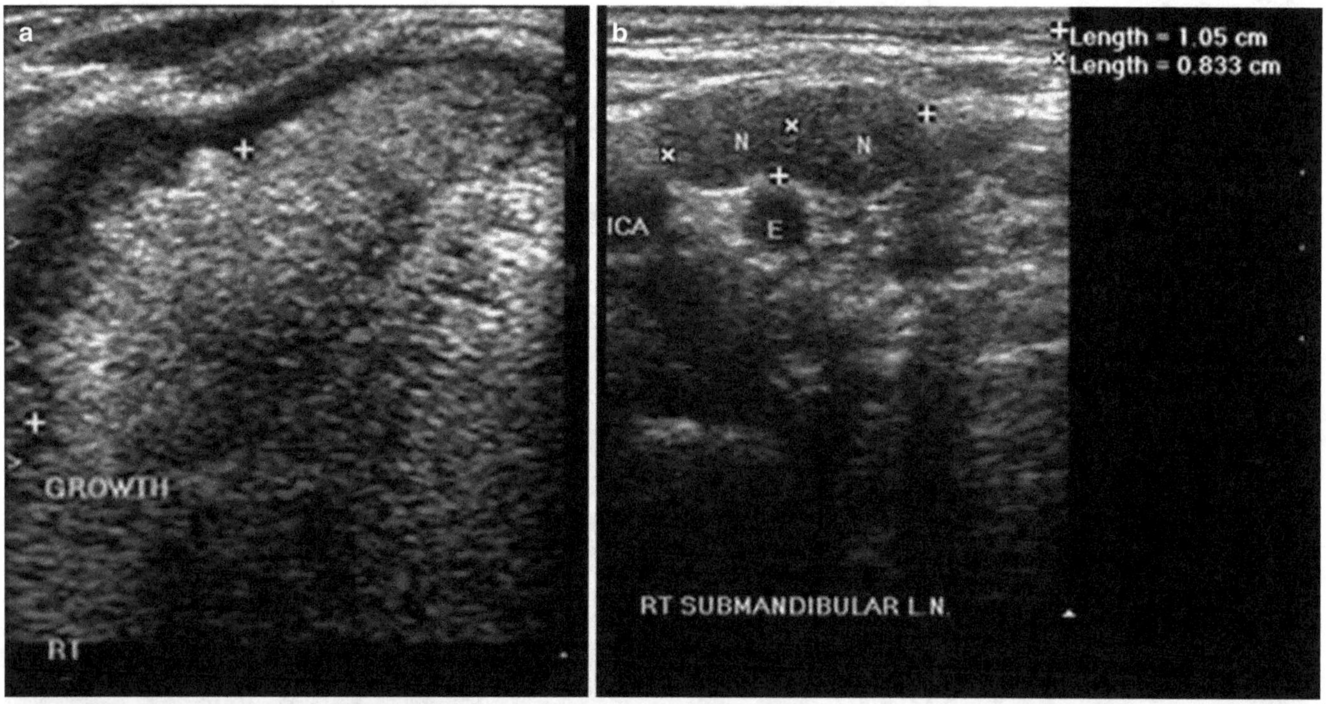




**Fig. 8.68** (**a**) and (**b**). Tongue malignancy against cheek wall. Irregular lesion along the Right anterolateral margin of the tongue by "Tongue touch" technique. Few enlarged lymph nodes are also noted with loss of hilar anatomy representing metastatic lymph nodes. (40 year old male, with complaint of swelling over the tongue)

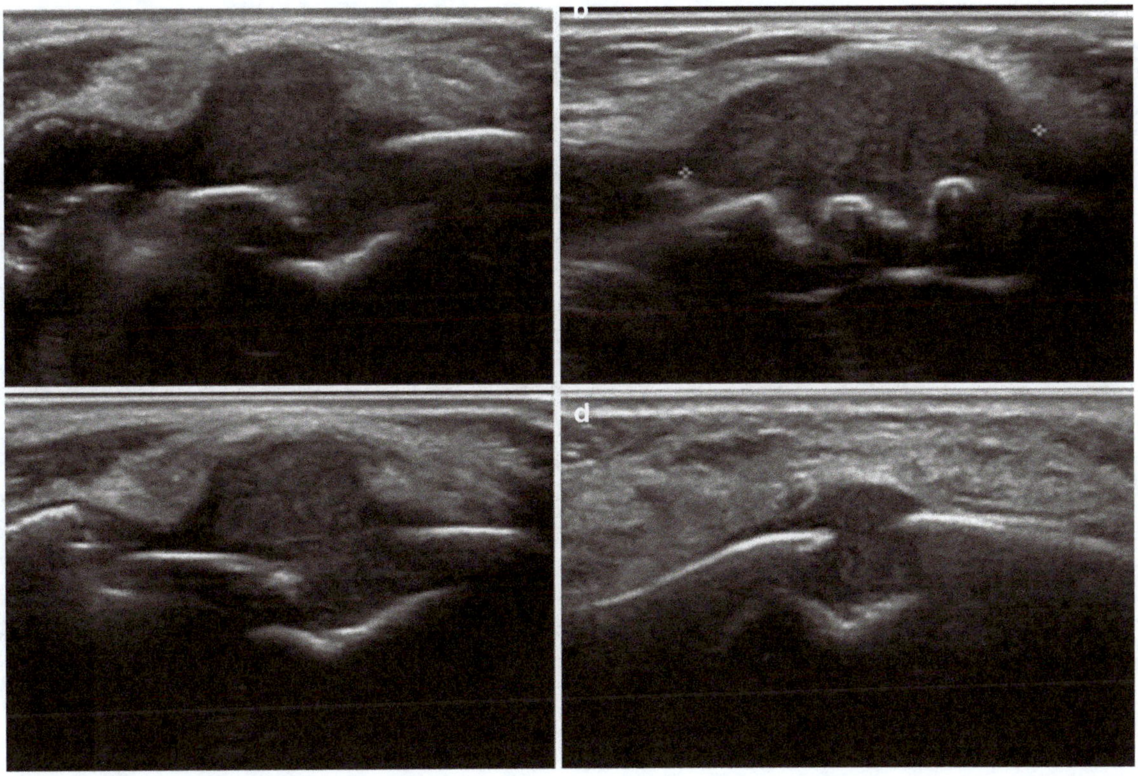



**Fig. 8.69** (**a, b, c,** and **d**) Buccal malignancy with mandibular infiltration. Heterogeneous mass lesion along the buccal mucosa extending into lower buccogingival sulcus with infiltration into submucosa and buccinator muscle. Focal cortical break is also noted in the mandibular bone with intraosseous infiltration. (48 year old male tobacco chewer presenting with right cheek swelling)

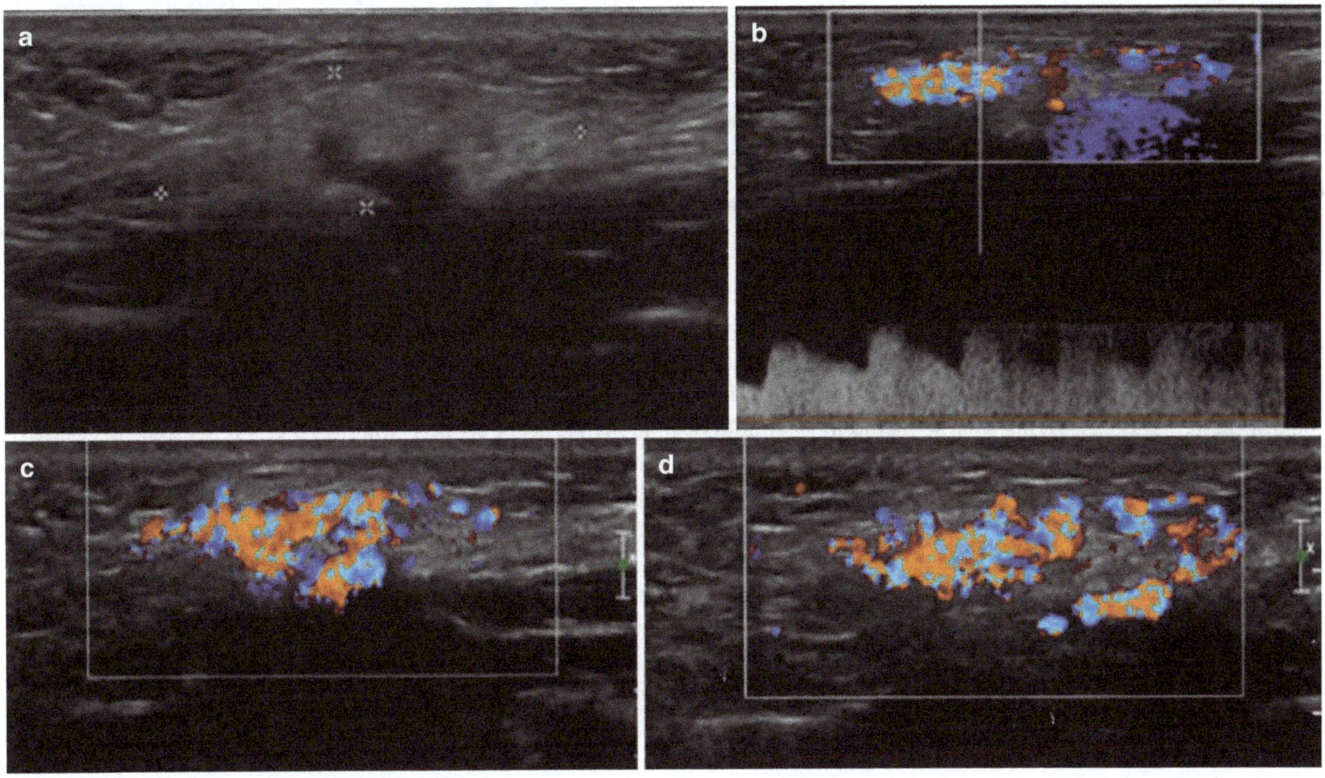



**Fig. 8.70** (**a, b, c,** and **d**) Arteriovenous malformation (AVM) cheek. Focal soft-tissue thickening with internal hypoechoic areas. Doppler study shows multiple vascular channels with high velocity, low resistance flow suggestive of AVM. (40 year old female presenting with history of swelling and intermittent pain)

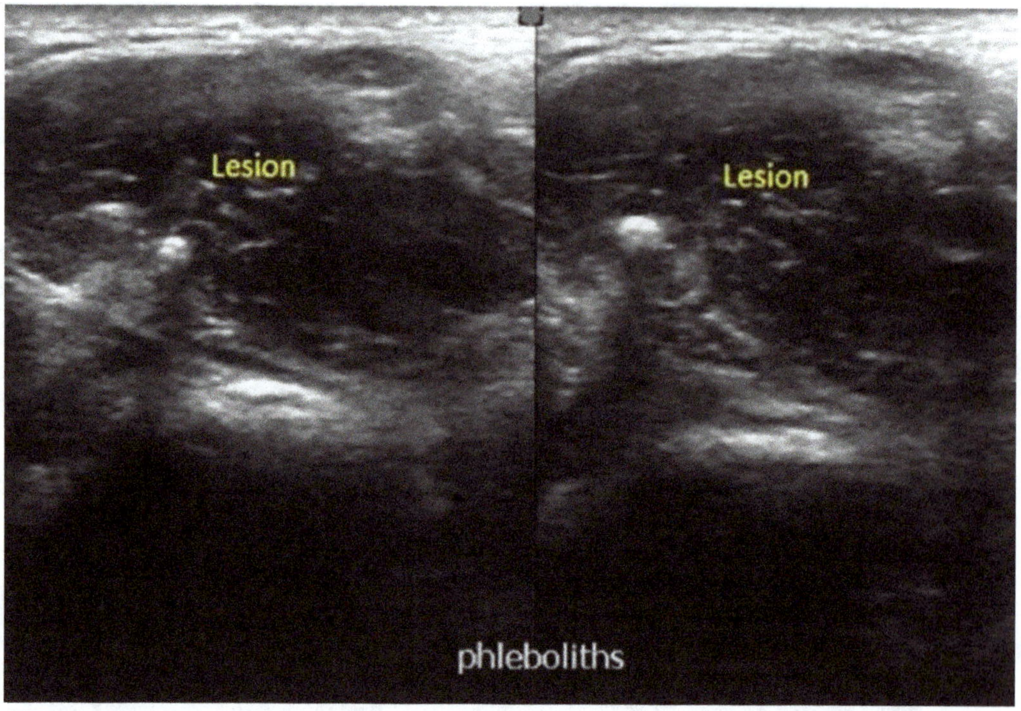




**Fig. 8.71** Cheek Hemangioma. Mixed echoic hemangioma with phlebolith. Absence of flow signals due to low-velocity flow

## 8.12 Conclusion

It is extremely difficult to limit radiology to a chapter and what has been written does not represent the whole of maxillofacial radiology. Only the relevant aspects and the bare minimum essentials of radiology for maxillofacial surgeons have been covered in this chapter. The entire range of radiology for maxillofacial surgeons, dealing with surgical problems pertinent to the maxillofacial region, would require more expansive and elaborate writing.

This chapter on radiology provides an outlook to the surgeon, who can proceed to applying radiology in his everyday surgical practice. In the event of encountering any lacunae in the book, the MFS must refer to the textbooks dedicated to maxillofacial radiology. Being a surgeon, the MFS should be aware of the use of the chest radiograph and its applications in his practice. The role of high-resolution ultrasonography has also been emphasized in this chapter. Dental radiology, both extra and intraoral, has not been included since all maxillofacial surgeons have extensive knowledge of the same in their surgical practice.

Since it is the MFS who is acquainted with the patient's clinical status, he must properly plan the imaging pathway for the patient. It is for this purpose that the MFS should be aware of the various imaging modalities as regards their nature, mode of image formation, their usefulness over other modalities, and their drawbacks. Radiation safety and cost effectiveness of a specific imaging modality also need to be kept in mind. The imaging method selected should be one that provides the required information within the shortest time possible, be the safest option for the patient, and be the most economical, while at the same time providing maximum information.

The MFS can commence with simple basic imaging methods like plain radiography or USG and later proceed to higher imaging methods in case the basic methods were not enough to satisfy the surgeon's needs for patient management. A recent costlier imaging method does not necessarily mean it is the best. Many times, it is the simpler basic imaging methods that provide more crucial findings that help in understanding complex disease processes.

**Acknowledgments** The authors would like to acknowledge & thank Dr Niranjan Kumar, M.Ch FRCS. ; Honorable Vice-Chancellor, Shri Dharmasthala Manjunatheshwara University for his valuable constructive suggestions and constant support towards this endeavour.

## References

1. Fusaro F, Constantinides F, Maglione M, Dalessadri D, Vettori E, Lenarda RDI. Comparison of orthopantomography (OPG) and computed tomography (CT) accuracy in predicting inferior alveolar nerve injury following lower third molar surgical extraction [Internet]. 2017 [cited 2019Jun3]. Available from: https://www.researchgate.net/publication/319548814_Comparison_of_orthopantomography_OPG_and_computed_tomography_CT_accuracy_in_predicting_inferior_alveolar_nerve_injury_following_lower_third_molar_surgical_extraction
2. Abramovitch K, Rice DD. Basic principles of cone beam computed tomography. Dent Clin N Am. 2014;58(3):463–84.
3. Lucas J.. What are gamma-rays? Available from: https://www.livescience.com/50215-gamma-rays.html
4. Ferreira RI, de Almeida SM, Boscolo FN, Santos AO, Camargo EE. Bone scintigraphy as an adjunct for the diagnosis of oral diseases. J Dent Educ. 2002;66(12):1381–7.
5. Appadurai R, Lingeshwar D, Venugopal S, Christina RD. Bone scintigraphy as a diagnostic tool in condylar hyperplasia [Internet]. 2017 [cited 2019Jun3]. Available from: http://www.joomr.org/article.asp?issn=2321-3841;year=2017;volume=5;issue=3;spage=84;epage=89;aulast=Appadurai
6. Griffeth LK. Use of PET/CT scanning in cancer patients: technical and practical considerations [Internet]. Proceedings (Baylor University. Medical Center). Baylor Health Care System; 2005 [cited 2019Jun4]. Available from: https://www.ncbi.nlm.nih.gov/pmc/articles/PMC1255942/
7. Williams N, O'Connell PR, McCaskie AW. Bailey and Love's short practice of surgery. 27th ed. New York: CRC Press; 2018.
8. Pooley RA. AAPM/RSNA Physics Tutorial for Residents Fundamental Physics of MR Imaging [Internet]. 2005 [cited 2019Jun3]. Available from: https://pubs.rsna.org/doi/pdf/10.1148/rg.254055027
9. Singh GP, Dogra S, Kumari E. Ultrasonography: maxillofacial applications. Annals of Dental Specialty. 2014;2(3):104–7.
10. Kumar V, Abbas AK, Aster JC. Robbins and Cotran pathologic basis of disease. 9th ed. Philadelphia: W.B. Saunders; 2015.
11. Fraser RS, Muller NL, Colman N, Pare PD. Fraser and Pare's diagnosis of diseases of the chest. 4th ed. Philadelphia: W.B. Saunders; 1999.
12. Christopoulos A. Mouth Anatomy [Internet]. Overview, Gross Anatomy: Oral Vestibule, Gross Anatomy: Oral Cavity Proper. 2015 [cited 2019Jun5].
13. Surgical fascial spaces [Internet]. online presentation [cited 2019 Jun 7];Available from: https://en.ppt-online.org/369373
14. La'Porte SJ, Juttla JK, Lingam RK. Imaging the Floor of the Mouth and the Sublingual Space [Internet]. RadioGraphics. 2011 [cited 2019Jun5]. Available from: https://pubs.rsna.org/doi/full/10.1148/rg.315105062
15. Joshi SK, Kamalapur MG, Joshi AS, Hallikeri K. Ultrasonographic evaluation of carcinoma of buccal mucosa: Ultrasound technique and evaluation of neoplastic conditions. J. Evid. Based Med. Healthc. 2016;3(34):1649–55.

# Part V

## Maxillofacial Surgery: Essential Concepts

9

# Infection Prevention and Surgical Protocols

Rishi Kumar Bali

## 9.1 Introduction

A study comprising data from 56 countries in 2004 stated that the annual major surgery volume was estimated to be 187–281 million operations, accounting for approximately one operation annually for every 25 human beings alive [1]. In subsequent studies, data were obtained from a total of 194 Member States of the World Health Organization for the years 2005–2012. According to these studies, 312.9 million operations took place in 2012, showing an increase from the 2004 estimate of 226.4 million operations. 6.3% and 23.1% of operations were carried out in *very-low* and *low*-expenditure countries representing only 36.8% (2573 million people) and 34.2% (2393 million people) of the global population of 7001 million people, respectively [2]. The incidence of postoperative infections reported among the developed countries like UK and USA was approximately 5% and 5–6%, whereas in developing countries like India it is much higher, accounting for approximately 10–25%. [3, 4].

The main problem encountered in the practice of surgical safety is that existing safety practices are not adequate in some countries. Lack of resources is the main reason behind this, particularly in developing countries. Good infection prevention and control is essential to ensure the safety of the patient undergoing any surgical procedure in the operating theater. The surgical site infections (SSIs) constitute 20% of the total hospital-acquired infections [4]. These infections cause substantial patient mortality and morbidity and burden healthcare systems with massive costs. Since these infections are primarily acquired during the operative procedure when the wound is still open, stringent protocols need to be followed at this point to minimize their onset.

R. K. Bali (✉)
Postgraduate Department of OMFS, DAV Dental college hospital, Yamunanagar, Haryana, India

## 9.2 Terminology

To establish surgical protocols, it is important to understand the basic concepts of sterilization, asepsis, and infection control. In this respect, the following terminologies are very commonly used:

**Antibiotics**
These agents are a by-product of certain microorganisms, which either have the capacity to destroy or inhibit the growth of other microorganisms at low concentrations.

**Anti-Infective**
A substance (or drug) capable of killing microorganisms or inhibiting their growth, in particular, pathogenic microorganisms. This is a general term used to encompass those drugs that specifically act on certain types of microorganisms, including antibacterial (antibiotics), antifungal, antiviral, and antiprotozoal agents.

**Antimicrobial Agent**
Any agent synthetically or naturally obtained that can destroy or attenuate the microorganisms.

**Antisepsis**
It is the process in which microbial agents on a living surface are either killed or their growth is arrested.

**Antiseptic**
These are the substances applied on the living tissues to reduce the possibility of infection, sepsis, and putrefaction by inhibiting the activity or growth of the microorganisms.

**Asepsis**
The state of being free from living pathogenic organisms.

**Aseptic**
Free of or using methods to keep free from microorganisms.

**Aseptic Processing**
It is defined as the processing and packaging of a sterile product into sterilized containers followed by proper sealing with a sterilized closure in a manner to control microbiological recontamination.

**Bactericide**
It is an antimicrobial agent that has the capacity to destroy both nonpathogenic and pathogenic organisms but may not destroy bacteria in spore form.

**Bacteriostatic**
It is an antimicrobial agent that inhibits the growth of microorganisms but is not capable of killing them.

**Bioburden**
The occurrence of viable microorganisms on a surface or object before the sterilization procedure.

**Biologic Indicator (BI)**
A standardized test preparation of bacterial spores used to demonstrate effective sterilizing conditions by providing a defined resistance to a specific sterilization process.

**Chemical Indicator**
These are agents or devices used to monitor or confirm the attainment of one or more of the parameters required for a satisfactory sterilization process or used in a specific test of the sterilization equipment.

**Chemisterilant**
It is an agent, chemical in nature with properties that kills all forms of microbial agents, including spores.

**Cleaning**
It is the process of removing all forms of foreign materials (from objects using detergents & water, soaps, and enzymes) by employing the mechanical action of washing or scrubbing the object.

**Contamination**
It is the process of entry of microbial agents into tissues or any aseptic environment.

**Crossinfection**
The spread of infection from one person, object or place to another.

**Decontamination**
The process by which a person or a surface is made free from all the agents that contaminate the surface and lead to the spread of infections. [5]

**Detergent**
It is a chemical agent with cleansing actions in dilute solutions, which, on combining with impurities and dirt, make them more soluble.

**Disease**
Disruption of the normal performance of the vital functions of a plant or animal by an infection.

**Disinfectant**
This is an agent, usually a chemical, applied on inanimate objects that destroys microorganism in the vegetative form but not the spores.

Chemical disinfectant agents are categorized into low level, intermediate, and high level (depending on the product claims and regulatory requirements in different parts of the world).

- High-level disinfection (HLD): It is a process in which a small number of spores or certain bacteria are killed by the use of certain antimicrobial agents at a specific temperature and appropriate concentration.
- Intermediate-level disinfection (ILD): It is a process in which vegetative forms of all microorganisms are destroyed but affect the activity of spores of certain bacteria.
- Low-level disinfection (LLD): It is a process in which vegetative forms of all microorganisms are destroyed having no activity on spores of bacteria at very low concentrations.

**Disinfection**
Antimicrobial process to remove, destroy, or deactivate microorganisms on surfaces or in liquids. Disinfection is often considered as a reduction of the numbers and types of viable microorganisms (or "bioburden") but may not be assumed to render the surface or liquid free from viable microbial contamination (in contrast to sterilization).

**Droplet Nuclei**
These are those particles of 1–10 μm that are implicated in the spread of airborne infections.

**Exogenous Infection**
The infecting microorganism comes from an external source.

**Fomites**
Any inanimate object that is capable of absorbing or transmitting infectious microorganisms from one person to the other.

**Fumigation**
The process of disinfecting or purifying an area or object with the fumes of certain chemical agents.

**Germicide**
Agents that are designed to kill and destroy pathogenic organisms on the surface of different things.

**Infection**
It is the process of invasion of the tissues by microorganisms and their multiplication in the body of the host to produce disease.

**Microorganisms or Microbe**
Microscopic organisms, which may exist in its single-celled form or in a colony of cells.

**Minimum Effective Concentration (MEC)**
The lowest concentration of a chemical or product, used in a specified process that achieves a claimed activity.

**Minimum Recommended Concentration (MRC)**
The lowest concentration of a chemical or product specified by the equipment manufacturer to be used in a process.

**Nosocomial**
This comes from two Greek words, i.e., "*nosus*" meaning "*disease*" and "*komeion*" meaning "*to take care of.*" Also known as "hospital-acquired infections." These are the infections originating or taking place in a hospital.

**Operating Room (OR)**
The operating room or operating theater is a facility within a hospital where surgical procedures are carried out in an aseptic environment.

**Pathogen**
A pathogen is a tiny living organism, such as a bacterium or virus that is capable of producing disease in an individual.

**Resistance**
It is the natural ability of the agent to oppose the effects of any harmful agents.

**Soil**
Natural or artificial contamination on a device or surface following its use or simulated use.

**Sterile Barrier System**
Packaging that prevents the ingress of microorganisms following a sterilization process, thereby preserving the sterile state.

**Sterilizer**
Equipment designed to achieve sterilization.

**Sterilizing Agent**
Physical or chemical agent (or combination of agents) that has sufficient microbicidal activity to achieve sterility under defined conditions.

**Septic**
Contaminated or infected.

**Spores**
These are the reproductive forms of some microorganisms that can survive harsh environmental factors and have the capability of developing into new viable microbes.

**Sterilization**
Sterilization is a process that destroys or removes all microbial life completely, including spores by means of certain chemical or physical processes.

**Sterile**
Free from living microorganisms.

**Sterilize**
Total destruction of all living forms.

**Vector**
It is an organism that does not cause disease itself but which spreads infection by conveying pathogens from one host to another.

**Virulence**
It is a pathogen's ability to infect, sustain, or spread infection in a living a host. Historical background of present day protocols is enumerated in Table 9.1.

## 9.3 Surgical Site Infections

Approximately 2–5% of all surgical patients tend to acquire surgical site infections (SSIs) [4]. In developed & high-income countries (HICs), SSIs are the second most common cause of healthcare-associated infections [6], whereas in Low- & Middle-Income Countries (LMICs) or underdeveloped & developing countries these infections are the most common ones. Thus, to reduce the risk of surgical site infections, a more systematic approach has to be adopted, based on proper knowledge regarding the status of the patient, type, & time of the operation, personnel involved and the health care facilities available during a surgical procedure. The main pathogenic source of surgical site infections is the endogenous flora (usually aerobic gram positive cocci) of the patient present in the skin, the mucous membranes, or the hollow viscera. The exogenous sources of infection include

**Table 9.1** Historical background leading to proper sterilization and disinfection protocols

| Year | Event |
|---|---|
| • First century BC. | *Varo and Columella* postulated that diseases were caused by invisible beings, "animals minutia," inhaled or ingested |
| • 500 AD | *Sushruta* instructed operating team members to clean and fumigate the operating theater with vapors of certain disinfectants prior to all surgical procedures |
| • 1493–1541 | *Paracelsus*, called the father of medicine, reformed pharmacopeia and introduced compositions of lead, copper, sulfur, iron, and mercury |
| • 1546 | *Fracastorious* proposed a "contagion vivum," as the possible cause of infectious diseases. |
| • 1827–1912 | *Joseph Lister*, "father of modern surgery," demonstrated that antisepsis could prevent infections; also known as "Listerian era" |
| • 1889 | *William Stewart Halsted* introduced rubber gloves for his scrub nurse |
| • 1882 | *Robert Koch* introduced the use of mercuric bichloride as antiseptic agents and isolated the bacilli of tuberculosis |
| • 1880s and 1890s. | Sterilization of instruments, hand washing, and the wearing of masks, caps, gloves, and gowns was introduced |

**Table 9.2** WHO: Ten essential objectives for safe surgery

(1) The operating team must ensure that the correct surgical procedure is to be carried out on the correct patient.
(2) The operating personnel should have adequate knowledge regarding the anesthesia, its methods of administration as well as its effects so that minimum pain is experienced by the patient.
(3) The operating personnel should be well prepared for any life-threatening conditions like loss of airway or respiratory function.
(4) The operating team should be prepared for risk of high loss of blood.
(5) The operating team should be well versed with the history of the patient in order to prevent or induce any allergic or adverse drug reactions that can cause a significant risk for the patient.
(6) Care must be taken to minimize the formation of surgical site infections by using proper measures.
(7) Proper care must be taken to not leave any instrument or any foreign material at the surgical site.
(8) All specimens should be carefully identified and secured for further investigations.
(9) Proper communication must be present among the operating team personnel for the safe conduct of the surgical procedure.
(10) A routine surveillance of the surgical volume, safety protocols, capacities, and the outcomes must be carried out by all the hospitals and the health care systems.

members of the surgical team, environment of the operating theater and tools, materials & instruments brought to the sterile zones during the surgical procedure. Various strategies employed to prevent or control the occurrence of surgical site infections include reducing the contamination by microorganisms on the sterile surgical instruments as well as the body of the patient, prophylactic preoperative antibiotic coverage, carrying out the surgical procedure carefully, proper handling of the operating room.

## 9.4 Surgical Safety

Surgical safety is of utmost importance in order to prevent major and life-threatening complications leading to undue loss of life and patient morbidity. Thus, a list of ten essential objectives with a surgical safety checklist have been elucidated by the WHO to be followed by all the personnel present in the operating room to reduce the risk of such complications [7] (Tables 9.2 and 9.3).

## 9.5 Environmental Control and Design

**Operating Room (OR)**

The operating room or operating theater is a facility within a hospital where surgical procedures are carried out in an aseptic environment. Since the operating theater is a highly sterile, aseptic, and restricted area in a hospital setting, it is mandatory for all the personnel concerned to have a proper understanding of the working of the operation theater abiding by certain laws, regulations, and professional guidelines. Integrated infection control in the operation theater is the key to decreasing morbidity and mortality among the patients undergoing surgery.

Following essentials must be present in an operating room:

– Adequate lighting
– Proper ventilation with 20 (ACH) air changes/hour
– Correct and sufficient instruments needed in the surgery
– Proper machines and equipment for monitoring the condition of the patients during the surgeries
– Emergency drugs and other items
– Separate rooms should be present to carry different procedures

• Location of the Operating Theater: The location of the operation theater should be such that adequate natural light and proper ventilation is present. For this, a two- or three-story building away from the general hustle and bustle of the hospital is preferred.
• Operation rooms: The standard recommended size of the operation theater is 6.5 m × 6.5 m × 3.5 m and can be modified as per requirement
• Doors and Windows: There should be separate entry and exit doors. The width of the door should be approximately

**Table 9.3** WHO's Surgical Safety Checklist

| Before induction of anesthesia | Before skin incision | Before patient leaves operating room |
|---|---|---|
| Sign in | Time out | Sign out |
| Patient has confirmed<br>• Identity<br>• Site<br>• Procedure<br>• Consent | Confirm all team members have introduced themselves by name and role | Nurse verbally confirms with the team<br>• The name of the procedure recorded<br>• The instrument, sponge, and needle counts are correct (or not applicable)<br>• How the specimen is labeled (including patient name)<br>• Whether there are any equipment problems to be addressed |
| Site marked/not applicable | Surgeon, anesthesia professional and nurse verbally confirm<br>• Patient<br>• Site<br>• Procedure | |
| Anesthesia safety check completed | Anticipated critical events<br>• Surgeon reviews: What are the critical or unexpected steps, operative duration, anticipated blood loss<br>• Anesthesia team reviews: Are there any patient -specific concerns<br>• Nursing team reviews: Has sterility (including indicator results) been confirmed? Are there equipment issues or any concerns? | Surgeon, anesthesia professional and nurse review the key concerns for recovery and management of this patient |
| Pulse oximeter on patient and functioning | Has antibiotic prophylaxis been given in the last 60 min?<br>• Yes / not applicable<br>Is essential imaging displayed<br>• Yes/not applicable | |
| Does patient have a known allergy<br>• No/yes<br>Difficult airway /aspiration risk<br>• No<br>• Yes, and equipment /assistance available<br>Risk of >500 ml blood loss (7 ml/kg in children)<br>• No<br>• Yes and adequate intravenous access and fluids planned | | |

1.2 to 1.5 m. Sliding doors are preferred than spring-loaded doors in order to minimize the generation of the air currents during the opening and closing of the doors. Windows made from glass are preferred, which are to be planned on one side only.

- The surface/flooring: The flooring must be such that it is nonslippery, strong, & with minimum joints to decrease the accumulation of dust and other tiny particulate matter within it.
- Walls: Washable light and soothing painted walls should be present
- Ceiling: Hard, impervious surface, plaster painted ceiling should be present.

### Different Zones of Operation Theater Complex

There are four different zones observed in any operating room complex described on the basis of type of cleanliness present, presence or absence of microorganisms, and the different procedures to be carried out in each zone (Fig. 9.1).

1. *Protective zone*: It includes
   - Changing room for all the concerned persons
   - Transferring passage for the materials, equipment, and the patient
   - Rooms for administrative staff
   - Storage & record maintenance
   - Pre- and postoperative
   - Intensive and Coronary Care Units
   - Storage rooms to keep the sterilized objects
2. *Clean zone*: Links the protective zone to the aseptic zone
   - Clean rooms
   - Storage room for equipment
   - Rooms designed for surveillance, maintenance, and firefighting
   - Exit areas in case of emergencies exists

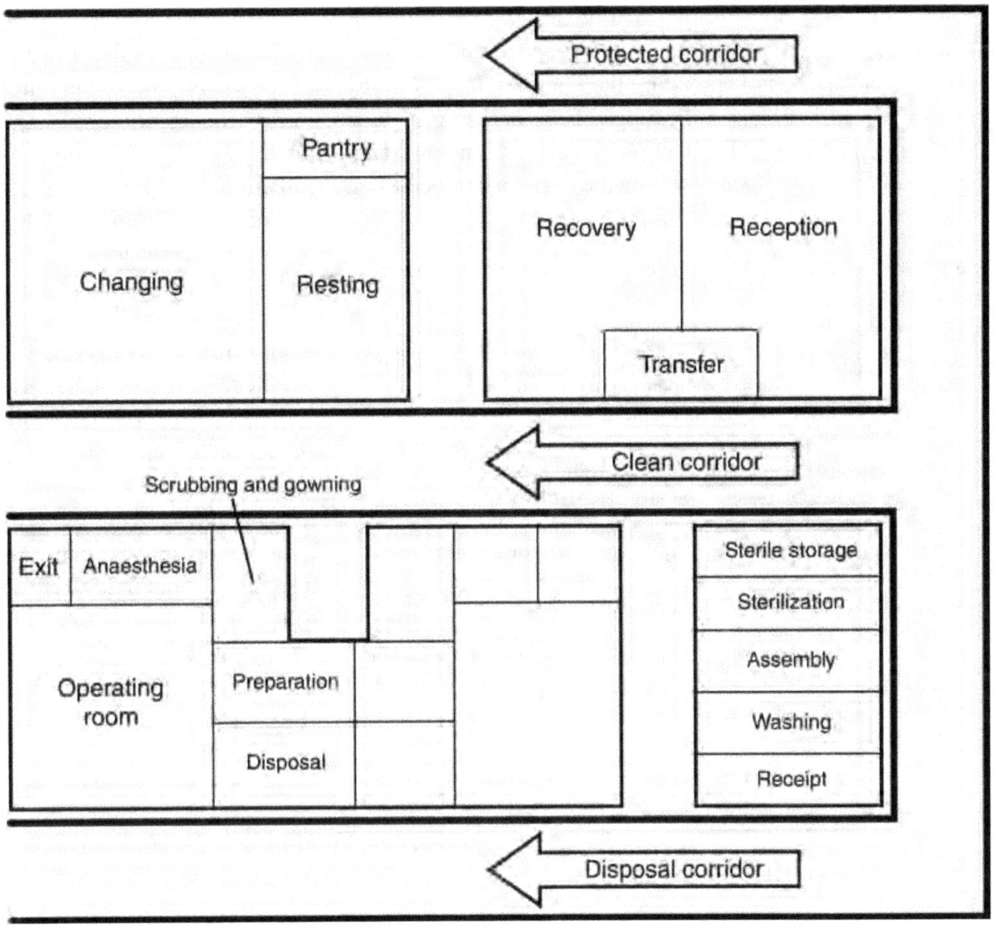


**Fig. 9.1** Different zones of operation theater complex

3. *Aseptic zone:* houses the operating rooms
4. *Disposal zone:* separate exit for disposing contaminated linen /used materials and instruments

**Important Points**

- The sterilized materials are transported from a sterile area to the operation theater on a covered cart, thus preventing any accumulation of the dust particles on their surfaces.
- Before entering the operation theater, all supplies/materials must be removed from their shipping or transported containers.
- All the blood-coated or soiled instruments/equipment must be transported in a covered wrap or container from the operating room to the decontamination or reprocessing area.
- Care must be taken that the soiled instruments/equipment must not to be stored with the sterilized goods.

**Maintenance in the Operation Theater**

- The machinery must be surveyed at least every week.
- Proper ventilation should be checked regularly and the filters should be changed as required.
- At the time of maintenance or inspection or observation of any fault in the working of the operation theater, the members of The Infection Control team should be informed. The theater should be thoroughly examined by the members of the team and appropriate measures must be taken to maintain the infection control protocols. The operation theater must only be functional after being carefully evaluated and cleared by the infection control team.
- Back-up facility for operation theater in all aspects should be present in any setup to provide any uninterrupted sessions at the time of maintenance or any fault observed.

## 9.6 Disinfection and Sterilization

Sterilization is the ultimate procedure in controlling the undesired activities of microorganisms that are outside of the human body. Its purpose in the operating field is to prevent the spread of infectious disease, and in surgery, it primarily relates to processing reusable instruments. Surgical instruments are an integral part of surgical field and, being reusable, have greater chances of spreading the microorganisms if any of the reprocessing steps fails. Steps of reprocessing include cleaning, repackaging, disinfection or sterilization, and reusing. Cleaning, being the first step in the cycle of reprocessing, is the major step in the removal of any organic matter present on the surface of the instruments. Any failure in the removal of the visible soil at the initial stage can create a discrepancy in the efficacy of the subsequent disinfection and sterilization procedures. Sterilization is more effective a process than disinfection. The process of disinfection is carried out with the use of various chemical agents. Chemical disinfecting agent necessarily does not kill all microorganisms or spores present on an inanimate object but instead reduces the number of microorganisms to a level that is not harmful to health. Depending on their potency against microbes, they are classified as *High-*, *Intermediate-*, or *Low-level* disinfectants.

**Table 9.4** Spaulding Classification of Medical Devices And Level of Disinfection

- Critical: An instrument that has a direct contact with sterile tissues or vascular system [8]; such items are to be sterilized and made free from all microorganisms. Examples are extraction forceps, scalpel blades, bone chisels, periodontal scalers, surgical burs, needles
- Semicritical: An instrument that does not usually penetrate the sterile tissues but does come in contact with intact mucous membrane. These items are made free from microorganisms by high-level disinfection. Examples include endoscopes, amalgam condensers, air/water syringe, impression trays, dental hand piece, dental mirrors
- Noncritical: An instrument that does not touch the patient directly or come in contact with the intact skin only. These items may be cleaned or disinfected by low-level disinfection. Examples include light arm/handles, dental chair, dental X-ray equipment, chair side computers, chair switches.

The type of the sterilization procedures to be carried out for an object depends upon the classification of the instruments based according to the Spaulding Classification of the medical devices, the type of material of which the object is made of, the microorganisms to be present on the object, and availability of the sterilization methods and equipment (Table 9.4).

**The Instrument Processing (Decontamination Steps)** (Fig. 9.2)

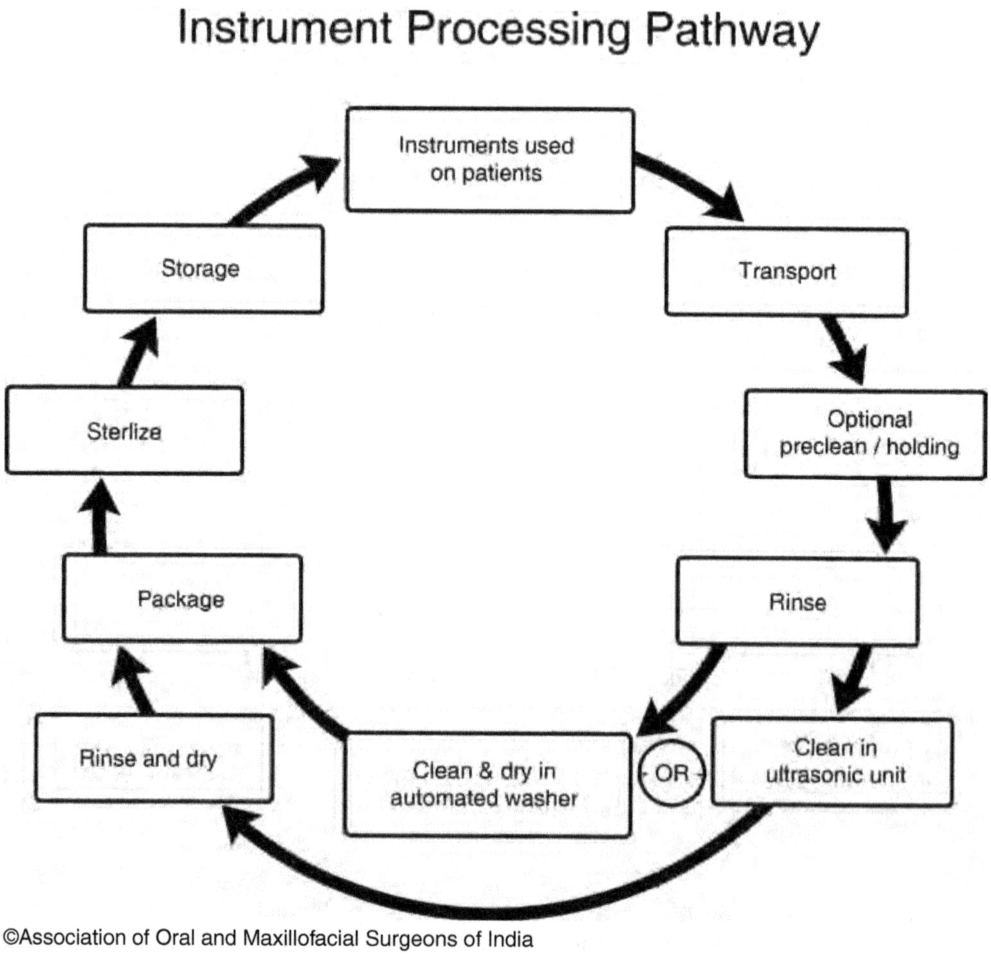


**Fig. 9.2** Instrument processing steps

Various methods of decontamination include.

- Physical cleaning.
- Water purification
- Ultrasonic cleaning
- Disinfection
- Antisepsis
- Sterilization

Processing of the clinical or surgical items is a two step procedure.

A. **Cleaning**, being the first step, is the most essential one, which is succeeded either by Disinfection or Sterlization
   - Cleaning is the process of removing all the foreign particles present on the surface of the object, which is accomplished by means of two main steps, i.e., cleaning by friction to remove foreign particles and rinsing away by fluids to remove the debris so cleaned.
   - If the objects to be sterilized, remain soiled with foreign materials, the microorganisms will be trapped in the organic matter and may interfere with the proper sterilization or disinfection procedure. Therefore, thorough cleaning should always precede the sterilization process.
   - Cleaning may be manual or mechanical and is normally accomplished by the use of water, detergents, and mechanical agents. Detergent is essential to dissolve proteins and oil that can reside on instruments and equipment after use.

1. *Mechanical cleaning*

   With the advancement in the sterilization equipment, most units are automated and there is very less handling of dirty equipment by the concerned staff. The equipment to be processed is placed in trays and is ready for washing.

   - *Washing machine*: It gives a cold rinse followed by a hot wash at 71 °C for 2 min. This is followed by a 10-second hot rinse at 80–90 °C and then by dry heat at 50–75 °C.
   - *Ultrasonicator*: The ultrasonicator is a device, which is extremely efficient in removing the debris. 0.44 W/cm$^3$ of power is used to remove the debris by the process of sonic waves produced. The solution used most often to clean is an enzymatic presoak (protease formula that dissolves protein).

2. *Manual cleaning*

   It is an active method that is carried out by thoroughly brushing the item with the help of a toothbrush under water to prevent the release of aerosols. The brush should be thoroughly cleaned after use and should be dried. The cleaned items are then dried and made ready for the proper sterilization procedure to be carried out depending upon the material of which they are made and the use they perform.

   Manual cleaning is necessary when:

   - Cleaning of instruments by mechanical means is not possible
   - Instruments to be cleaned are delicate in nature
   - Objects to be cleaned have a narrow lumen (Fig. 9.3)

3. *Soaking of instruments prior to cleaning:*

   There are times when cleaning alone cannot remove the debris present on the surface of the objects as the items become highly soiled with foreign materials. For this, it is sometimes necessary to soak instruments/objects prior to cleaning. A container having a deeper base is filled with detergent & water and all the instruments are kept in it for 3–5 min. The solution prepared is agitated by shaking it vigorously. The cleaned instruments are now removed from the container and placed over a tray for air drying.

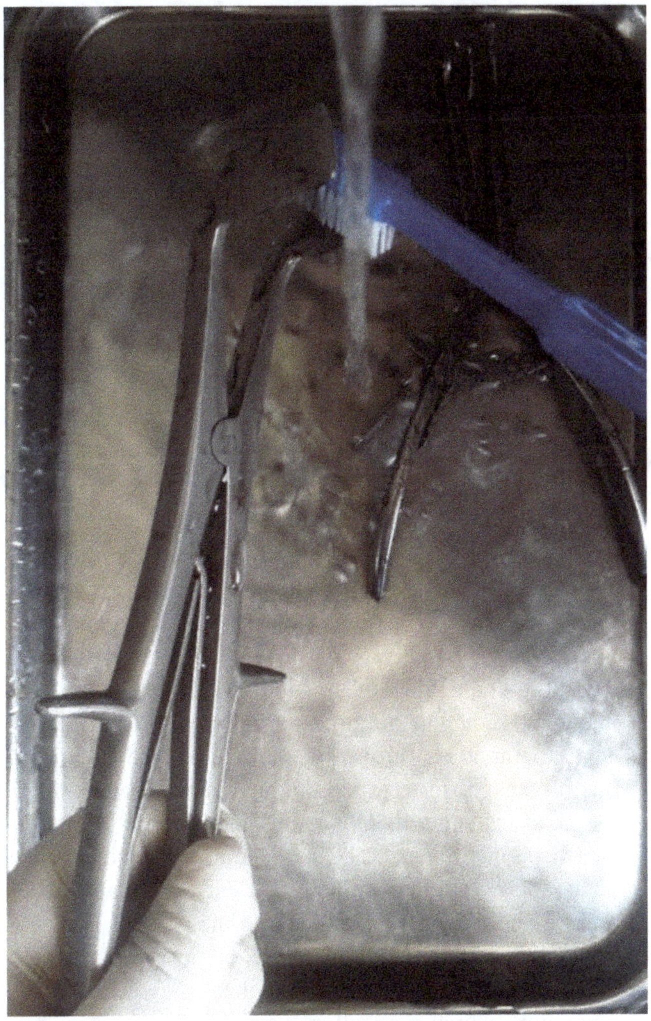



**Fig. 9.3** Manual Cleaning

B. **Disinfection and Sterlization**

- *Disinfection* can be achieved by either thermal or chemical processes. The thermal disinfection procedure is more easily controlled, more reliable, nontoxic and leaves no residue on the surface and is preferred more than chemical disinfection procedures. The main indication of chemical disinfectant use is the heat-sensitive objects. Chemical High-level disinfection (HLD):
  (a) Most commonly used for heat-labile instruments/objects (e.g., endoscopes) where single use is not cost effective.
  (b) Disinfectants used for this purpose are
    - Glutaraldehyde: 2% for 20 min.
    - Hydrogen peroxide: 6%–7.5% for 20–30 min.
    - Per acetic acid: 0.2–0.35% for 5 min.
    - Ortho-phthalaldehyde (OPA) for 5–12 min.
  (c) Steps:
    - All items to be disinfected are cleaned and dried.
    - Fresh disinfectant solution should be made each day in a sterile container. If a previously prepared solution is to be used, an indicator strip is dipped in the solution to check for the effectiveness of the solution.
    - Open all hinged instruments and disassemble whichever possible.
    - Place all items in the solution completely submerged in the container.
    - The container is covered and the instruments are allowed to soak in for 20 min.
    - Remove the items using dry, high-level disinfected pickups.
    - Rinse thoroughly with boiled water.
    - Air-dry by placing on disinfected tray.
    - Items disinfected are covered in a disinfected container and used within a week.

*Sterilization*

Sterilization is a method by which an article, medium, or surface is made free from all microbial invasions, including spores. The main aim of sterilization of instruments is proper delivery of sterilized instruments at the operating field, thereby maintaining a sterile environment and reducing the spread of infections from one person to another. Proper handling of the sterilized instruments is done by appropriate wrapping and storage of the instruments, thereby increasing the shelf life of the sterilized instruments. The instruments should be bagged or wrapped in a muslin cloth or clear pouches or paper before and after the procedure and the wrapping should be sealed with tape. No pin, staple, or any paper clips are to be applied on the wrapping as these may create small openings, which may allow entry of microorganisms, thereby hampering the process of sterilization. Sterilization is accomplished by:

1. *Steam sterilization (autoclaving):-*
   - This is the most simple and efficient means of sterilizing instruments. It is also commonly called steam sterilizing or autoclaving.
   - The steam autoclaves best suited for outpatient practice are usually made to operate in the following range.
     - Temperature 121 °C (250 °F) at a pressure of 15 pounds per square inch (psi) for 15 min.
     - Temperature 134 °C (270 °F) at a pressure of 30 psi for 3 min. This process termed "flash sterilization" has practical use in the operating room where fast sterilization of instruments may be necessary.
   - This combination of moisture and heat provides the bacteria-destroying power currently most effective against all forms of microorganisms.
   - Mainly used for items that are wrapped or porous.
   - Autoclaves are either classified as horizontal or vertical (based on design) and gravity displacement or vacuum type (based on functioning).
   - Autoclaves can also be classified as Type "N" and Type "B."
   - Type "N" autoclaves are the ones that do not remove air from the sterilization chamber with the help of a vacuum pump. These are used for solid loads.
   - Type "B" autoclaves remove air from the sterilization chamber with the help of a vacuum pump. Wrapped and hollow instruments, which can be sterilized and used later, are to be sterilized by this type of autoclave.
   - Importance of bagging the instruments for sterilization.
     - The main aim of bagging or wrapping the instruments prior to sterilization procedure decreases the chances of contamination of the items after the sterilization procedure is complete.
     - Two-layer wrapping of objects should be preferred and the materials used for this can be cotton fabric or muslin, paper, newspaper (Fig. 9.4).
   - Monitoring of sterilization.
   - Sterilization monitoring is a process by which adequate sterile environment and the effectiveness of the procedure is determined by assessing the biological, mechanical, and chemical parameters.
   - The most widely used and accepted parameter of assessing the sterilization procedures is the use of biological indicators (BIs) that directly inhibit the growth of highly resistant microorganisms, rather than merely testing the physical and chemical conditions necessary for sterilization. Since the spores present in a biological indicator are in a much higher number and are highly resistant by nature compared to the other and common microorgan-

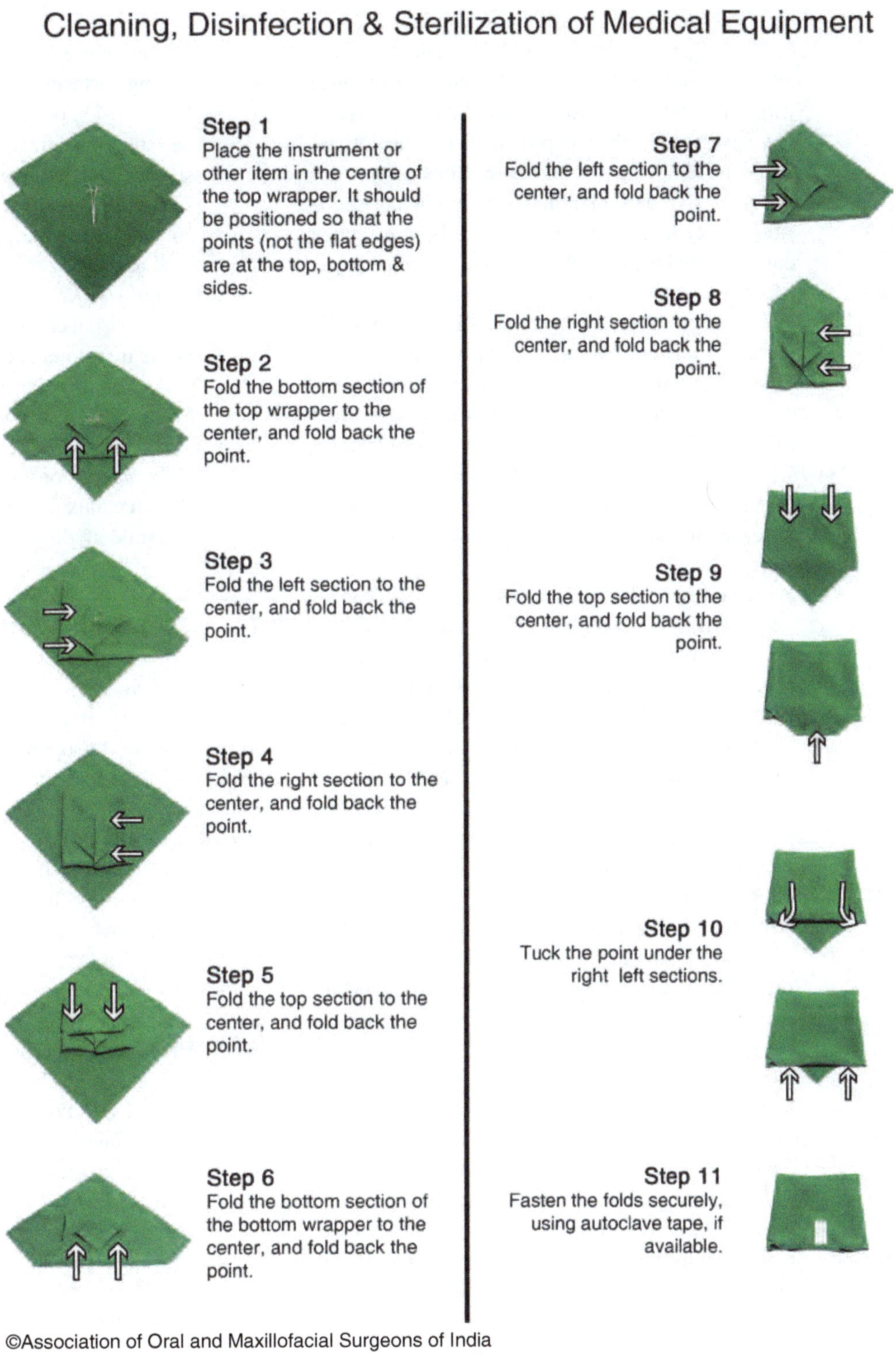


**Fig. 9.4** Diagram depicting the way the instruments are wrapped for sterilization

isms found on items used for the patient, an inactivated biological indicator indicates that the other microorganisms are killed depicting an effective sterilization procedure. A control BI, from the same lot as the test indicator and not processed through the sterilizer, should be incubated with the test BI; the control BI should yield positive results for bacterial growth.

- Assuring the temperature & the cycle time, and observing the gauges or display for the pressure on the sterilization equipment for each set of items to be sterilized come under the mechanical monitoring of sterilization.
- Certain chemical agents are used to check the efficacy of the sterilization procedure being carried out by undergoing chemical changes in their properties on

being exposed to the sterilizing conditions. These chemical agents are called the chemical indicators and these include TST (Time-Steam-Temperature) Strip. This TST strip is to be placed in a big surgical wire basket and when exposed to a critical time, steam, and temperature it undergoes a change in color from yellow to dark blue indicating complete sterilization procedure. Another strip is to be used when double-layered packing of instruments in crepe paper is done to assess the parameters inside the sterilizer.

- Another form of sterilizing monitor is the use of the external indicators. These are usually in the form of Tapes. The main indication of the complete sterilization procedure is the change in color of the strips of the tape from yellow to dark brown or black.
- *How to store the sterilized instruments/objects*
  - There must be a separate area for storing of the sterile instruments and single-use (disposable) products.
  - The storing of the bagged sterilizer objects can be depicted either by the date on which they are sterilized or the procedure for which it is to be used or an event causing it to become contaminated.
  - All the packed items must be carefully inspected before using to verify the integrity of the outer covering and the condition of the packing (dry/wet).
  - Once the packing is assessed and if any breach is seen in the packing, the wrapping should be replaced and the instruments again sent for the sterilization procedure.
  - All the sterilized instruments must be kept in covered drawers.
- Care must be taken that all instruments should be placed away from the place where chances of getting wet are higher.
- *Expiry of the sterilized instruments*
- The expiry of the materials and objects undergoing the sterilization procedure depends on the type and time of the sterilization process, the efficacy of the process, and the handling of the sterilized instruments.
- Once all the sterile conditions are met, 4 weeks is the maximum time for which the items are considered sterilized and safe for use. However, the contaminated instruments are preferred processing and sterilization prior to every procedure.

2. *Ethylene oxide:*
   - It is used for sterilization of heat-labile and moisture-sensitive items, supplies, and equipment.
   - The operating cycle ranges from 2–24 h and it is a relatively expensive process.
   - It can be used for glass, paper surfaces, clothing, plastics and metals, food stuffs, and dental equipment.
   - It is unsuitable for fumigating rooms because of its explosive property.
3. *Dry heat:*
   - It may be used for sterilization of instruments with cutting surfaces.
   - No corrosion occurs with this method of sterilization.
   - Dry heat sterilization, which usually occurs consists of hot air oven has typical cycles of 1 h at 171 °C or 2 h at 160 °C.
   - Air is a poor conductor of heat and requires a long time for getting the instruments effectively sterilized.
4. *Chemical sterilization and disinfection:*
   - This is also a choice for some limited circumstances.
   - Some instruments cannot be subjected to high temperatures and in a field environment chemical sterilization may have to be used.
   - The disinfectant must remain in contact with the surface for appropriate time.
   - Disinfectants include Chlorine solutions, 2–3.2% glutaraldehyde, iodophors, and phenols.

## 9.7 Operating Room Decorum

1. *Hand hygiene:*

Hand hygiene by operation theater persons is the most efficient way to reduce the risk of spread of infections.

2. *Surgical hand wash:*
   - Surgical hand wash or surgical hand rub should be carried out prior to the procedure in order to decrease the residing flora of the hand.
   - Steps:
     - All jewellery from wrists and hands must be removed.
     - The temperature of water is to be adjusted so that it is slightly warm. Hands and forearms are to be washed 5 cm above the level of the elbows to remove any particles of dirt.
     - Before performing the first scrub of the day, a nail cleaner is used to clean the fingernails and the nail beds.
     - The nails should be cut short and no nail polish should be used.
     - Antimicrobial agent is to be applied on the hands and in circular motion; lathering should begin at the finger tips of one hand and between the fingers, continuing from the fingertip to 5 cm above the elbow. The same process is to be repeated for other arm and hand.
     - The rubbing should be done for a period of 3–5 min.
     - Each arm is to be washed separtely at the level of elbow, starting at the fingertips.
     - One side of the sterile towel is used to dry the fingertips up to the elbow of one hand and the other side is used to dry the same on the other hand.

3. *Barrier techniques:*
   Barrier techniques are useful where the chances of spread of infection are higher.
   (a) Head Cover
   Prior or during the procedure, all facial and head hair should be tied properly and covered by means of head covers. Ideally head covers should be disposable and made of soft, nonporous cloth like material. If one has long hair, the hair should be tied in a bun. In situations where tying a bun is not possible, use of helmets or hoods or headgears is of utmost significance.
   (b) Masks
   - Tuberculosis is one of the most common infectious diseases that can spread through airborne route,
   - The main aim of using a mask is the prevention of transmission of infectious agents from the member of the operating team to the patient's wounds and also protecting the operating team members from the splashes and sprays from the patient.
   - The masks, which are disposable in nature, are always preferred.
   - The mask should be made of synthetic fibers, must be flat with two or three pleats that expand to cover the area up to chin, and should have filters of polypropylene or polyester (Fig. 9.5).

   (c) Scrub suits and cover gowns
   These are the pair of garments to be worn over, or instead of regular clothing of the persons involved in the surgical procedures to protect the transmission of any infectious agent present on the regular clothing from the operating personnel to the patient or any other personnel. These should have a simple design, should be comfortable, should be easy to clean and wash, should be economical, easily replicable if damaged and should have minimal place for the contaminants to hide.
   (d) Surgical gowns
   These are a loose pair of clothing to be worn over the scrub suits or cover gowns at the time of the surgery to protect both the patient and the operating personnel from transfer of microorganisms, blood or body fluids, and another particulate matter.
   Steps of wearing gown:
   - Dry the hands completely and hold the gown in such a manner that it is at the least risk of contamination.
   - Slip arms into the sleeves through the armholes, keeping at the shoulder level and away from the body.
   - Hold arms out and slightly up.
   - The circulating person must pull the gown over the shoulders touching only inside of the gown.
   All the belts and loops are to be tied securely (Fig. 9.6).

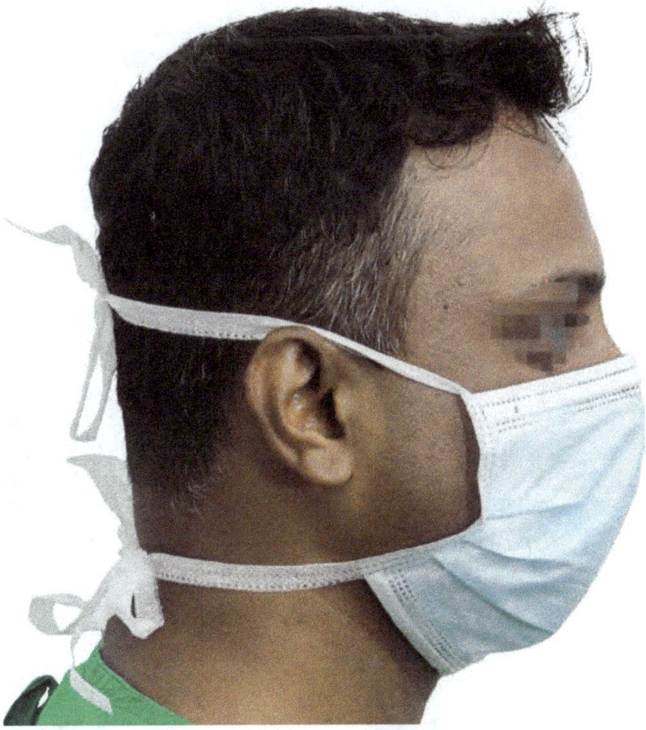



**Fig. 9.5** Surgical Mask

   (e) Gloves
   They help to protect the operator from infection by bacteria and viruses from patient's blood. Gloving is essential to protect both the surgeon and the patient from blood-borne viruses and to prevent wound from becoming contaminated with the surgeon's skin flora. The "open gloving" and "closed gloving" technique of donning the gloves should be employed for wearing gloves.
   - Steps in wearing gloves by Open Gloving Technique
     - Handwashing must be performed under aseptic conditions.
     - Inspect the outer covering for the integrity. Open the first nonsterile packaging by peeling it completely off the heat seal exposing the inner sterile wrapper, but without touching it.
     - The inner sterile packing is kept on a dry area, without touching the outer surface. Open the package and fold it toward the bottom so as to unfold the paper and keep it open.
     - By using index finger and thumb of one hand, the folded edge of the glove is grasped.
     - In a single movement the other hand is slipped into the glove.
     - The second glove is picked by using the cuff of the other glove and sliding the fingers of the gloved hand into it.

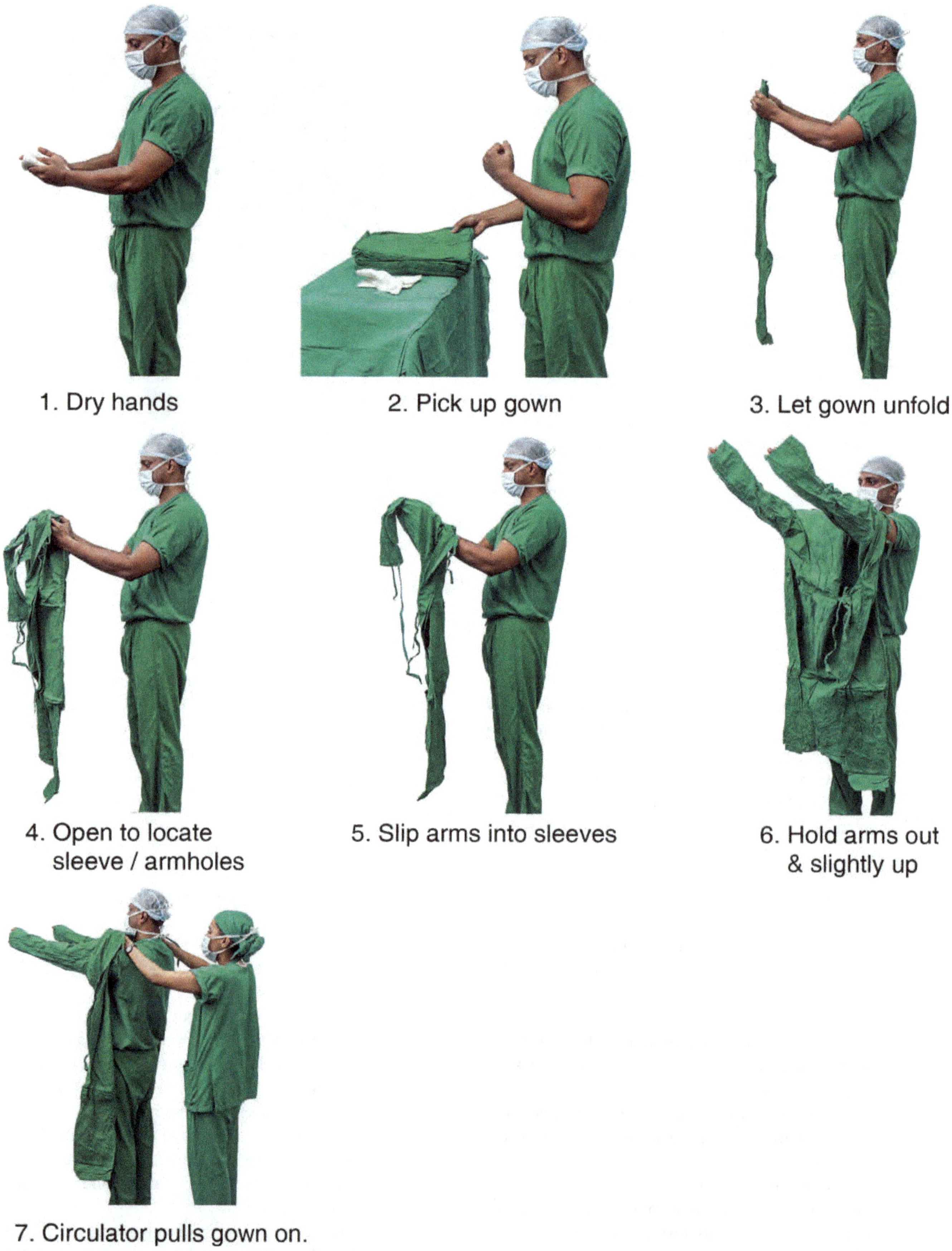



**Fig. 9.6** Putting on the sterile gown

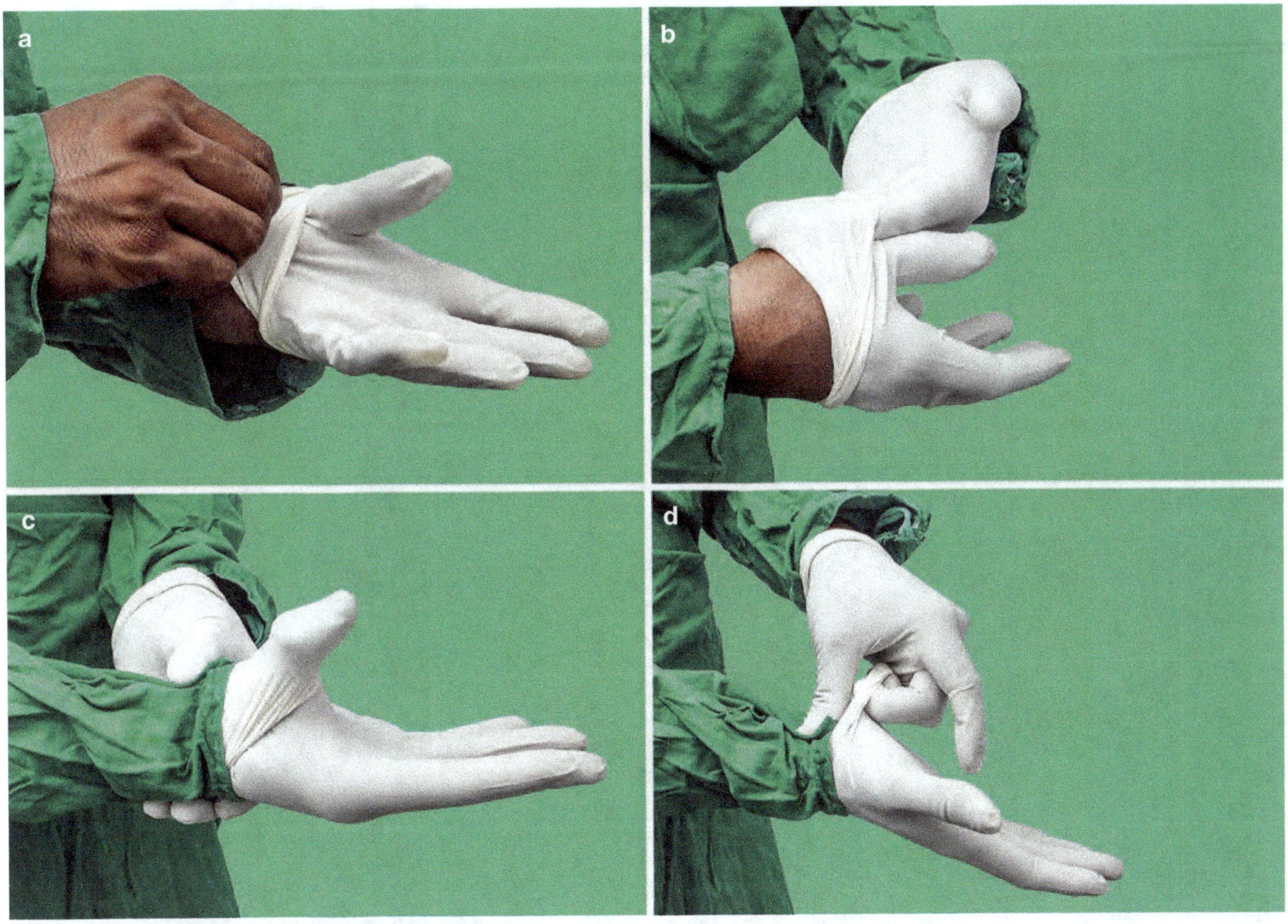




**Fig. 9.7** Putting on sterile gloves by open gloving technique

- In a single movement, slip the second glove on to the ungloved hand while avoiding any contact/resting of the gloved hand on surfaces other than the glove to be donned (Fig. 9.7).
- Steps of wearing gloves by closed gloving technique
  - If the cuffs are not fitting, a tuck is taken in each gown.
  - The circulating person should open the outer covering of the glove and should flip them onto the sterile field.
  - The inner packing containing the gloves is opened carefully and the glove is picked up by the folded cuff edge with the hand covered by the sleeve.
  - The glove is placed on the sleeve of the opposite gown, the palm facing downwards, with the fingers of the glove pointing toward the shoulder.
  - The gloves should be placed in such a manner that the rolled cuff edge of the gloves connects the sleeve to the gown cuff. Bottom cuffed and rolled edge of the glove is grasped at the bottom with the index finger and thumb.
  - With the opposite hand, the outermost edge of the cuff of the gloves is held taking care that the uncovered fingers are not exposed by it.
  - Stretch the glove over the hand
  - By using the opposite hand covered with sleeve, both the cuffs of the sleeve and the glove are seamed and the glove is pulled over the hand.
  - The same procedure is to be followed for the other hand. The fingers are adjusted to properly fit in the glove (Fig. 9.8).

4. The role of drapes:

   Drapes are used during surgical procedure to protect the contacting of the unprepared surfaces/areas and maintaining the sterility of environmental, equipment, and the surrounding of the patients.

   The different drapes available are:-

   - Towel drapes, which are used for squaring off the operative site, wrapping syringes & small instruments, and

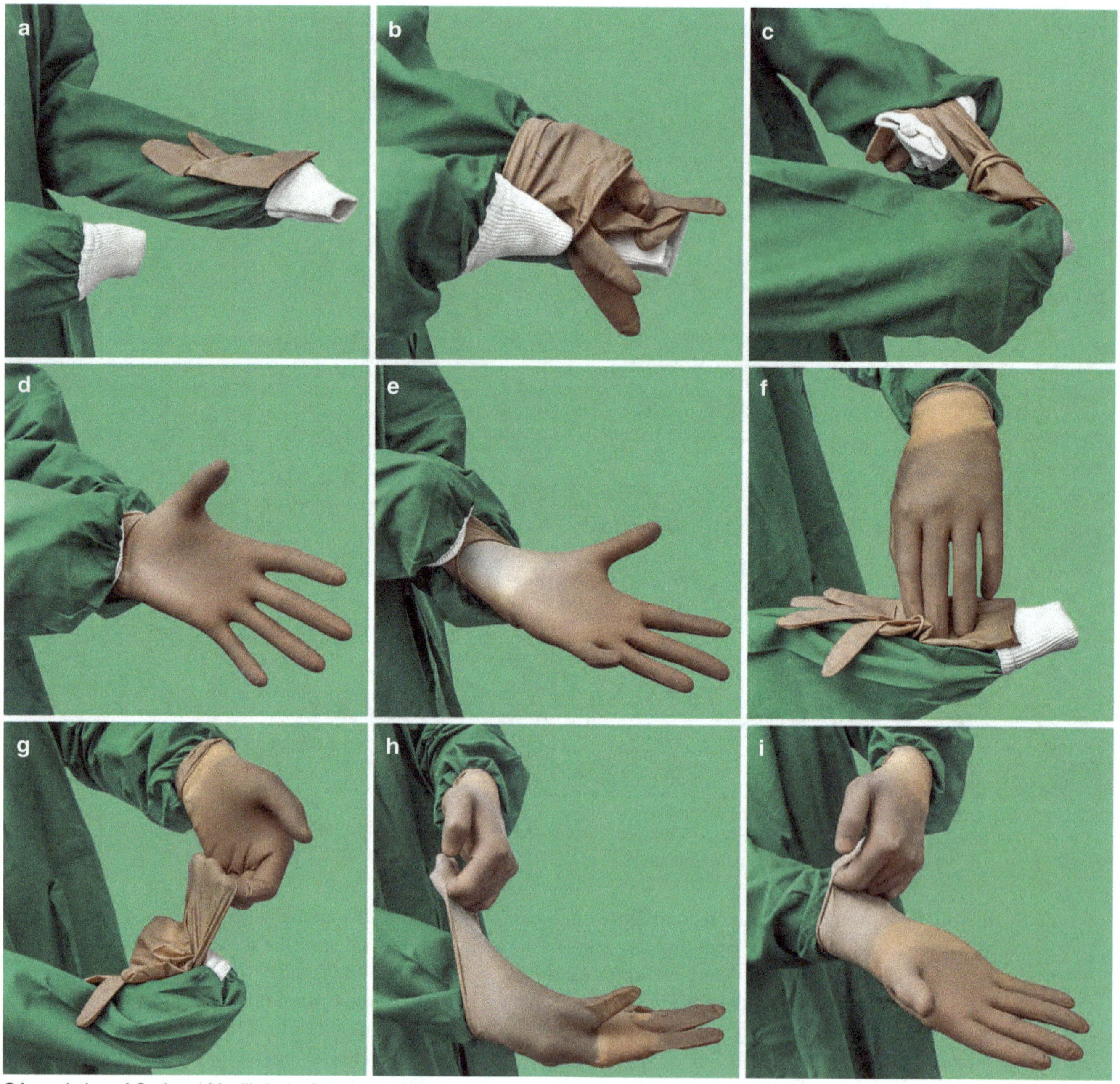




**Fig. 9.8** Putting on sterile gloves by closed gloving technique

drying of the hands. These must be more resistant to water and must be made of cotton compared to linen.

- Lap sheets are used for covering the patient. They are large and long, usually made of lightweight cotton, and provide limited protection and coverage to the patients or staff or the surface areas.
- Site drapes are made of cotton and have a circular opening in the center that is placed over the prepared operative site. These drapes are primarily intended for use with minor surgical procedures (Fig. 9.9).

## 9.8 Classification of Surgical Wounds

A widely used classification of surgical wounds is based on an estimate of likelihood of bacterial contamination of the operative site. In 1964 [9], National Academy of Sciences/National Research Council defined five general classes of operations:

1. *Refined-Clean:* Elective operations not drained and primarily closed.

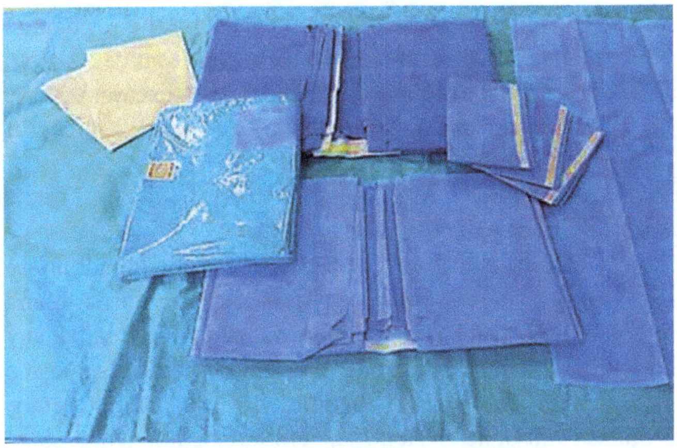



**Fig. 9.9** Different types of drapes

2. *Other-Clean:* Clean cases other than refined clean.
3. *Clean-Contaminated:* Oral cavity, gastrointestinal, or respiratory tract entered without significant spillage, entrance of genitourinary tract in presence of infected urine, entrance of biliary tract in presence of infected bile or minor break in technique.
4. *Contaminated:* Major break in operative techniques (e.g., surgical entrance of unprepared bowel without gross spillage of bowel contents); acute bacterial inflammation without pus; fresh, traumatic wound from a relatively clean source.
5. *Dirty:* Presence of pus or perforated viscous (prior to operation), old traumatic wound, or traumatic wound from a dirty source.

Currently, this classification has been condensed into four groups for general use, without a subdivision of the clean category and in the modified form it is categorized into four categories [10]

1. *Clean sites (wounds):*
   - Elective (not urgent or emergency).
   - Primary closed.
   - No acute inflammation or transection of tracheobronchial, biliary, gastrointestinal, oropharyngeal tracts.
   - No technique breaks.
2. *Clean-contaminated sites (wounds):*
   - Emergency or urgent cases that are otherwise "clean."
   - Elective procedures.
   - Reoperation via "clean incision" within 7 days.
   - Blunt trauma, intact skin, and negative exploration.
3. *Contaminated sites (wounds):*
   - Acute nonpurulent inflammation.
   - Major technique break or major spill from hollow organs.
   - Entrance of genitourinary or biliary tracts in presence of infected urine or bile, respectively.
   - Penetrating trauma less than 4 h old.
   - Chronic open wounds to be grafted or covered.
4. *Dirty sites (wounds):*
   - Purulence or abscess.
   - Preoperative perforation of tracheobronchial, biliary, gastrointestinal, oropharyngeal tracts.
   - Penetrating trauma more than 4 h old.

## 9.9 Risk Factors Affecting the Rate of Postoperative Wound Infections

*"Cut Well, Sew Well, Heal Well"* is an axiom favored by surgeons but is not always destined to be true. Altemeir and Culbertson (1965) [11] depicted that the risk of infection varies:

(a) The risk of infections is proportional directly to the dose of contamination to bacteria.
(b) The microbial virulence is also directly proportional to the risk of infections.
(c) The patient's ability to control and inhibit the resistance is proportional inversely. [12]

These factors interact in a complex way to fasten the development of infection. Since the days of Altemeier, clinical and epidemiologic studies have identified the risk factors that affect the rate of postoperative surgical site infection. This can be best explained by the classical epidemiological triangular model, i.e., model of interaction between agent host and environment resulting in disease (Fig. 9.10).

The risk of postoperative wound infection also depends on the patient factors, pre and intraoperative factors (Table 9.5). Haley et al. (1985), in the Study of the Efficacy of Nosocomial Infection Control "(SENIC)," [13] identified four independent and additive risk factors for postoperative wound infection. These factors are operation on the abdomen, operation lasting for more than 2 h, contaminated or dirty wounds (NRC CLASSIFICATION), and the presence of more than three discharge diagnoses.

- Hair removal should not be performed on routine basis to decrease the risk of surgical site infection. Razors should not be used to remove the hair as they increase the chances

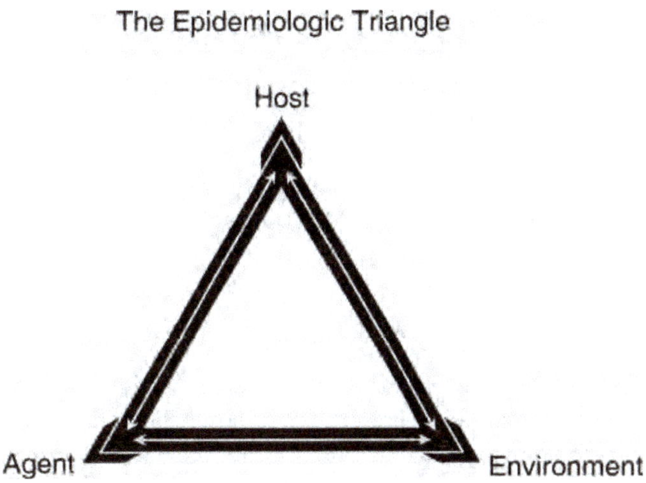




**Fig. 9.10** Classical Epidemiological triangle

**Table 9.5** Factors that predispose a patient to infection

| *Patients factors* | Preoperative factors | Intraoperative factors |
|---|---|---|
| *Age*<br>• Malnutrition<br>• Obese persons<br>• Underlying diseases<br>• Hidden infections<br>• Immunosuppressive therapy<br>• Any recent surgery<br>• Longstanding illness | • Longer duration of hospital admission<br>• Improper scrubbing prior to procedure<br>• Removal of hair<br>• Preoperative prophylactic coverage | • Contamination at the time of procedure<br>• Longer duration of the procedure<br>• Any foreign object<br>• Transfusion reactions occurring at the time of the procedure |

of infections [14]. Electric clippers with disposable heads must be used only for removing hair few hours prior to the surgical procedure.

- The treatment protocols and the condition of the patient during the hospital stay make them more prone to the spread of infections.
- Wound dressings: Cover surgical incisions with an appropriate interactive dressing at the end of the operation.

## 9.9.1 Factors Influencing the Development of Nosocomial Infections

### 9.9.1.1 The Microbial Agent

Hospital infections occur as a result of a variety of microorganisms. The microorganisms causing the disease may be divided into the following categories:

1. Conventional pathogens are the ones that are capable of causing a disease in normal and healthy person.
2. Conditional pathogens are the ones that initiate the onset of a disease in persons who have decreased immunological response to infection or when implanted directly into sterile area or tissues.
3. Opportunistic pathogens are the ones that normally do not harm its host but can cause disease when the host's resistance to the microorganisms is low.

During the stay in a hospital, the patient comes in contact with various kinds of microbial agents (such as viruses, fungi, parasites, and bacteria), which are the main cause of the occurrence of infections in a patient. This exposure is not the only reason for the development of hospital-acquired infections. The other possible reasons are the host's natural defense mechanisms (healthy/compromised/immunosuppressed), conditions present in a hospital environment, microbiology of the microbial agents (characteristic features), infective material present on the microbial agent, resistance to the antimicrobial agents, and other factors. The hospital-based infections may be a result of the spread of infection from one person to the other or by the residential flora of the patient or from any contaminated sources or from sources of the external origin (e.g., airborne diseases).

Following are the factors that are the main sources of spread of hospital-based infections:

### 9.9.1.2 Susceptibility of the Patient

Patient factors that lead to the occurrence of infection are age, host's immune response, presence of any disease, and interventions, which either help in diagnosing or treating any condition. Patients, either infant or older individuals, are at a higher risk of acquiring infections. Patients having a compromised immune system, undernourished, having some underlying chronic disease (AIDS, leukemia, malignant tumors, renal failure, diabetes mellitus, etc.), undergoing irradiation therapy, all at the highest risk of being infected by the hospital-based infections. Certain processes like catheterization, biopsy, intubations, etc. make the patient more vulnerable to these infections.

### 9.9.1.3 Resistance of the Bacteria

Resistance of bacteria to antimicrobial agents is seen with the prolonged or prophylactic use of these agents. The microbial agents present normally in the human flora have both sensitive and resistant strains. Some antimicrobial agents have their action on sensitive strains by suppressing their activity, whereas the resistant strains are still active. These active resistant strains are the major cause of the development of resistance against the antimicrobial agents. Examples of resistant microbial agents are Multiresistant Klebsiella, strains of pneumococci, staphylococci, etc. In low-income or middle-income countries, this is the major problem faced due to unavailability and unaffordability of the better drugs.

### 9.9.1.4 Month of Operation

The possible explanation for increased infection rates in summer is the relatively high environmental temperature leading to humid climate, resulting in excessive sweating. In addition, excessive sweating results in the displacement of bacteria lodged in skin appendages to the surface.

### 9.9.1.5 Use of Electric Cautery

The use of electric cautery for cutting and coagulation during surgery causes more inflammation; more necrosis and abscess than the conventional use of scalpel and thus it increases the susceptibility of tissue for infection. Soballe et al [15], in their experimental study, found that electric cautery lowers the contamination threshold for infection of laparotomies and concluded that electric coagulation current should be used only when the need for meticulous hemostasis outweighs the considerably increases risk of infection.

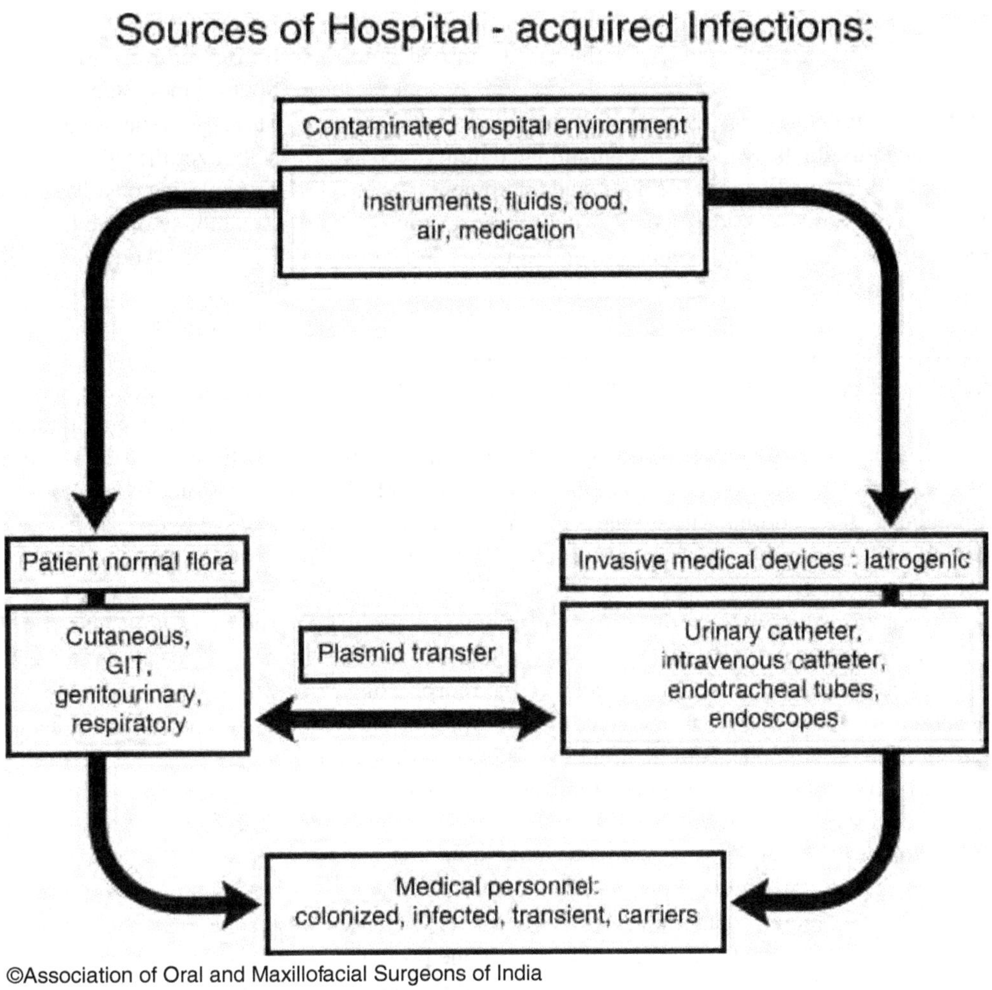


**Fig. 9.11** Sources of hospital-acquired infections

#### 9.9.1.6 Duration of Operation

There is a direct correlation between the infection rate and time taken for the procedure. This may be the result of the more complicated operations being of longer duration, increased wound contamination from airborne bacteria, increased damage to the tissues due to large exposure of the wound, and increased manipulation; moreover, local resistance of tissue is reduced due to drying.

#### 9.9.1.7 Spread of Infection

The microbial agents are spread by different ways in a health care setup. The different ways with which the agents can spread are contacting, droplets, airborne route, via vehicle, and vector-borne (Fig. 9.11).

Sources of the infectious agents are either external, i.e., from one person to the other, or from the hospital's environment; or internal, i.e., within the patient himself.

- *Contacting* is the most frequent and important route of spread of infections. It is further of two types, i.e.
  - *Direct* contacting is the spread of infection directly from the person infected from the infection to other normal who has increased chances of being infected. It also occurs among two patients where one acts the source of microbial agents and the other becomes the one to receive the infection.
- *Indirect* contacting is the spread of infection indirectly from one person/object to the other. It involves contact of a susceptible host with a contaminated intermediate object. Droplets spread results due to generation of droplets from the source person mainly during coughing, sneezing, and talking, and during the performance of certain procedures such as bronchoscopy, which can travel a shorter distance via air and get deposited on the body of the other susceptible person.
- *Airborne transmission* results from spreading of small particulate matter (approximately 5 pm or smaller in size) through the air, which remain suspended in the air for a longer period of time. These particles are passed from one individual to the other by the process of inhalation of

these particles. The main diseases to be spread via the airborne route are Tuberculosis, Influenza, Common cold, etc.

- *Vehicle spread* is the spread of infectious microbial agents to the individuals by means of contaminated items such as food, water, medications, devices, and equipment.

*Vector*-borne transmission occurs when vectors such as mosquitoes, flies, rats, and other vermin transmit microorganisms.

## 9.10 COVID 19 and Maxillofacial Surgery

The occupational risk of acquiring viral diseases has been well known in Maxillofacial Surgery [16]. The WHO announced the Corona virus pandemic also known as COVID-19 as a public health emergency of international concern on January 30, 2020.

Coronaviruses are RNA viruses infecting many species of animals including humans, name coronavirus was derived from corona meaning crown like because of the morphology observed for these viruses in the electron microscope. This family of viruses includes Middle East Respiratory Syndrome (MERS-CoV), Severe Acute Respiratory Syndrome (SARS-CoV), and novel Coronavirus (n CoV).

Coronavirus is enveloped having round, spherical, or sometimes pleomorphic structure, with size ranging from 80 to 120 nm in diameter, containing a positive-strand RNA. The virus is made up of lipid bilayer envelop, membrane protein, and nucleocapsid, these structures also protect the virus when the virus is outside the host cell. The lipid bilayer forms the viral envelop which anchors the membrane protein, envelop protein, and the spike protein. The spike protein (S-protein) is responsible for the crown-like structure of the coronavirus as it forms the protrusions from the surface which bind to the host cells.

### 9.10.1 Mode of Transmission of SARs-CoV 2

Human to human transmission is due to respiratory droplet transmission and contact transmission. Spread occurs through coughing, sneezing, spitting, contacting the body fluids of the infected patient. The COVID-19 can remain infectious on inanimate surfaces from 2 h to 9 days, depending on the humidity, temperature, surface type, and viral load [17]. It has become an occupational threat to health care providers worldwide.

Some of the known routes of spread of infection to health care providers are:

- Manual ventilation with a bag and mask
- Intubation
- Open endotracheal suctioning
- Bronchoscopy
- Cardiopulmonary resuscitation
- Sputum induction
- Surgery on the lungs
- Nebulizer therapy
- Noninvasive positive pressure ventilation (BIPAP, CPAP)
- An autopsy on the lungs
- High-speed devices such as those used for surgery, post-mortem
- Dental procedures

Aerosols generating procedures (AGP) create widespread environmental contamination and therefore pose a greater risk of transmission of infection to healthcare workers. Oral and maxillofacial surgeons are particularly vulnerable to this transmissible disease by way of the droplet or aerosol transmission due to the area of work and the type of instrumentation [18].

The incubation period is long and unpredictable ranging from 0 to 27 days with a mean of 6.4 days. Recent studies have shown that asymptomatic patients and those within the incubation period are also potential spreaders of the disease [19].

### 9.10.2 Symptoms

Symptoms may range from mild symptoms to severe respiratory distress and some patients may be asymptomatic.

- Common symptoms may include fever, cough, fatigue, shortness of breath, loss of taste, and smell.
- Less common symptoms may include myalgia, headache sore throat, and chills.
- Rare symptoms may include nausea, vomiting, nasal congestion, diarrhea, palpitation, and chest congestion.

### 9.10.3 Radiographic Findings

- **Chest X-ray** may show findings that of atypical pneumonia showing bilateral consolidations in lateral lower lobes, bronchovascular thickening.
- **Chest CT** ground-glass opacity and areas of consolidation laterally.

### 9.10.4 Testing and Laboratory Findings

The real time polymerase chain reaction (RT-PCR) of respiratory secretions from bronchoalveolar lavage, endotracheal aspirate, and nasopharyngeal or oropharyngeal swab is the definitive test.

Other laboratory findings include lymphopenia, increased prothrombin time, and mildly raised CRP and ESR.

### 9.10.5 General Preventive Measures

COVID 19 has shifted the focus on teleconsulting which includes tele screening, telemedicine, and triage. Telemedicine should be practiced whenever possible to decrease the footfall.

Thorough history should be obtained from the patient regarding COVID 19 illness and elective procedures should be postponed and only emergent conditions should be taken up for surgery.

Patient should be called on the basis of appointments, time between two appointments should be sufficient enough to perform all necessary sanitization measures and ensure minimal patient to patient overlap. In the waiting area, posters should be displayed to encourage hand hygiene and the wearing of masks and the area should be well ventilated. A minimum of 2 m distance should be maintained between the individuals.

Extraoral radiographs should be preferred as an alternative to intraoral periapical radiographs.

In the operatory there should be minimum personnel present, Air Conditioners should be avoided, doors and windows are advised to be kept open. The operating room should be spacious with adjoining two rooms for donning and doffing of the PPE's. No touch sensor-based sanitizer dispenser should be installed at the entry and exit of OR [20].

All the surfaces of equipment like OR table, motor drills etc., should be covered with plastic sheets and sheets to be changed after every patient.

OT's should be equipped with HEPA filter (0.1 micron efficiency) and high frequency of air changes (ideally 25 per hour) should be ensured to reduce the viral load [20].

High-volume suctions should be used with one-third of suction jars prefilled with povidone-iodine solution.

The Povidone Iodine solution has been shown to have significant viricidal activity up to 3 h and it has been advised to coat the oral cavity and nasal passages of both the patient and the operating team before the surgery [21, 22].

Fogger machines with 0.5% sodium hypochlorite can be used for sterilization of dental chairs, tables, doors, doorknob, etc. [20]. One-minute contact of the chemical ensures viral kill.

### 9.10.6 Personal Protective Equipment

- Masks including three-ply surgical masks, N95, N99 (FFP3), and the Powered air-purifying respirators (PAPR's) provide viral filtration in the increasing order. It is important to mention that N95 masks were not found to be adequate to prevent transmission in Chinese surgeons and PAPR's had to be used to prevent transmission from COVID patients [23].
- Surgical gloves.
- Goggles and cover all gowns.
- Triple protection gowns and face shield protect the surgeon from exposure to any kind of infected aerosols, body fluids of the patient. Disposable gowns are made of nonwoven material and protect from liquid penetration. Personal protective equipment like basic kit 45 GSM, medium kit 70 GSM for surgery, and advance kit for ICU 180 GSM are recommended to be worn [20].

### 9.10.7 Specific Precautions to Be Taken During Surgery

- Surgery on COVID patient should be performed in a negative pressure theater or in airborne infection isolation room [20].
- Focus should be on minimally invasive techniques whenever possible which could reduce the time of surgery and/or reduce aerosol generation.
- Local anesthesia with appropriate sedation should be preferred over GA.
- The surgeon should enter the theater after 20 min following intubation with complete PPE to minimize the exposure to aerosols [23].
- Scalpels should be preferred over cautery.
- Use of high-power drills, oscillating saw, and forceful irrigation should be avoided.
- Absorbable sutures should be used to avoid unnecessary trips of the patient [18].

As the COVID-19 situation is a dynamic evolving one and there is no definitive treatment available proper planning and implementation of infection control protocols are key to preventing transmission of the disease in the Maxillofacial settings.

## 9.11 Control of Nosocomial Infections

CDC elucidated certain guidelines to check the nosocomial infections in the Study on efficacy of nosocomial infection control (SENIC). These guidelines have decreased the emergence of hospital-acquired infections by a greater number. However, any breach in the infection control procedures can lead to spread of such infections.

Certain conditions leading to improper infection control and spread of such infections are:

1. Improper sterilization and disinfection procedures.
2. Presence of contaminants in the food or water

3. Environment of the health care setup.
4. Untrained and inadequate personnel
5. Insufficient knowledge of Infection control principles and practices among the staff.
6. Antibiotic abuse both in the community and in the hospital.

### 9.11.1 Prevention from Nosocomial Infections

Following are the steps that can be taken by the staff in a hospital setup to prevent the spread of such infections:

- Isolation rooms for persons suffering from contagious diseases such as COVID 19 and tuberculosis.
- Hand-scrubbing practices prior to performing any procedure.
- Disinfecting all the areas in a health care setup.
- Adequate sterilization and disinfection protocols to be followed everywhere.
- The wound dressings should be changed at an appropriate time with the use of proper agents.
- The antimicrobial agents should be carefully used. Prolonged use should be avoided whenever possible to avoid the emergence of the resistance.
- Proper management of the biomedical waste.

## 9.12 Conclusion

Preventing and controlling infections is the key factor in improving care and ensuring safety of both the patient and the health care worker. Infection control addresses factors related to the spread of infections within the operation theater complex (whether patient-to-patient, from patients to staff and from staff to patient, or among staff), including prevention (via hand hygiene/hand washing, cleaning/disinfection/sterilization, vaccination, monitoring).

Integrated infection control in the operation theater has various aspects, ranging from its designing ,environmental cleaning , management of biomedical waste and adherence to theatre attire. Use of Personal Protective Equipment (PPE) including gloves, gowns, face masks ,respirators and full face visors are essential to minimize risks of occupational infections. Whether in developed or developing country, where resources are limited, thorough knowledge about the principles of infection control and a little ingenuity will suffice to solve the problem of hospital-acquired infections.

Surgical site infections are a result of microbial invasion in a sterile atmosphere. The main sources of microbial invasion in the operating theater include the atmosphere of the operating theater, the medical and the paramedical staff present at the time of the procedure, surgical instruments, and the patient at times also. Proper designing of operation theater, appropriate microbiological monitoring, proper sterilization, and strict adherence to barrier techniques form the basis to prevent infections in an operating environment.

## References


1. Weiser TG, Regenbogen SE, Thompson KD, Haynes AB, Lipsitz SR, Berry WR, Gawande AA. An estimation of the global volume of surgery: a modelling strategy based on available data. Lancet. 2008 Jul 12;372(9633):139–44.
2. Weiser TG, Haynes AB, Molina G, Lipsitz SR, Esquivel MM, Uribe-Leitz T, Fu R, Azad T, Chao TE, Berry WR, Gawande AA. Size and distribution of the global volume of surgery in 2012. Bull World Health Organ. 2016 Mar 1;94(3):201.
3. Bali R, Sharma P, Nagrath S, Gupta P. Microbial isolations from maxillofacial operation theatre and its correlation to fumigation in a teaching hospital in India. Journal of maxillofacial and oral surgery. 2014 Jun 1;13(2):128–32.
4. de Lissovoy G, Fraeman K, Hutchins V, Murphy D, Song D, Vaughn BB. Surgical site infection: incidence and impact on hospital utilization and treatment costs. Am J Infect Control. 2009 Jun 1;37(5):387–97.
5. Block SS. Definition of terms. Disinfection, sterilization, and preservation. Philadelphia: Lippincott Williams & Wilkins. 2001:19–28.
6. Bratzler DW, Houck PM, Workgroup SI. Antimicrobial prophylaxis for surgery: an advisory statement from the National Surgical Infection Prevention Project. Am J Surg. 2005 Apr 1;189(4):395–404.
7. Safety WP, World Health Organization. WHO guidelines for safe surgery: 2009: safe surgery saves lives. Geneva: World Health Organization; 2009.
8. Petersen BT, Chennat J, Cohen J, Cotton PB, Greenwald DA, Kowalski TE, Krinsky ML, Park WG, Pike IM, Romagnuolo J, Rutala WA. Multisociety guideline on reprocessing flexible gastrointestinal endoscopes: 2011. Gastrointest Endosc. 2011;73(6):1075–84.
9. B'erard F. Postoperative wound infections: the influence of ultraviolet irradiation of the operating room and of various other factors. Ann Surg. 1964;160(1):1–92.
10. Knight R, Charbonneau P, Ratzer E, Zeren F, Haun W, Clark J. Prophylactic antibiotics are not indicated in clean general surgery cases. Am J Surg. 2001 Dec 1;182(6):682–6.
11. Altemeier WA, Culbertson WR, Hummel RP. Surgical considerations of endogenous infections—sources, types, and methods of control. Surg Clin N Am. 1968 Feb 1;48(1):227–40.
12. Cheng H, Chen BP, Soleas IM, Ferko NC, Cameron CG, Hinoul P. Prolonged operative duration increases risk of surgical site infections: a systematic review. Surg Infect. 2017 Aug 1;18(6):722–35.
13. Haley RW, Culver DH, Morgan WM, White JW, Emori TG, Hooton TM. Identifying patients at high risk of surgical wound infection: a simple multivariate index of patient susceptibility and wound contamination. Am J Epidemiol. 1985;121(2):206–15.
14. Edmiston CE, Lee CJ, Krepel CJ, Spencer M, Leaper D, Brown KR, Lewis BD, Rossi PJ, Malinowski MJ, Seabrook GR. Evidence for a standardized preadmission showering regimen to achieve maximal antiseptic skin surface concentrations of chlorhexi-

dine gluconate, 4%, in surgical patients. JAMA Surg. 2015 Nov 1;150(11):1027–33.
15. Soballe PW, Nimbkar NV, Hayward I, Nielsen TB, Drucker WR. Electric cautery lowers the contamination threshold for infection of laparotomies. Am J Surg. 1998 Apr;175(4):263–6.
16. Bali R, Sharma P, Garg A. Incidence and patterns of needlestick injuries during Intermaxillary fixation. Br J Oral Maxillofac Surg. 2011;49:221–4.
17. Kampf G, Todt D, Pfaender S, Steinmann E. Persistence of coronaviruses on inanimate surfaces and their inactivation with biocidal agents. J Hosp Infect. 2020;104(3):246–51.
18. Bali RK, Chaudhry K. Maxillofacial surgery and COVID-19, The pandemic!! J Maxillofac Oral Surg. 2020;19(2):159–61.
19. Meng L, Hua F, Bian Z. Coronavirus disease 2019 (COVID-19): Emerging and future challenges for dental and oral medicine. J Dent Res. 2020;99(5):481–7.
20. Datarkar A, Purohit S, Tayal S, Bhawalkar . Operating room protocols in OMFS during Corona virus (Covid-19) pandemic. J Maxillofac Oral Surg. 2020;19(3):327–31.
21. Eggers M, Koburger-Janssen T, Eickmann M, Zorn J. In vitro bactericidal and virucidal efficacy of povidone-iodine gargle/mouthwash against respiratory and oral tract pathogens. Infect Dis Ther. 2018;7:249–59.
22. Kirk-Bayley J, Challacombe S, Sunkaraneni V, Combes J. The use of povidone iodine nasal spray and mouthwash during the current COVID-19 pandemic may protect healthcare workers and reduce cross infection. Br Dent J. 2020;228(12):902.
23. https://aocmf3.aofoundation.org/#o=News%20Date%20Facet,Descending. Accessed 30 Mar 2020

# 10

# Role of Pharmacology and Pharmacotherapy in OMS

Latha P. Rao

> The human fascination—and sometimes infatuation—with chemicals that alter biological function is ancient and results from long experience with, and dependence on, plants. Many plants produce harmful compounds for defense that animals have learned to avoid and humans to exploit [1]

## 10.1 Introduction

With phenomenal increase in the knowledge about mechanism of action of chemical compounds and rapid introduction of new drugs, pharmacology—the science of drugs—has become increasingly important to all health professionals. Practice of maxillofacial surgery utilizes drugs either as primary treatment modality or as a facilitator of surgical procedures. A detailed description of the pharmacodynamics & pharmacokinetics of these drugs is beyond the scope of this chapter. The readers are encouraged to refer to the standard textbooks of pharmacology for the same.

## 10.2 Antimicrobial Agents

Infections caused by microorganisms have threatened human life since time immemorial. Some of the organisms had the potential to spread from one infected person to another at an alarming rate causing worldwide pandemics and epidemics. With the discovery of the first antibiotic, "the magic bullet"—Penicillin, patients could effectively be cured of many life- threatening infections [2].

Antimicrobial agents are of the few classes of drugs that effectively treat the etiology of conditions and not simply alleviate the symptoms of the diseases.

L. P. Rao (✉)
Department of craniomaxillofacial surgery, Aster Medcity, Kochi, Kerala, India

### 10.2.1 Definition

The term antibiotic was first used by Selman Waksman et al. to describe any substance produced by a microorganism that is antagonistic to the growth of other microorganisms in high dilution [3]. This definition excluded substances like gastric juices and hydrogen peroxide that kill bacteria but are not produced by microorganisms. It also excluded synthetic antibacterial compounds like the sulfonamides. In current usage, however, the term "antibiotic" is applied to any medication that kills bacteria or inhibits their growth, regardless of whether that medication is produced by a microorganism or not.

### 10.2.2 Classification

The antibiotics have been classified in many ways, based on their chemical nature, mechanism of action, type of organisms against which primarily active spectrum of activity, etc. (Table 10.1). The antibiotics exert their remarkably specific action on the microorganisms, sparing the host, due to their selectivity for target components, which are either absent or not very important in humans. Among these targets are bacterial and fungal cell wall synthesizing enzymes, the bacterial ribosome, the enzymes required for nucleotide synthesis and DNA replication, etc.

### 10.2.3 Oral Microflora

The infectious diseases associated with the oral and maxillofacial region have unique microbiological features because of the abundance and variety of microorganisms in this region. The normal flora of the oral cavity consists of up to $10^{11}$ bacteria per gram of tissue, with anaerobic bacteria predominating [4]. Although the subtypes and proportions of organisms differ, the general pattern of the indigenous

**Table 10.1** Different classes of antibiotics—based on their chemical structure and mechanism of actions

| Class of antibiotics | Common examples | Mechanism of action | Bacteriostatic / Bactericidal |
|---|---|---|---|
| *Beta lactams*—most widely used | (a) Penicillins<br>(b) Cephalosporins | Inhibit bacterial cell wall synthesis | Bactericidal |
| *Sulfonamides*—first commercial antibiotics | (a) Sulfanilamide<br>(b) Sulfadiazine<br>(c) Sulfizoxazole | Prevent bacterial growth and multiplication | Bacteriostatic |
| *Aminoglycosides* | (a) Streptomycin<br>(b) Neomycin<br>(c) Kanamycin<br>(d) Paramomycin | Inhibit bacterial protein synthesis | Bactericidal |
| *Tetracyclines*—more chances of resistance formation | (a) Tetracyclines<br>(b) Doxycycline<br>(c) Oxytretracycline | Inhibit bacterial protein synthesis | Bacteriostatic |
| *Chloramphenicol*—first line of drug only in conjunctivitis | | Inhibit bacterial protein synthesis | Bacteriostatic |
| *Macrolides*—second most prescribed | (a) Erythromycin<br>(b) Clarithromycin<br>(c) Azithromycin | Inhibit bacterial protein synthesis | Bacteriostatic |
| *Glycopeptides*—last-resort drugs | (a) Vancomycin<br>(b) Teicoplanin | Inhibit bacterial cell wall synthesis | Bactericidal |
| *Ansamycins*—have antiviral activity also | (a) Geldanamycin<br>(b) Rifamycin<br>(c) Naphthomycin | Inhibit bacterial RNA synthesis | Bactericidal |
| *Quinolones*—rapid development of resistance | (a) Ciprofloxacin<br>(b) Levofloxacin<br>(c) Trovafloxacin | Inhibit bacterial cell wall synthesis | Bactericidal |
| *Streptogramins* - two groups of antibiotics that act synergistically | (a) Pristinamycin I A<br>(b) Pristinamycin II A | Inhibit bacterial protein synthesis | Bactericidal |
| *Oxazolidinones*—potent last-resort drugs | (a) Linezolid<br>(b) Posizolid<br>(c) Tedizolid<br>(d) Cycloserine | Inhibit bacterial protein synthesis | Bacteriostatic |
| *Leptopeptides*—instances of resistance rare | (a) Daptomycin<br>(b) Surfactin | Disrupt multiple cell-membrane functions | Bactericidal |

microflora is similar in healthy individuals. However, systemic diseases and concurrent use of medications result in the presence of unusual organisms as part of the normal flora and an increase in diseases caused by normal organisms that usually are considered to have low pathogenicity. Usually, the microorganisms are held in check by the body's defense mechanisms. When these mechanisms are impaired, infection may result from an otherwise minor bacterial exposure.

The pathobiology of mixed odontogenic infection is relatively clear. The early cellulitis is the result of streptococci, the moderate-to-severe infection is caused by a combination of aerobic and anaerobic bacteria, and the well- circumscribed chronic abscess is caused primarily by anaerobic bacilli alone [5]. A complex mix of strict anaerobes and facultative anaerobes account for most of the odontogenic infections. Empirical antibiotic choices can be made in this situation where the microbiological pattern is well established (Table 10.2).

### 10.2.4 Guidelines to the Therapeutic Use of Antibiotics

Understanding that infections are ultimately dealt by the host's immune systems, and antibiotics play only an adjunctive role, is critical. Antibiotic therapy should be reserved for those with clearly established infection. Surgical treatment of the infection also should be initiated as early as possible.

Antibiotics help in preventing infections after a contamination has happened or they can abort a developing infection, if administered early. Antibiotics should not be used as a substitute for the needed surgical treatment.

In most clinical situations, it is easy to determine whether a patient has an infection—local and systemic findings would point to the diagnosis. Diagnostic difficulty arises when a patient who has had a maxillofacial procedure performed, during the second or third day after surgery, develops swelling and pain. Similarly, elevated temperature and white blood cell count also may be found. Surgical insult and

**Table 10.2** Efficacy of commonly used antibiotics against head and neck pathogens and dosage

| Antibiotics | Aerobes | Staphylococcus | Anaerobes | Dose |
|---|---|---|---|---|
| Penicillin | Excellent | No action | Guarded against prevotella, porphyromonas, fusobacterium, bacteroides | Penicillin G- 6,00,000 – 1,200,000 u q4h im/iv<br>Penicillin V – 250-500 mg q6h orally |
| Amoxycillin / clavulanate | Excellent | Active | Guarded against prevotella, porphyromonas, fusobacterium, bacteroides | 375-625 mg q8h orally<br>1.2 g q8h im/iv |
| Cefuroxime | Excellent with all except guarded action against capnocytophaga and no action against eikenella | Active | No action against prevotella, porphyromonas, fusobacterium, bacteroides | 1.5 g q8h im/iv |
| Erythromycin | Good, guarded against capnocytophaga & eikenella | Active | Guarded action against fusobacterium, no action against prevotella, porphyromonas, bacteroides | 250-500 mg q6h orally<br>1-4 g /day in divided doses q6h iv for severe infections |
| Clindamycin | Excellent | Active | Active | 150–300 mg q8h orally<br>1200–2400 mg /day in divided doses q8h for severe infections |
| Ciprofloxacin | Good | Guarded action | Guarded action | 500 mg q12h orally<br>400 mg q12h iv |
| Metronidazole | No action | No action | Active | 400 mg q8h orally<br>500 mg q8h iv |

prolonged general anesthesia often result in these symptoms. Clinical judgment is important in making the diagnosis, and the clinician should weigh all information available before making the diagnosis of infection.

There are a few basic guidelines to be followed in the administration of antibiotics (Table 10.3).

### 10.2.5 Consistency in Route of Administration

In severe infection, parenteral antibiotics are needed to get adequate blood levels. But with an initial response within couple of days, one is always tempted to switch to oral administration. When this is done, the infection may recur because blood levels achieved with oral dose are suboptimal. Maintenance of peak blood levels of antibiotic, until eradication of bacteria, is important, which may take 5–6 days. After the fifth day of parenteral administration, the blood levels achievable with oral administration are usually sufficient.

### 10.2.6 Cross-allerginicity between Penicillins & Cephalosporins

A frequently asked question about penicillin allergic patients is whether the cephalosporins can be used safely. Overall the frequency of crossallergenicity between the two groups of drugs is low (7–18%) [10, 11]. Cross-allergenicity appears to be most common among penicillin, aminopenicillins, and early-generation cephalosporins, which share similar R-1 side chains; this is thought to increase the risk of cross-reactivity. Patients with a history of anaphylaxis to penicillins should not receive first- or second-generation cephalosporins, while third- and fourth-generation cephalosporins should be administered with caution, preferably in a monitored setting.

### 10.2.7 Patient Monitoring

The patient should be monitored for the response to treatment and any deterrent should be identified and rectified. A second empirical choice should be avoided, if at all possible because the likelihood of success is substantially less. Repeat cultures may also be attempted.

In some cases, the patient may respond well to the empirical antibiotics, but the culture and sensitivity report would reveal that the organisms isolated are resistant to the antibiotics being used. The combined surgical and antibiotic treatment, along with natural host defenses, would have resulted in resolution of infection. The antibiotic may or may not have played an important role. The antibiotic that was clinically effective for the patient should be continued despite the contradictory data.

## 10.3 General Considerations in the Prophylactic Use of Antibiotics

The original guidelines for timing and use of antibiotics to prevent infection postoperatively were established by Burke and Miles et al.'s experimental observations [12, 13]. They

**Table 10.3** Guidelines for the use of antibiotics

1. *Empirical therapy*
2. *Identification* of the organisms—obtain culture & sensitivity in
   (a) Compromised host defenses
   (b) Persistence of infection in spite of appropriate antibiotics & surgical therapy.
   (c) Postoperative infection
   (d) Suspected cases of actinomycosis, osteomyelitis
3. Use of *specific narrow-spectrum antibiotic*—to prevent/ minimize bacterial resistance [6] & superinfections [7].
4. Reserve *combination therapy* for:
   (a) Patient with life-threatening sepsis of unknown cause
   (b) Increased bactericidal effect against a specific organism is required
   (c) Prevention of rapid emergence of resistant bacteria—e.g., tuberculosis
   (d) Empiric treatment for certain odontogenic infections—that are rapidly progressing posteriorly around the neck space
5. Use of antibiotics with proven history of success
6. Use of the least toxic antibiotic
7. Use of a *bactericidal* rather than a bacteriostatic drug
8. *Proper administration*: Dose, time interval, route of administration, & consistency in the route of administration
9. Cost of the antibiotics
10. *Patient compliance*—decreases with increasing number of pills [8]
11. *Patient monitoring*—initially a subjective sense of feeling better, then look for reduction in swelling, pain, & temperature [9]
12. *Causes of failure of antibiotic therapy*:
    (a) Inadequate surgical intervention –
        (i) Failure to drain pus,
        (ii) Increasing pressure inside tissue spaces,
        (iii) Retained nonvital tissue or foreign body.
    (b) Other sources of infection—IV catheter, Foley's catheter
    (c) Reduced or compromised host defenses—immunocompromised, malnourished, dehydrated patients
    (d) Mistakes in antibiotic administration
        (i) Improper route of administration,
        (ii) Inadequate dosage,
        (iii) Patient noncompliance,
        (iv) Incorrect carrying out of physician's orders.
    (e) Wrong culture report or misinterpretation of the culture report

noted that antibiotics must be given within 4 h after injection of bacteria into a surgical site to prevent the aggressive level of infection that occurs when no antibiotics are administered.

Antibiotic prophylaxis entails administering the antibiotic appropriate for the potential microbial contamination before the surgical insult, at a high enough dosage to establish an appropriate bacteriologic titer [14].

1. *Indications for antibiotic prophylaxis* [15, 16] are given in Table 10.4.
2. *Condition & bacterial contamination of the surgical area*: Surgical wounds are generally classified into clean, clean–contaminated, contaminated, and dirty/infected [16–18] (Table 10.5).

   With judicious use of antibiotics, the infection rates are known to be lesser [16, 18].

**Table 10.4** Indications for antibiotic prophylaxis

1. Compromised host defenses
   (a) Physiological—old age, obesity, malnutrition
   (b) Disturbances in circulation—massive transfusion, recent surgery
   (c) Disease related—poorly controlled diabetes, cancer, leukemia, alcoholic cirrhosis, end-stage renal diseases
   (d) Compromised immunity—multiple myeloma, total body irradiation, splenectomy
   (e) Immunosuppressants—cytotoxic drugs, glucocorticoids, azathioprine, cyclosporine
2. Potential for bacterial contamination of a sterile field
3. Procedures with high infection rate
4. Surgical procedures in which there is a high mortality / morbidity rate following infection
5. When a foreign body is inserted into the tissues

**Table 10.5** Classification of surgical wounds

| Type | Incidence of infection (values given for general surgical cases) | Examples for the types of surgical wounds in maxillofacial surgery |
|---|---|---|
| Clean | 1-5% | Temporomandibular joint surgery, facial cosmetic surgery |
| Clean–contaminated | 3-11% | Orthognathic procedures, extractions |
| Contaminated | 10-17% | Maxillary fracture with active maxillary sinusitis |
| Dirty wound | >27% | Mandibular fracture through an infected third molar socket |

**Table 10.6** Need for postoperative antibiotics

| | |
|---|---|
| 1 | Compromised immunity |
| 2 | Inflammation at the surgical site |
| 3 | Evidence of wound dehiscence |
| 4 | Active periodontal disease |
| 5 | Poor oral hygiene |
| 6 | Inadequate surgical skill |
| 7 | Prolonged surgery |
| 8 | Wound contamination during surgery |

3. The *selected antibiotic should be bactericidal* against the most common microorganisms that cause infection in the oral cavity. The bactericidal antibiotics rely less on the host defense mechanisms providing faster results [18].
4. The *concentration of antibiotics* in the tissue should be sufficient to fight the bacteria that may enter the surgical wound at incision or during the course of surgery. To achieve a blood concentration of *three-four fold that of minimum inhibitory concentration*, the antibiotic is typically given at twice the treatment dose *1 h prior to surgery* [14, 16].
5. Usually antibiotics can be administered as a single preoperative dose. In cases where the surgeon feels that postoperative infection is a high possibility, the drug can be *extended postoperatively as deemed necessary* [19] (Table 10.6).

One must be vigilant in identifying cases where antibiotics are required for the success of surgery, as antibiotic usage and overusage have considerable risks [6, 7, 20, 21]—gastrointestinal disturbances, toxicity reactions, antibiotic resistance and superinfections, anaphylaxis, pseudomembraneous colitis, etc.

### 10.3.1 Prophylactic Uses of Antibiotics in Maxillofacial Surgery

Infection, one of the most common postoperative complications, can be prevented by the timely use of appropriate antibiotic. In spite of many studies in literature, a definitive conclusion cannot be made regarding the need for antibiotic prophylaxis in maxillofacial surgery and, if needed, the dose required. The antibiotic prescription pattern is still hugely based on personal preferences and shows wide regional variation, which many a time is inappropriate. The drugs would be initiated either at an incorrect time, or would be continued beyond the time required, and this has greatly contributed to the emergence of resistant bacteria [6].

Prophylactic use of antibiotics should be evidence based taking into consideration the effectiveness and the possible adverse outcomes of antibiotic therapy. Moreover, a thorough knowledge of the likely organisms involved in the infection is needed to prevent the prescription of unsuitable antibiotics. Antibiotics, if needed, should have a spectrum of activity that involves streptococci, anaerobic Gram-positive cocci, and anaerobic Gram-negative rods, which are considered the most pathogenic for oral infections and should be bactericidal and the least toxic agents available - amoxicillin being the most common choice of the clinicians [12, 18].

The need for antibiotic prophylaxis and the preferable drugs for wisdom teeth removal, orthognathic surgery, dental implants, maxillofacial trauma, and in special circumstances like patients with diabetes mellitus, patients—pre- and post-organ transplant, rheumatic heart disease—valve replacements, oncological surgery & reconstruction, cleft surgeries, etc. are mentioned in the following sessions.

### 10.3.2 Antibiotic Prophylaxis in the Surgical Removal of Wisdom Teeth

Though one of the most commonly performed minor oral surgical procedures, the reported infection rate with the removal of mandibular third molars is ≤10% [22]. However, the rate can be as high as 25% when the patient's immunity is compromised [20]. The infection rate associated with the corresponding procedure in maxilla is quite low, <1% [20, 22]. The higher rate of postoperative infection in relation to mandibular third molar has been attributed to the reduced vascularization and the gravity-induced pooling of bacterial-rich saliva.

The prophylactic use of antibiotics in wisdom teeth removal had been an issue of many debates. There are studies for [20, 23] and against [24, 25] the practice of antibiotic prophylaxis in third molar removal. Considering the potentially contaminating oral environment in which the third molar removal is carried out, it is reasonable to favor antibiotic prophylaxis. Moreover, since the postoperative infection and alveolar osteitis, an inflammatory response whose etiology could be traced to bacterial contamination and fibrinolysis of the socket blood clot, cause debilitating pain and severe functional impairment, it is only prudent to consider the use of prophylactic antibiotics.

Studies have shown that preoperative administration of antibiotics reduces the postoperative infection when administered 1-2 h prior to the procedure [26, 27]. Amoxicillin/amoxicillin—clavulanic acid is the widely used antibiotic in the prophylaxis for the surgical removal of impacted teeth [28] and when given as a single dose preoperatively is found to reduce postoperative infection and alveolar osteitis [21]. But certain other studies have failed to show a considerable difference between amoxicillin, clindamycin, metronidazole, and placebo in terms of postoperative infection rates [25]. Studies have found topical tetracycline [29], chlorhexidine irrigation [30],& metronidazole dressings [31]into the mandibular third molar sockets, effective in reducing the postoperative infection & the incidence of dry socket. Review of literature does not give definite indication to use of antibiotics as prophylaxis in healthy patients or asymptomatic impacted teeth and in case of the removal of maxillary wisdom teeth [22].

Studies have advocated the use of antibiotic prophylaxis in immunocompromised patients to prevent infection after surgical removal of impacted teeth [22].

Two recent meta-analyses [28, 32] summarize the antibiotic prophylaxis in wisdom teeth removal (Table 10.7).

### 10.3.3 Antibiotic Prophylaxis in the Placement of Dental Implants

Dental implants play a crucial role in the successful restoration of missing dentition. The success rate of dental implants is high, with only 0-10% of reported failure rates [33]. However, risk of failure is high during the first year after implant placement [34]. The implant surfaces can become colonized by oral and perioral microorganisms during surgery (perioperative contamination) [35]. This can lead to pain, swelling, bone loss, and eventually failure of implants. The failure of the dental implants is multifactorial (Table 10.8).

**Table 10.7** Antibiotic prophylaxis in wisdom teeth removal—Key points

| | |
|---|---|
| 1 | Factors influencing the rate of postoperative infection [20, 32] *may need to consider postoperative antibiotics*<br>History of pericoronitis<br>Smoking<br>Old age<br>Poor oral hygiene<br>Duration of surgery<br>Amount of bone removal<br>Presence of foreign bodies—hemostats or devitalized bone fragments<br>Operator skill |
| 2 | Amoxicillin & Amoxicillin—clavulanic acid equally effective [28] |
| 3 | Systemic administration more effective [32] |
| 4 | Single preoperative dose: 30–90 min prior to procedure [18, 32] |
| 5 | Usually double the usual strength is given preoperatively [18, 26] |
| 6 | Antibiotics reduce incidence of alveolar osteitis [21]. |
| 7 | Topical tetracycline [29], chlorhexidine [30], & metronidazole [31] effective in reducing the infection rate |
| 8 | Preoperative and extended postoperative doses may be required in immunocompromised patients [22] |
| 9 | No antibiotic prophylaxis required in removal of asymptomatic mandibular third molars and maxillary third molars in healthy individuals [22] |

**Table 10.8** Factors affecting the survival of implants [33, 34]

| | |
|---|---|
| Local factors | 1. Pre-existing infections<br>2. Quality & quantity of bone<br>3. Bone grafts—autogenous vs allogenic<br>4. Ill-fitting prostheses<br>5. Bad oral hygiene<br>6. Irradiated bone |
| Systemic factors | 1. Immunocompromised diseases<br>2. Diabetes<br>3. Long-term steroids<br>4. Malnutrition<br>5. Elderly patients<br>6. Smoking |
| Surgical factors | 1. Incorrect instruments<br>2. Overheating during placement<br>3. Lack of attention to sterility.<br>4. Increased duration of the procedure [20]<br>5. Operator skill [20] |

Hence all these local, systemic, surgical, and procedural factors contributing to implant failure should be eliminated before considering infection as the reason for failure [33].

Because of the morbidity associated with infection of the implants, antimicrobial therapy is routinely used with the aim of prevention of surgical site infection. Though by definition, dental implant placement is a clean-contaminated surgery with 3–11% chances of infection, the infection rate can be brought down to about 1% by proper patient selection, attention to surgical details, and by judicious use of antibiotics [18].

There are studies supporting antibiotic use to reduce implant failures [33, 34] and studies that fail to show any added benefits of antibiotics against implant failurte [36]. Few other studies have observed similar failure rates for the implants with a single preoperative dose and routine use of antibiotic for 7 days [37].

The currently advocated dose of antibiotic prophylaxis for implant surgery is 2–3 g of amoxicillin 2 h prior to multiple implant placement, especially along with bone graft [33]. If the patient is allergic to penicillin group, 600 mg clindamycin should be given 1 h before surgery. For sinus augmentation, 1.2 g of amoxicillin/clavulanic acid starting day before the surgery is the prophylaxis of choice [33]. Chlorhexidine gluconate mouth rinses have been known to reduce the number of pathogenic microorganisms, by lysing the bacterial cell membranes, and by virtue of its substantivity, can get retained in the oral soft tissues and get released slowly for up to 12 h [30, 33]. The key points in the antibiotic prophylaxis for dental implants are given in Table 10.9.

### 10.3.4 Antibiotic Prophylaxis in Orthognathic Surgery

Orthognathic surgical procedures aim to correct the facial deformities and malocclusion, thereby improving the functional disorders of the stomatognathic system. It is an elective procedure, usually carried out in young healthy adults. It is considered as a clean-contaminated procedure with a reported infection rate of 3–11% [18, 39]. But certain studies have reported the rate of infection after orthognathic surgery to be as high as 6–33.4% [39]. The postoperative infection was found to be related to poor oral hygiene and the habit of smoking.

The surgical site infections (SSIs) that develop can be incisional SSIs and organ and space SSIs [40]. Both types of SSIs can occur after orthognathic surgery and may develop within the first few weeks after surgery. The development of SSIs increased the total length of hospital stay and expenditure. Though the potential for postoperative infections after orthognathic surgery is known for a very long time, a consensus has not yet been achieved with regard to the drug that is useful, the dose, and the duration of administration.

The specific orthognathic procedure that has been associated with higher infection rate was mandibular sagittal split osteotomy, especially where a transbuccal approach had been adopted for fixation [38]. Increased rate of infection associated with mandibular procedures has been attributed to the diminished vascularity of mandible in comparison with maxilla and pooling of food and saliva along the vestibular incision line in the mandible. Till the incision seals off, oral microflora can freely enter the deeper tissues from the pooled saliva. Though concomitant extractions, especially of partially erupted mandibular third molars had been implicated as a risk factor for the development of postoperative infec-

**Table 10.9** Antibiotic prophylaxis in dental implants—Key points

*Care to be taken* [35]:
Through oral prophylaxis & measures to improve oral hygiene
Stabilize oral focus of infection
Procedure in a well-monitored aseptic environment—disinfection, draping, hand scrubbing, sterile gowns & gloves, sterile instruments
Prevent contamination of implants with contact with skin, infected oral mucosa, & sinus lining
Bactericidal antibiotic with coverage against pathogenic oral microflora [12, 18, 33]
Preoperative administration of antibiotics—1 h before the procedure, twice the therapeutic dose [18, 33]—Amoxicillin 2gm, / clindamycin 600 mg 1 h prior to surgery
Chlorhexidine gluconate rinses—hugely effective in controlling the immediate local infection [30, 33].

1 *Only Chlorhexidine 0.12% rinse twice daily in healthy individuals* [33]
(a) Simple implant,
(b) Short duration,
(c) No bone graft,
(d) Sterile environment is ensured..

2 *Single preoperative dose + Chlorhexidine 0.12% rinse twice daily in healthy individuals* [33]
(a) Multiple implants with minimal tissue reflection,
(b) Immediate extraction & implant placement,
(c) Socket bone grafting.

3 *Single preoperative dose + 3 doses / day X 3 postoperative days + Chlorhexidine 0.12% rinse twice daily in healthy individuals* [33]
(a) Multiple implants with extensive tissue reflection,
(b) Multiple extractions & implant placement,
(c) Bone grafting—allografts,
(d) Long duration.

4 *Single preoperative dose + 3 doses / day X 5 postoperative days + Chlorhexidine 0.12% rinse twice daily* [33]
(a) In medically compromised patients,
(b) Extensive tissue reflection,
(c) Full arch implants,
(d) Block bone grafting—autografts,
(e) Indirect sinus floor lift procedures,
(f) Active periodontal disease.

5 *Loading dose on the previous day + 3 doses / day X 5 postoperative days + Chlorhexidine 0.12% rinse twice daily* [33]
In sinus lift procedure

tion, studies were not able to support or refute this [38, 41] Longer surgeries involving multiple/segmental procedures also show a higher rate of infections [12, 18, 38].

Use of various antibiotics has been proposed—penicillin [42], ampicillin [43], amoxicillin with or without clavulanate [43], clindamycin [42], or a member of the cephalosporin group [19, 41]. Literature fails to report a significant difference in the infection rate when using a penicillin or nonpenicillin group of antibiotics or among the various types of penicillins [18, 19, 44]. Based on the bacteriological studies, penicillin, amoxicillin, or amoxicillin—clavulanic acid or cephalosporins is commonly recommended in the preoperative antibiotic prophylaxis for orthognathic surgery [19, 38, 41–44].

The preoperative single dose of antibiotic increases the level of the drug in circulation prior to incision. Whether short-term antibiotics (single dose or dose × 24 h) [ 42] or extended-term antibiotics (for more than 24 h) [ 41, 43] is beneficial in the prevention of postoperative infection after orthognathic surgery is still a debatable question [19, 38, 41, 44].

### 10.3.5 Is Antibiotics Needed when Bone Plates and Screws Are Being Inserted?

One question that keeps on surfacing is whether prophylactic antibiotics are needed in cases where bone plates and screws are used to hold the bony segments together. Any foreign body inserted into the body, be it a medical device or implant, may elicit a foreign body reaction. Moreover, the microorganisms can colonize on the implant surface in a biofilm, while they are being inserted, and as the physical presence of the implants may compromise the blood supply to the region, thereby reducing the delivery of body's immune cells to the region and resulting in infections at the host –implant interface by normal flora with low virulence [45, 46]. The oral biofilm and its toxins, adhered to the surface of titanium plates and screws used for stabilization of osteotomy segments, could be a source of local or regional infectious complications [19]. Hence, the use of antibiotic prophylaxis is justified.

*Take-home points regarding antibiotic prophylaxis in orthognathic surgery are mentioned in* Table 10.10.

### 10.3.6 Antibiotic Prophylaxis in Maxillofacial Trauma

In today's world of fast-moving vehicles and expressways, hundreds of thousands of people get involved in road traffic accidents. Head and face are among commonly injured body parts. Both the soft and hard tissues of the face may be involved in the trauma. Firearms, contact sports, and interpersonal violence are other reasons for facial injuries. The management of these injuries should follow protocols and be done in a systematic manner. With advances in anesthetic and surgical techniques and availability of better implant materials with favorable metallurgy, open reduction and internal fixation (ORIF) has become the norm. The re-establishment of form, function, & cosmesis is of paramount importance. To arrive at this goal, the probable complications of ORIF need to be prevented or managed correctly. Of the various complications reported, none has generated more interest and controversy than the occurrence of postoperative infection. By adhering to the standard surgical protocols and strict aseptic techniques, the occurrence of postoperative

**Table 10.10** Antibiotic prophylaxis in orthognathic surgery—Key points

1. Risk factors for SSIs [47, 48]
   (a) Longer surgery;
   (b) Short-term antibiotic prophylaxis;
   (c) Extraction of a third molar during surgery;
   (d) Greater number of osteotomies performed;
   (e) Older age;
   (f) Smoking;
   (g) Poor oral hygiene;
   (h) Compromised immune system.
2 Orthognathic surgery - clean–contaminated wound—with the osteotomized maxilla / mandible exposed to oral / nasal / antral cavities [48].—Antibiotics needed
3 Need for antibiotics in presence of bone plates & screws [45, 46].
4 Loading dose of double strength 1 h prior to incision [18].
5 Confusion between—single loading dose + short-term doses × 24 h vs long-term antibiotics for more than 24 h [19, 44].
Commonly isolated organisms—aerobic bacteria—streptococci (43%) & anaerobic bacteroides (50%) [18, 39]
6 Amoxicillin / amoxicillin—clavulanic acid—best suited [19, 42–44].
7 Higher infection rate—mandibular osteotomies with transbuccal approach for fixation [38].
8 Longer procedures & segmental osteotomies—more prone for infection [38].
9 Concomitant removal of mandibular third molars does not increase the risk for postoperative infection [39], though may cause issues with fixation.

infection can be brought down considerably. But the presence of the microorganisms in the oral cavity and facial skin and possible contamination from environment necessitate the consideration of antibiotics in the maxillofacial trauma management.

Though prophylactic antibiotics were considered essential in the management of maxillofacial trauma for many years [18], the evidence for this preventive intervention was weak and confusing. Among facial fractures, mandibular fractures are most commonly studied, because of the compound nature of the fractures, except in the ramus—condyle unit, where the fractures usually do not communicate with the external environment. Fractures of the mandibular condyles or Lefort fractures of maxilla are rarely infected when compared with the fractures involving mandibular angle, body, or symphysis [49, 50].

The decision to use antibiotic prophylaxis depends on whether the fracture is an open or closed type and whether it is going to be managed with open or closed reduction. Open procedures were four times more commonly prone to postoperative infections according to a few studies [41, 51, 53, 54], whereas certain other studies reported no difference between the patients treated with closed reduction and maxillomandibular fixation and those who underwent open reduction and internal fixation [54]. The microbiology of the infected fractures was mixed and responded to beta-lactam antibiotics well.

**Table 10.11** Antibiotic prophylaxis in maxillofacial trauma—Key points

1. Risk factors for SSIs [22, 32, 51, 56]
   (a) Longer surgery;
   (b) Older age;
   (c) Smoking;
   (d) Poor oral hygiene;
   (e) Compromised immune system.
2 Mandibular fractures/ fractures of the teeth-bearing area—open / compound fractures.—Antibiotics needed [49, 50, 53, 54].
3 Need for antibiotics in presence of bone plates & screws [45, 46]
4 Loading dose of double strength 1 h prior to incision [18, 56].
5 Beta-lactam antibiotics—preferred [56].
6 Higher infection rate—in fractures involving mandibular teeth–bearing areas [49]
7 Longer duration of antibiotics in immunocompromised patients [49, 52].
8 Chances of infection more with open reduction than in those treated with closed reduction with no antibiotic prophylaxis [16, 50, 51]. But with single dose of perioperative antibiotics, no significant difference between closed & open reduction [51, 54]
10 Delayed healing and increased infection rate with tobacco smoking [51].

Studies have shown that single dose of preoperative antibiotic prophylaxis is sufficient to prevent wound infection [51, 54]. If the surgery extends beyond the half-life of the antibiotic, the antibiotic can be redosed [51]. The need for postoperative antibiotics in the maxillofacial trauma too has been extensively studied [16, 49, 53, 55, 56]. These studies reported no statistically significant difference in the development of SSIs between the patients who had received perioperative antibiotics and those who had received extended antibiotics in the postoperative period.

Longer antibiotic usage has been advocated in the immunocompromised patients [32, 52, 56]. The habit of tobacco smoking was found to have a deleterious effect on the healing of mandibular fractures by inducing hypovascularity and prolonged inflammation [54]. The other major factors, which contribute to the occurrence of SSIs, are poor oral hygiene, extremes of age and malnutrition [22, 32].

*Important points mentioning the need for antibiotics in the management of maxillofacial trauma are given in* Table 10.11.

### 10.3.7 Diabetes Mellitus & Antibiotic Prophylaxis in Maxillofacial Surgery

Diabetes mellitus is a metabolic disorder resulting in elevated glucose levels, due to inadequate insulin secretion (type I) or reduced insulin secretion with an accompanying insulin resistance (type II). Diabetic patients pose a special challenge to the surgeon as the balance between the insulin they can secrete and the hyperglycemia induced by surgical stress-adaptive hormones catecholamines, cortisol, growth hormone, and glucagon is lost. Patients, who are nondiabetic, usually are able to handle this glucose overload effectively, whereas diabetic patients may have issues resulting in cardiovascular complications, infection, and reduced rates of wound healing. Moreover, the defective polymorphonuclear leukocytes function and macro- and microvascular dysfunction resulting in compromised local circulation increases the susceptibility to infections [57]. With the vast microbiological colonization of the oral cavity, it has always been assumed that maxillofacial surgical procedures carry a high risk of infection and prolonged or delayed wound healing. The guidelines as to the prophylactic use of antibiotics in diabetic patients had been vague as "....are more prone to infection necessitating routine antibiotic prophylaxis for all maxillofacial procedures" [58].

In many of the literature surveys, authors have noted that well-controlled diabetic patients are at no increased risk of postoperative infection than normal healthy patients and delayed wound healing is not a pressing concern due to the rich vascularity of the region [59, 60]. Antibiotic prophylaxis is warranted only in conditions where a normal patient also would benefit from it. Poorly controlled diabetic patients would require normalization of their hyperglycemic state prior to elective procedures. In emergency situations, antibiotic prophylaxis prior to the surgical incision is desirable and attempts should be made to control the glycemic level during the peri- and postoperative period [58–60].

### 10.3.8 Antibiotic Prophylaxis in Head and Neck Oncology

Head and neck oncology patients usually require a major surgical procedure +/− with radiation therapy. The surgical site tends to be large, the surgical time and postoperative immobilization period longer. The surgical management attempts at removal of the tumor, clearance of the neck nodes, and involves an additional surgical site from where flap is harvested for reconstruction—either microvascular flaps or pedicled ones [61]. The large wound area exposed to local flora of the oral cavity and the skin is at risk of wound contamination and infection. Nosocomial infections are known to run a protracted course and pre-existing general comorbidities further increase the morbidity and, thus, the hospital expenses associated with these surgeries.

The reasons for increased infection rate are mainly the number of procedures carried out in the same operation (excision, neck dissection, tracheostomy, and distant flap harvest), the pooling of saliva due to difficulty in swallowing, leading to aspiration, and the inability in obtaining a watertight closure when the flap is inset in the recipient bed leading to salivary leak and contamination of neck wounds with saliva [62, 63].

**Table 10.12** Key points in oral oncology & antibiotic prophylaxis

| Key points |
|---|
| Increased risk of SSIs [62]<br>Multiple procedures done at a single operation,<br>Large wound area,<br>Long procedure,<br>Tobacco & alcohol abuse<br>Immunocompromised patients |
| Probable pathogens [62] - Escherichia spp. & staphylococcal spp |
| Preferred antibiotic [62] - ampicillin & sulbactum |
| Bartella et al. (2017) [62] - Statistically significant reduction in infectious complications with postoperative antibiotics |

The need for antibiotic prophylaxis is well established in the oncologic surgery, but the need for a long postoperative course of antibiotics is still debated upon. There are studies, which have shown benefits of prolonged antibiotics in preventing postoperative infections like pneumonia, urinary tract infections, sepsis, and SSIs in patients who had oral squamous cell carcinoma [64], and there are studies, which have shown no extra benefits of prolonged postoperative antibiotics [63, 64].

Escherichia spp. and Staphylococcus spp. are predominantly responsible for the infections and in 72% were sensitive to ampicillin & sulbactum [62].

*A few key points, which would be beneficial in making a decision, are given in* Table 10.12.

### 10.3.9 Antibiotic Prophylaxis in Cleft Surgeries

Orofacial clefting is one of the more common congenital anomalies and cleft lip & palate deformity is the most common among them. Management of cleft lip & palate deformity involves staged procedures and spans over 12–16 years. The management aims at correction of the deformity so that function and cosmesis are restored as much as possible and the psyche of the individual is minimally scarred. Postoperative infections can result in wound breakdown, poor speech & esthetics, and nasal regurgitation of food in cleft lip and palate patients.

Various authors had reported on obtaining swabs from nose and oral cavity to identify the possible pathogens and using antibiotics according to the culture reports before cleft lip and palate repair [65–67]. The pathogenic bacteria isolated from the swabs were Staphylococcus aureus and beta hemolytic streptococci [67]. But later studies demonstrated that there were not many differences between the group that underwent swab acquisition and corresponding antibiotics therapy and the group that didn't receive any antibiotics in terms of postoperative complications [68]. The rate of complications was found to be independent of the potential pathogens in the mouth [65].

*Factors, which have been implied as contributing factors to wound dehiscence, are given in* [66, 67] Table 10.13.

**Table 10.13** Factors contributing to wound dehiscence in cleft surgeries

| |
|---|
| Wide clefts |
| Closure under tension |
| Bilateral clefts |
| Long duration of surgery |
| Poor technique—traumatized nasal mucosa |
| Independent of potential oral pathogens |

In a recent prospective study, Azner et al. (2015) noted a statistically significant reduction in the incidence of palatal fistulas with 5 days of postoperative antibiotics [69]. But 80% of their control group, who had received no postoperative antibiotics, too healed without any complications. Both study and control groups had received a single dose of cefuroxime 30 mg / kg body weight, before incision. The use of one dose of antibiotics before incision has been advocated by other authors also and may be more effective in preventing complications related to wound infection than a prolonged course of postoperative antibiotics [68].

### 10.3.10 Organ Transplant and Antibiotic Prophylaxis

The concept of organ donation had always excited mankind. Twentieth century saw developments that made the dream of replacing a diseased organ with a healthy one a reality. Understanding the human immunology and the development of powerful immunosuppressant drugs laid the foundation for modern transplant medicine, making transplantation of kidney, liver, lungs, and heart a successful treatment option. As the transplant science advanced, so did the numbers and life span of transplant patients and their need for dental/maxillofacial surgical procedures. As these patients are on immunosuppressants, they are more prone to opportunistic infections and their sequel. Hence, care must be given to treat or remove the existing/potential sources of infection before the transplant procedures.

In a pretransplant patient, the need for maintaining oral hygiene should be stressed upon. The treating physician should be consulted with regard to the fitness to undergo the planned procedures and the safety of using any drugs if required. Drugs, which have a hepatic metabolism or renal clearance, should be used with caution in patients with compromised liver or kidney function. The selection of antibiotics is made after careful evaluation of the existing pathology and the chances of spread of infection with the planned dental treatment.

In the immediate post-transplant period—the first 3 months post-surgery, the graft, and the patient are very vulnerable to any insult—graft anastomoses are susceptible to endarteriris due to bacterial colonization as they are not yet

**Table 10.14** Key points—organ transplant and antibiotic prophylaxis

| |
|---|
| Pretransplant patients—stress on<br>1. Elimination of potential focus of infection,<br>2. Oral hygiene,<br>3. Liver / kidney friendly drugs. |
| Post-transplant patients: |
| Immediate postop:<br>1. Only emergency procedures,<br>2. Aggressive management of infections. |
| 3 months postop—noninvasive elective procedures |
| 6 months postop—invasive elective procedures under antibiotics |
| Beta-lactam antibiotics - relatively safer to be used in renal and hepatic transplant patients [72] |
| No consensus on minimally invasive procedures in patients with meticulous oral hygiene [71] |

fully epithelialized. Hence, only emergency procedures should be done. Any acute orofacial infection developing should be managed aggressively, surgical drainage, culture and sensitivity of the organism, and appropriate antibiotics would be required [70]. After 3 months, elective, noninvasive procedures can be carried out. Since the patients who have undergone organ transplantation are immunosuppressed and are at high risk of infection, prophylactic antibiotics need to considered for any invasive dental procedures, even after 6 months. Beta-lactam antibiotics are relatively safer to be used in renal and hepatic transplant patients [71]. But for those with meticulous oral hygiene, there is no consensus regarding the need for antibiotic prophylaxis for minimally invasive procedures [71]. The decision to use antibiotics should be done on a case-to-case basis.

*Important points to be kept in mind while contemplating antibiotic prophylaxis in organ transplant patients are given in* Table 10.14.

## 10.4 Infective Endocarditis

Bacterial endocarditis, a rare but life-threatening condition, was initially described by Lewis & Grant in 1923 [72]. They suggested that bacteria released into the blood stream after a dental procedure colonize on the heart valves or the endocardium. The bacteremia associated with infections of skin and soft tissues, genitourinary tract, and gastrointestinal tract are also known to result in infective endocarditis (IE). Bacteria can gain direct access to the bloodstream through the indwelling catheters. The American Heart Association (AHA) came up with the first guidelines to reduce the risk of IE following invasive procedures in 1955 [73]. The AHA guidelines have been updated regularly since then and the latest one was released in 2007 [74]. The 2007 guidelines categorized cardiac conditions into having a low risk, moderate risk, and high risk of developing IE and advocated the use of antibiotic prophylaxis only in

**Table 10.15** High-risk cardiac conditions, which require antibiotic prophylaxis [75]

| |
|---|
| Prosthetic cardiac valves |
| Congenital heart diseases—unrepaired, with palliative shunts or conduits or repaired with prosthetic material or those repaired, but with residual defects |
| Previous IE |
| Cardiac transplants who have developed valvulopathy |

high-risk-category patients (Table 10.15) who were to undergo dental procedures that involved the manipulation of gingival tissues or the periapical region of teeth or incision of the oral mucosa.

The guidelines prescribed a single dose of antibiotic 30-60 minutes prior to the procedure—Amoxicillin 2 g PO, Cephazolin/Cephtriaxone 1gm IV/IM, or Clindamycin 600 mg PO/IM/IV, depending on whether the patient is unable to take oral preparations or is allergic to penicillin or not [74]. The reason for the revision of the antibiotic policy was predominantly the observation that IE is more likely to result from transient bacteremias caused by routine daily activities, like chewing food, and by regular oral hygiene care. The authors concluded that maintaining optimal oral hygiene is more important in reducing the risk of IE and the adverse effects of antibiotics exceeded the benefits of antibiotic prophylaxis. The British Society for Antimicrobial Chemotherapy (BSAC) also recommend antibiotic prophylaxis only in those who have a history of healed IE, prosthetic heart valves, and surgically constructed conduits [75]. The advice to the patient is to concentrate on achieving and maintaining meticulous oral hygiene as this has been found to reduce the risk of IE. Similar observations were made by the National Institute for Health and Care Excellence (NICE) [76] and the European Society of Cardiology (ESC) [77].

There has been a rising concern over the potential for an increased incidence of IE and a worse prognosis for the diseased since the guideline changes by the AHA, NICE, ESC, BSAC. Several studies have been carried out to assess the impact of these changes on the disease incidence in adults and pediatric population. Whereas earlier studies showed not much difference pre- and post-guideline changes in incidence [78], recent studies have noted a definite increase in the incidence of IE post-guideline changes [79]. Sakai et al. in 2017, though noting no change in the incidence and severity of IE in pediatric patients, pre- and post- guideline changes, reported an increase in the viridans group streptococci (VGS)–induced IE in older age group [79]. The data from these studies point to the need for further investigation into the effectiveness of 2007 guidelines, though it has been argued that the increase in IE incidence may be related to the increasing life span of the patients with congenital heart diseases and prosthetic devices and increase in the number of invasive procedures being performed on them.

## 10.5 Postoperative Pain Management in Maxillofacial Surgery

The International Association for the Study of Pain (IASP) defines pain [80] as: "an unpleasant sensory and emotional experience associated with actual or potential tissue damage or described in terms of such damage."

Pain is the most debilitating postoperative symptom and its control or elimination is usually the primary goal in postoperative management of a patient. Inadequate pain control resulting in patient distress is the most common cause of an increased length of hospital stay. The postoperative pain, inflammatory in character, is a temporary one persisting only until healing. But severe, acute, repetitive, postoperative pain increases the risk of the pain becoming chronic and may lead to allodynia and hyperalgesia [81]. Orthognathic surgery patients may continue to feel the pain even after 1 year of surgery [82]· Hence, appropriate pain management is critical to achieving a successful surgical outcome. Prevention of pain is more efficient than the treatment of pain. For this, an understanding of basic pathophysiology behind pain mechanism is important.

## 10.6 Pathophysiology of Postoperative Pain

Pain is initiated by the excitation of nociceptors, receptors that respond to noxious - mechanical, thermal, and chemical stimuli. Sensory nociception is disproportionately greater in the head and oral cavity when compared with other parts of the body. Often a patient's overanxiety about undergoing an elective surgery would result in an increased intensity of the perceived pain [83].

Surgical insult results in tissue trauma and initiates a chain of inflammatory events, causing a release of chemical substances responsible for nociceptor excitation. Trauma releases tissue phospholipids, which are converted into arachidonic acid due to the action of phospholipase A2 and the consequent conversion of this substance into prostaglandins, prostacyclins, and leukotrienes due to the action of cyclooxygenase (Cox) and lipoxygenase enzymes. These locally released chemical mediators sensitize the nociceptors and cause vasodilatation, with a consequent increase in cell permeability and edema. Trismus after a maxillofacial surgery is a sequela to the postoperative edema around the masticator muscles and is aggravated by pain [84]. The physiological responses to tissue trauma, pain & edema, can be managed successfully by inhibiting the pathways that produce the chemical mediators, before the occurrence of surgical trauma (Fig. 10.1).

Similarly, mechanisms, which enhance the endogenous pain inhibition and anxiolysis and patient education, can

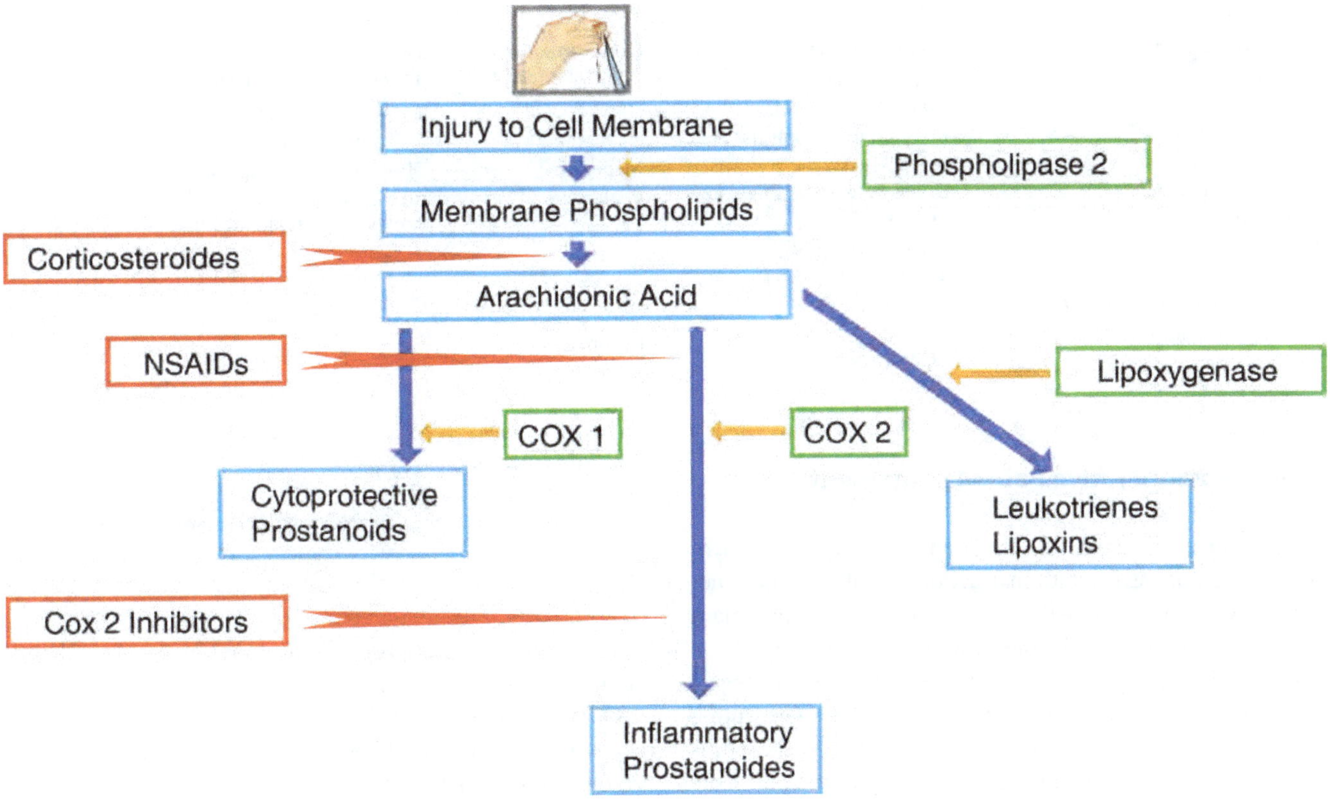


**Fig. 10.1** Pharmacologic interventions in arachidonic acid metabolism

modify cortical processing of pain perception [85]. All these measures collectively lead to an efficient postoperative pain management.

### 10.6.1 Pre-Emptive Analgesia

Postoperative pain has a protective function as it allows for undisturbed healing of the operated tissue by restricting movements. The aim of postoperative pain management is to reduce pain significantly, but not to eliminate it completely [86]. Overall postoperative pain experience could be reduced by paying attention to lessening of the pain during the surgical procedure itself. Pre-emptive analgesia is defined as an antinociceptive treatment that is started preoperatively and is active during surgery, reducing the physiological consequences of nociceptive transmission [87]. Since the introduction of the concept of pre-emptive analgesia by Woolf in 1983, many attempts to reduce the pain by using analgesics and adjunctive measures, such as the administration of long-acting local anesthesia, corticosteroids, and intraoperative nitrous oxide analgesia, have been reported [88]. These should be given before the surgical incision and should be timed so that the maximum plasma concentration of the drug is reached at the time of surgical incision. This will prevent the release of the inflammatory mediators, giving immediate analgesic effects. The use of IV analgesia has an added benefit over oral administration, as following oral administration analgesics reach maximum concentration after 1.5 h, whereas intravenous administration results in maximum concentration in a short period.

Numerous studies have shown beneficial effects of the preoperative administration of ibuprofen with paracetamol [89] piroxicam [90], ketorolac [91], meloxicam [92], parecoxib [93], and dexamethasone with rofecoxib [94]. There had been contradictory reports also in which the authors fail to find a clear-cut benefit for pre-emptive NSAIDS [95, 97]. The authors state that the pre-emptive intake of analgesics should not be used in all patients as a general rule. They base their recommendations on the lack of enhanced analgesic effects and on the potential adverse effects such as increased intraoperative bleeding [95].

Despite the confusion regarding the effectiveness of the pre-emptive analgesia, it has been strongly advised to start systemic analgesics before the local anesthesia effect wears off and/or give a nerve block with long-acting agent like bupivacaine [86].

**Table 10.16** Predictors of postoperative pain

| Patient-related factors | Surgical indicators |
|---|---|
| Age [98, 99] | Major surgeries—long duration |
| Female sex [98] | Bony surgery > soft tissue surgery [100] |
| Anxiety & apprehension, fear of the procedure | Bi-jaw surgery vs single jaw surgery |
| Pre-existing or chronic pain | Mandibular surgery > maxillary surgery |
| Preoperative use of opioids / neuropathic analgesics [98] | Oncological surgery |
| | Emergency procedures [101] |

## 10.6.2 Postoperative Pain Management

Postoperative analgesia has traditionally been achieved by prescribing analgesics with instructions to take as and when necessary. Experience with this approach was that many patients would not take the medication until the onset of significant pain. This practice earned the maxillofacial surgery the reputation of being an extremely painful one. The truth is that the postoperative pain management can be successfully achieved by carefully planning the delivery of the pain control measures at the appropriate time in the peri- and postoperative periods.

Pain perception is a subjective feeling, which is amplified by many factors and identification of the patients who are "at risk" for the development of severe postoperative pain would help in charting out an individualized management plan [97] (Table 10.16).

Identifying predictors of postoperative pain in patients before surgery, educating patients at the preoperative visit regarding the expected pain, and presenting the postoperative pain management plan will prepare patients better and relieve some of their anxiety regarding the procedure. An increased awareness of the importance of the psychological factors will allow more effective pain management.

## 10.6.3 Pharmacological Management of Postoperative Pain

The postoperative pain management is usually done with opioids and nonsteroidal class of anti-inflammatory drugs.

### 10.6.3.1 Opioids

Opioids have been in use for moderate-to-severe pain relief for a long period. References to opium poppy can be found in Sumerian and Egyptian culture, as back as 300 BC. The opium poppy, Papaver somniferum, gives rise to more than 20 different alkaloids [100]—morphine and codeine being the main ones (Table 10.17).

**Table 10.17** Opioid analgesics

| Drug name | Dose |
|---|---|
| Codeine | 15–60 mg orally q4-6h |
| Hydrocodone | 5–10 mg orally q3h |
| Oxycodone | 5–7.5 mg orally q6h |
| Meperidine | 50–150 mg orally q3–4h |
| Pentazocine | 50 mg orally q3–4h |
| Tramadol | 50-100 mg q4–6h, max 400 mg /day |

**Table 10.18** Side effects of opioid analgesics

| |
|---|
| Respiratory depression |
| Sleepiness |
| Constipation |
| Nausea & vomiting |
| Addictive potential [102] |
| Drug overdose death [103] |
| Pharmacological tolerance ➔ opioid-induced hyperalgesia [102, 104] |

Opiate alkaloids exert their action by acting on the opioid receptors- μ, κ, δ (mu, kappa, and delta), which otherwise provide sites for activation of endogenously released opioid substances - beta-endorphins, enkephalins, and dynorphin compounds, which produce endogenous central analgesia. Opiate agonists produce analgesia by inhibiting excitatory neurotransmission of substance P, acetylcholine, noradrenaline, and dopamine.

Unfortunately, opioid use, even when prescribed for short periods, comes with certain risks (Table 10.18).

For these reasons, most opioid agents used in outpatient postsurgical pain management are formulated in combination with non-narcotic analgesics [104]. This formulation potentiates the analgesic effects of the individual agents within the formulation while minimizing the side effects of pure opioid administration [105].

### 10.6.3.2 Tramadol

Tramadol, a synthetic substance with both opioid and non-opioid properties, is structurally related to codeine. It exhibits antidepressant and anxiolytic-like effects, in addition to analgesic action. It is considered safe for long-term use unlike NSAIDs with their potential for impairment of renal function and gastrointestinal complications, and with respect to other opioid medications for its low addiction rate and favorable safety profile. The most common adverse effect of tramadol is nausea and vomiting, especially with oral administration. Tramadol is contraindicated in patients with poorly controlled epilepsy because of its excitatory serotonergic effects. It is available either as a single drug or in combination with acetaminophen. Submucosal injection of tramadol at the extracted site of third molars has been proven effective in reducing the postoperative pain [106]. It suffers no side effects of systemic administration.

#### 10.6.3.3 Nonsteroidal Anti-Inflammatory Drugs (NSAIDs)

NSAIDs have been in use for the treatment of pain, fever, and inflammation since late 1800 [107]. The anti-inflammatory and analgesic properties of these drugs without the side effects and the addictive potential of opioids have made this class of drugs the first choice in ambulatory dentoalveolar procedures (Table 10.19).

They are a group of chemically heterogeneous compounds with several similar pharmacologic actions like anti-inflammatory, antipyretic, analgesic, and antiplatelet actions. They primarily act at the site of tissue injury by inhibiting the synthesis of prostaglandins within the endoperoxide pathway (Fig. 10.1).

**Table 10.19** Nonsteroidal anti-inflammatory drugs

| Drug name | Action | Analgesic Dose |
|---|---|---|
| Salicylic acid derivative—Acetyl salicylic acid | Analgesic, anti-inflammatory, antiplatelet, antipyretic—Nonselective cox inhibitor | 325-650 mg orally q4h / 1000 mg orally q6h. |
| Propionic acid derivative—Ibuprofen | Analgesic, anti-inflammatory, antipyretic—Nonselective cox inhibitor | 400–600 mg orally q4–6h |
| Propionic acid derivative—Naproxen | Analgesic, antipyretic—Nonselective cox inhibitor | 550 mg orally initially, then 275 mg orally q6–8h |
| Acetic acid derivative—Keterolac | Analgesic, antipyretic—Nonselective cox inhibitor | 30 mg IV or 60 mg IM q6h / 20 mg orally initially, then 10 mg orally q4–6h |
| Acetic acid derivative—Diclofenac | Analgesic, anti-inflammatory—Nonselective cox inhibitor | 50–75 mg orally/IV q12h |
| Oxicams—Piroxicam | Analgesic, anti-inflammatory—Nonselective cox inhibitor | 10-20 mg orally q 12 h |
| N- phenyl—anthranilates—Mefenamic acid | Analgesic, anti-inflammatory—Nonselective cox inhibitor | 500 mg load, then 250 mg q6h orally |
| Celecoxib | Cox 2 inhibitor | 200 mg orally q24h / 100 mg orally q12h |

Historically, majority of the NSAIDs were nonselective COX inhibitors with side effects related to the blockade of cytoprotective prostanoids - gastric irritation, increased bleeding time, and renal impairment. Over the past few years, selective COX2 inhibitors have been developed, which block the COX-2–mediated prostaglandins while maintaining the physiologically beneficial effects of the COX-1 isoenzyme [108].

Overall, NSAIDs are safe drugs to be used in the management of acute/postoperative pain. Parenteral use of NSAIDs has shown to be more effective in pain control [109]. About 60% of the patients would respond to the first NSAID, and the rest would show benefit with another NSAID. Ibuprofen is a widely used NSAID, with proven efficacy [110]. About 5% people experience "aspirin-sensitive asthma," probably due to the inhibition of Cox enzyme. Because of the probable mechanism of inducing asthma, it is felt that selective Cox 2 inhibitors may not cause asthmatic attacks [111].

#### 10.6.3.4 Paracetamol

Paracetamol or acetaminophen is a widely available analgesic with an antipyretic action. It acts by inhibition of the COX-3 isoenzyme, reducing the production of prostanoids in the central nervous system. This central inhibition explains the antipyretic action of paracetamol. Paracetamol shows an excellent result in relieving mild-to-moderate pain relief and fever [112]. When used in combination with other analgesics, it shows superior analgesic power, thereby reducing the dose of opioids required [96].

### 10.6.4 Guidelines to the Use of Analgesics

Since there is no definitive evidence or clear algorithms, the selection of NSAIDs, to a large extent, depends on clinical experience and side effects. Patient convenience and cost also play a minor role in the selection of analgesics.

Laskarides (2016), in his review on control of dental pain, puts forward his observations (Table 10.20) [113].

#### 10.6.4.1 Analgesic Ladder

WHO initially described the concept of "pain ladder" in their guidelines for the use of drugs for the management of cancer pain [114]. The concept has been now accepted in the management of all types of pain [104]. The concept is based on the use of first line of drugs for the mild-to-moderate pain and then climb the ladder to more potent drugs if pain still persists. Please see chapter on postoperative care, to view the analgesic ladder.

**Table 10.20** Key points in using analgesics

| | |
|---|---|
| 1 | Care to administer correct dose of opioids [100–103] |
| 2 | Opioids + NSAIDs—centrally acting - + peripherally acting analgesia ➔ moderate-to-severe pain relief |
| 3 | Tramadol—opioid & nonopioid properties—safe for long-term use [106]. |
| 4 | Ibuprofen—excellent analgesia, transition drug to wean off form opioids [110, 113]. |
| 5 | Use NSAIDs with caution—cardiovascular conditions & gastric irritation. |
| 6 | Paracetamol, tramadol, & short-acting opioids—drugs of choice [113]. |
| 7 | NSAIDs drug interactions – Sulfonyl urea & other hypoglycemic agents<br>Oral anticoagulants<br>Phenytoin<br>Sulfonamides |
| 8 | Paracetamol + NSAIDs—superior analgesic power [89, 112]. |
| 9 | Maximum daily dose of paracetamol 4 g decides the dose of combination therapy [113]. |

### 10.6.4.2 Preventive /Protective/Multimodal Analgesia

Pain is multifactorial in origin and multiple techniques and drugs may be required to achieve control over it. The simultaneous use of different classes of analgesics and techniques has been called preventive, protective, or multimodal analgesia [115]. This approach uses a combination of drugs that act at different sites of action on the nervous system by different mechanisms to prevent peripheral and central sensitization of pain. It results in additive analgesia, but with lowered side effects than the single agents when used alone. Intraoperative local anesthesia followed by a range of analgesic drugs have been found to be effective in controlling the pain in day cases and reduces the need for opioid analgesics [116].

The complex surgeries involving multiple surgical sites as in head and neck oncological cases and craniofacial surgeries would gain hugely from the administration of multimodal analgesia. Multimodal analgesia can be successfully achieved by combining the currently available analgesic modalities (Table 10.21).

**Table 10.21** The analgesics and adjuncts that can be used in multimodal analgesia [117]

| Drugs | Examples | Mechanism of action |
|---|---|---|
| A. Opioids [102]. | Codeine, Hydrocodone Tramadol | Inhibits excitatory neurotransmission of substance P, acetylcholine, noradrenaline, & dopamine. |
| B. Local anesthesia [86, 118] techniques. | Bupivacaine, levobupivacaine & ropivacaine—nerve blocks & infiltration | Blocks the pain transmission |
| C. Acetaminophen [112]. | Weak analgesic | IV administration raises the plasma & CSF concentration rapidly to achieve adequate analgesia |
| D. Nonsteroidal anti-inflammatory drugs (NSAIDs) [108, 110]. | Ibuprofen, Diclofenac, Mefenamic acid, nasal spray of ketorolac | Blocks arachidonic acid metabolism |
| E. Cyclooxygenase (COX)-2-specific inhibitors [108]. | Celecoxib | Cox 2 inhibitor |
| F. Adjuncts. | | |
| 1. *Steroids* [80]. | Dexamethasone, hydrocortisone | Blocks lipoxygenase & cox pathways |
| 2. N-methyl-d-aspartate *(NMDA). Antagonists* [97, 115, 117] | Ketamine | Effects on central sensitization & neural modulation |
| 3. *Alpha – 2 agonists* [97, 115, 117]. | Clonidine, Dexmedetomidine | Sedative and analgesia-sparing effects via central actions in the locus ceruleus and in the dorsal horn of the spinal cord, respectively |
| 4. *Anticonvulsants* [97, 115, 117]. | Gabapentin, pregabalin | Inhibits central sensitization through presynaptic or postsynaptic inhibition of calcium influx, which inhibits the release of neurotransmitters |

### 10.6.4.3 Patient-Controlled Analgesia (PCA)

Patient-controlled analgesics are intravenous agents, delivered through a microprocessor-controlled infusion pump, in which a predetermined dose can be delivered by the press of a button, and a lockout time can be set, so that patient cannot overdose himself [119]. PCA is usually used in patients who are distressed at the thought of postoperative pain. Fentanyl, morphine, & combinations are the usually used medications. Though PCA was initially thought to reduce the patient pain perception, thereby reducing the length of stay (LOS), studies have failed to show any statistically significant difference in the pain score and the LOS between the PCA group & non-PCA group of patients after orthognathic surgery [119, 120]. This could be attributed to the fact that the subjects in the PCA group were predominantly bijaw surgery patients for whom the surgical time was longer and the surgical procedure resulted in more tissue injury. But from patient's perspective, PCA is the preferred method, as they feel in charge of their own pain control [121].

## 10.7 Corticosteroids in Maxillofacial Surgery

When tissue damage occurs as a result of injury, body's natural defense mechanism is inflammation and body tries to heal. But overt inflammation results in pain, edema, and limitation of movement, trismus. These symptoms may not be evident immediately, but peak after the second day, returning to normal by seventh postoperative day [122]. Corticosteroids suppress the inflammation (Fig. 10.1) by interfering with the capillary dialatation, fluid transduation, fibrin deposition, leukocyte migration, and phagocytosis. Under normal nonstressful conditions, the body produces approximately 15 to 30 mg of hydrocortisone/cortisol per day. During stressful situations, 300 mg of hydrocortisone per day can be produced. Generally speaking, to suppress inflammation, the dose of exogenous corticosteroids must exceed the normal physiological amounts of hydrocortisone released [123].

The first reported clinical use of the anti-inflammatory properties of corticosteroids was in the treatment of rheumatoid artritis [124], following which its efficacy was tried in maxillofacial surgical procedures. The use of steroids and their effectiveness have been extensively studied in the third molar surgeries—the most commonly performed maxillofacial surgical procedure [125]. Markiewicz et al. noted that postoperative findings of swelling, trismus, and pain were significantly lower in the group who received corticosteroids, than in the control group in the immediate postoperative period (1–3 days) [126].

The use of dexamethasone and methyl prednisolone, in controlling the postoperative sequel of third molar surgery when these drugs are administered via parenteral [127], oral [128] submucosal [129, 130] and topical [131] routes, has been reported.

*Studies have evaluated different formulations, dosages, and routes and sites of administration of corticosteroids, without any consensus.* (Table 10.22).

Dexamethasone has a longer duration of action than methylprednisolone and is considered more potent. Intralesional/intramasseteric injection of dexamethasone is found to be better than the intravenous or parenteral administration in controlling postoperative edema & trismus and has an additional benefit of being given through an already-anesthetized area [130, 132].

Almeida et al. (2019) [133] failed to note any benefit of submucosal injection of steroid at the local site. Authors gave the reason for this as the displacement of the medicine from the local site when mucoperiosteal flap is reflected to expose the tooth. Similarly, the merits of intravenous administration of steroids perioperatively in major surgeries have been questioned by a group of authors [134]. Kainulainen et al. [134] reported infectious complications—pneumonia, gastrostomy site infections, & surgical site infections in oncological cases.

Though the reduction of edema brings about some reduction in discomfort, steroids alone do not have a clinically significant analgesic effect [130, 135] This has been attributed to the inability of the steroids to block the production of neurotransmitters by the injured tissues and central sensitization to pain. The combination of dexamethasone with tramadol or diclofenac sodium has been proven more effective in controlling postoperative pain and trismus, as opposed to corticosteroids alone [136]. Alexander & Throndson [127] summarized few salient points with regard to usage of steroids, based on their review (Table 10.23).

**Table 10.22** Commonly used steroids with their anti-inflammatory potency& equivalent dose and commonly used doses [1]

| Drug | Duration of action | Anti-inflammatory potency | Equivalent dose | Dose |
|---|---|---|---|---|
| Dexamethasone | Long acting | 25 | 0.75 mg | 0.5–5 mg /day PO, 4–20 mg /day IV |
| Betamethasone | Long acting | 25 | 0.75 mg | 0.5–5 mg /day PO, 4–20 mg /day IV |
| Prednisolone | Intermediate acting | 4 | 5 mg | 5–60 mg /day PO<br>10–40 mg / day IM or IV |
| Methyl prednisolone | Intermediate acting | 5 | 4 mg | 4–32 mg /day PO |
| Triamcinolone | Intermediate acting | 5 | 4 mg | 4–32 mg /day PO<br>5–40 mg intra-articular |
| Hydrocortisone | Short acting | 1 | 20 mg | 100 mg IV/IM bolus |

**Table 10.23** Summary of corticosteroid use in maxillofacial surgery

| | |
|---|---|
| 1 | Preoperative intralesional / parenteral administration of steroids to reduce the inflammation associated with surgery [125, 132]. |
| 2 | No adrenal suppression with small doses [125] |
| 3 | Long-term use—adrenal suppression interference with immune system & infection [126] |
| 4 | Usually tapering of dose is not required for short-term uses [137] |
| 5 | Contraindications [138]:<br>Active tuberculosis<br>Active viral / fungal infections<br>Active acne vulgaris<br>Primary glaucoma<br>Patients with psychoses |
| 6 | Use with care [138]:<br>Diverticulitis<br>Peptic ulcers<br>Cushing's syndrome<br>Renal insufficiency<br>Uncontrolled hypertension<br>Uncontrolled diabetes mellitus<br>Pregnancy & lactation<br>Chronic infections<br>Myasthenia gravis |
| 8 | Exogenous steroid dose > endogenous cortisol level [123, 138] |

## 10.8 Conclusion

Maxillofacial surgical practice involves use of many therapeutics to facilitate the treatment or promote healing. A careful evaluation of these drugs or reported literature, a detailed knowledge about their side effects, interactions with other chemicals, and how any alterations in the patient's physiology enhance or suppress the mechanism of action of these drugs is needed before their use or prescription. It is always prudent to remember that no medicine is without side effects and the benefits of using them should be weighed against the risks involved.

## References


1. Dandon RH, Brual LL. Goodman & Gilman's manual of pharmacology and therapeutics. 2nd ed. New York: McGraw Hill Education; 2014.
2. Gaynes R. The discovery of penicillin—new insights after more than 75 years of clinical use. Emerg Infect Dis. 2017;23(5):849–53.
3. Waksman SA. What is an antibiotic or antibiotic substance? Mycologia. 1947;39(5):565–9.
4. Salit IE. Diagnostic approaches to head and neck infections. Infect Dis Clin N Am. 1988;2:35–55.
5. Kuriyama T, Karasawa T, Nakagawa K, Saiki Y, Yamamoto E, Nakamura S. Bacteriologic features and antimicrobial susceptibility in isolates from orofacial odontogenic infections. Oral Surg Oral Med Oral Pathol Oral Radiol Endod. 2000;90:600–8.
6. Paterson SA, Curzon MEJ. The effect of amoxicillin versus penicillin V in the treatment of acutely abscessed primary teeth. Br Dent J. 1993;174:443–9.
7. Chang C, et al. Overview of penicillin allergy. Clinic Rev Allerg Immunol. 2012;43:84–97.
8. Raz R, Elchanan G, Colodner R, et al. Penicillin V twice daily vs four times daily in the treatment of streptococcal pharyngitis. Infect Dis Clin Pract. 1995;4:50–4.
9. Martin MP, Longman LP, Hill JB, et al. Acute dento alveolar infections: an investigation of the duration of antibiotic therapy. Br Dent J. 1997;183:135–7.
10. DePestel DD, et al. Cephalosporin use in treatment of patients with penicillin allergies. J Am Pharm Assoc. 2008;48:530–40.
11. Kelkar PS, Li JT. Cephalosporin allergy. N Engl J Med. 2001;345:804–9.
12. Burke JF. The effective period of preventative antibiotic action in experimental incisions and dermal lesions. Surgery. 1961;50:161–8.
13. Miles AA, Miles EM, Burke J. The value and duration of defense reaction of the skin to the primary lodgment of bacteria. Br J Exp Pathol. 1957;38:79–96.
14. Classen DC, Evans RS, Pestotnik SL, et al. The timing of prophylactic administration of antibiotics and risk of surgical-wound infection. N Engl J Med. 1992;326:281–6.
15. Pallasch TJ. Antibiotic prophylaxis: the clinical significance of its recent evolution. J Calif Dent Assoc. 1997;25(619–24):26–32.
16. Kamolratanakul P, Jansisyanont P. A review of antibiotic prophylaxis protocols in oral and maxillofacial surgery. J Oral Maxillofac Surg Med Pathol. 2018;30:395–404.
17. Garner JS. CDC guideline for prevention of surgical wound infections, 1985. Supersedes guideline for prevention of surgical wound infections published in 1982. (originally published in November 1985). Revised. Infect Control. 1986;7:193–200.
18. Peterson LJ. Antibiotic prophylaxis against wound infections in oral and maxillofacial surgery. J Oral Maxillofac Surg. 1990;48:617–620.
19. Tan SK, Lo J, Zwahlen RA. Perioperative antibiotic prophylaxis in orthognathic surgery: a systematic review and meta-analysis of clinical trials. Oral Surg Oral Med Oral Pathol Oral Radiol Endod. 2011;112:19–27.
20. Sancho-Puchades M, Herraez-Vilas JM, Berini-Aytes L, Gay-Escoda C. Antibiotic prophylaxis to prevent local infection in Oral surgery: use or abuse? Oral Med Oral Patol Oral Cir Bucal. 2009;14:E28–33.
21. Lewis MAO, McGowan DA, Macfarlane TW. Short – course, high-dosage amoxicillin in the treatment of acute dento-alveolar abscess. Br Dent J. 1986;161:299–302.
22. Lodi G, Figini L, Sardella A, Carrassi A, Del Fabbro M, Furness S. Antibiotics to prevent complications following tooth extractions. Cochrane Database Syst Rev. 2012;11:CD003811.
23. Figueiredo R, Valmaseda-Castellon E, Formoso-Senande MF, Berini-Aytes L, GayEscoda C. Delayed-onset infections after impacted lower third molar extraction: involved bacteria and sensitivity profiles to commonly used antibiotics. Oral Surg Oral Med Oral Pathol Oral Radiol Endod. 2012;144:43–8.
24. Sekhar CH, Narayanan V, Baig MF. Role of antimicrobials in third molar surgery: prospective, double blind, randomized, placebo-controlled clinical study. Br J Oral Maxillofac Surg. 2001;39:134–7.

25. Adde CA, Soares MS, Romano MM, et al. Clinical and surgical evaluation of the indication of postoperative antibiotic prescription in third molar surgery. Oral Surg Oral Med Oral Pathol Oral Radiol. 2012;114(5 Suppl):S26–31.
26. Lacasa JM, Jimenez JA, Ferras V, Bossom M, Sola-Morales O, Garcia-Rey C, et al. Prophylaxis versus pre-emptive treatment for infective and inflammatory complications of surgical third molar removal: a randomized, double-blind, placebo-controlled, clinical trial with sustained release amoxicillin/clavulanic acid (1000/62.5 mg). Int J Oral Maxillofac Surg. 2007;36:321–7.
27. Pasupathy S, Alexander M. Antibiotic prophylaxis in third molar surgery. J Craniofac Surg. 2011;22:551–3.
28. Menon RK, Gopinath D, Li KY, et al. Does the use of amoxicillin/amoxicillin–clavulanic acid in third molar surgery reduce the risk of postoperative infection? A systematic review with meta-analysis. Int J Oral Maxillofac Surg. 2018;48(2): 263–73.
29. Poeschl PW, Eckel D, Poeschl E. Postoperative prophylactic antibiotic treatment in third molar surgery–a necessity? J Oral Maxillofac Surg. 2004;62:3–8. Discussion 9
30. Larsen PE. The effect of chlorhexidine rinse on the incidence of alveolar osteitis following the surgical removal of impacted mandibular third molars. J Oral Maxillofac Surg. 1991;49:932–7.
31. Lyall JB. Third molar surgery: the effect of primary closure, wound dressing and metroniadazole on postoperative recovery. J R Army Med Corps. 1991;137:100–3.
32. Ren Y-F, Malmstrom HS. Effectiveness of antibiotic prophylaxis in third molar surgery: a meta-analysis of randomized controlled clinical trials. J Oral Maxillofac Surg. 2007;65(10):1909–21.
33. Resnik RR, Misch C. Prophylactic antibiotic regimens in oral implantology: rationale and protocol. Implant Dent. 2008;17:142–50.
34. Rasmusson L, Roos J, Bystedt H. A 10-year follow-up study of titanium dioxide-blasted implants. Clin Implant Dent Relat Res. 2005;7(1):36–42.
35. Friberg B. Sterile operating conditions for the placement of intraoral implants. J Oral Maxillofac Surg. 1996;54:1334–6.
36. Esposito M, Coulthard P, Oliver R, Thomsen P, Worthington HV. Antibiotics to prevent complications following dental implant treatment. Cochrane Database Syst Rev. 2003:CD004152.
37. Hossein K, Dahlin C, Bengt A. Influence of different prophylactic antibiotic regimens on implant survival rate: a retrospective clinical study. Clin Impl Dent Rel Res. 2005;7(1):32–5.
38. Davis CM, Gregoire CE, Steeves TW, et al. Prevalence of surgical site infections following orthognathic surgery: a retrospective cohort analysis. J Oral Maxillofac Surg. 2016;74:1199–206.
39. Chow LK, Singh B, Chiu WK, Samman N. Prevalence of postoperative complications after orthognathic surgery: a 15-year review. J Oral Maxillofac Surg. 2007;65:984–92.
40. Horan TC, Gaynes RP, Martone WJ, Jarvis WR, Emori G. CDC definitions of nosocomial surgical site infections, 1992: a modification of CDC definitions of surgical wound infections. Infect Control Hosp Epidemiol. 1992;13(10):606–8.
41. Danda AK, Ravi PE. Ectiveness of postoperative antibiotics in orthognathic surgery: a meta-analysis. J Oral Maxillofac Surg. 2011;69:2650–6.
42. Posnick JC, Choi E, Chavda A. Surgical site infections following bimaxillary orthognathic, osseous genioplasty, and intranasal surgery: a retrospective cohort study. J Oral Maxillofac Surg. 2017;75:584–95.
43. Danda AK, Wahab A, Narayanan V, Siddareddi A. Single-dose versus single-day antibiotic prophylaxis for orthognathic surgery: a prospective, randomized, double-blind clinical study. J Oral Maxillofac Surg. 2010;68:344–6.
44. Brignardello-Petersen R, Carrasco-Labra A, Araya I, Yanine N, Cordova Jara L, Villanueva J. Antibiotic prophylaxis for preventing infectious complications in orthognathic surgery. Cochrane Database Syst Rev. 2015;1:CD010266.
45. Mangram AJ, Horan TC, Pearson ML, et al. Guideline for prevention of surgical site infection, 1999. Centers for Disease Control and Prevention (CDC) hospital infection control practices advisory committee. Am J Infect Control. 1999;27:97–132.
46. Peel TN, Buising KL, Choong PF. Prosthetic joint infection: challenges of diagnosis and treatment. ANZ J Surg. 2011;81:32–9.
47. Fridrich KL, Partnoy BE, Zeitler DL. Prospective analysis of antibiotic prophylaxis for orthognathic surgery. Int J Adult Orthodontics Ortho Surg. 1994;9(2):129–31.
48. Laskin DM. The use of prophylactic antibiotics for the prevention of postoperative infections. Oral Maxillofac Surg Clin North Am. 2003;15:155–60.
49. Abubaker O, Rollert MK. Postoperative antibiotic prophylaxis in mandibular fractures: a preliminary randomized, double-blind, and placebo-controlled clinical study. J Oral Maxillofac Surg. 2001;59:1415–9.
50. Haug RH, Assael LA. Infection in the maxillofacial trauma patient. In: Topazian RG, Goldberg MH, Hupp JR, editors. *Oral and Maxillofacial Infections*. Ed 4. Philadelphia: PA, Saunders; 2002. p. 359–80.
51. Andreasen JO, Jensen SS, Schwartz O, Hillerup Y. A systematic review of prophylactic antibiotics in the surgical treatment of maxillofacial fractures. J Oral Maxillofac Surg. 2006;64:1664–8.
52. Dillon JK, Christensen B, McDonald T, et al. The financial burden of mandibular trauma. J Oral Maxillofac Surg. 2012;70:2124–34.
53. Shridharani SM, Berli J, Manson PN, et al. The role of postoperative antibiotics in mandible fractures: a systematic review of the literature. Ann Plast Surg. 2015;75:353–7.
54. Gaal A, Patel Y, Smiley N, et al. Limiting antibiotics when managing mandible fractures may not increase infection risk. J Oral Maxillofac Surg. 2016;74:2008–18.
55. Baliga SD, Bose A, Jain S. The evaluation of efficacy of postoperative antibiotics in the open reduction of the zygomatic and mandibular fracture: a prospective trial. J Maxillofac Oral Surg. 2014;13:165–75.
56. Miles BA, Potter JK, Ellis E. The efficacy of postoperative antibiotic regimens in the open treatment of mandibular fractures: a prospective randomized trial. J Oral Maxillofac Surg. 2006;64:576–82.
57. Goodson WH III, Hunt TK. Wound healing and the diabetic patient. Surg Gynecol Obstet. 1979;149:600–8.
58. Zoeller GN, Kadis B. The diabetic dental patient. Gen Dent. 1981;29:58–61.
59. Rahimi-Nedjat RK, Sagheb K, Pabst A, et al. Diabetes and hyperglycemia as risk factors for postoperative outcome in maxillofacial surgery. J Surg Res. 2017;217:170–6.
60. Ramaraj PN, Cariappa KM. Is there a need for antibiotic prophylaxis after routine dental extraction in diabetic patients? Br J Oral Maxillofac Surg. 2006;44:421.
61. Lee DH, Kim SY, Nam SY, Choi SH, Choi JW, Roh JL. Risk factors of surgical site infection in patients undergoing major oncological surgery for head and neck cancer. Oral Oncol. 2011;47:528–31.
62. Bartella A, Kamal M, Teichmann J, et al. Prospective comparison of perioperative antibiotic management protocols in oncological head and neck surgery. J Cran-Max-Fac Surg. 2017;45:1078–82.
63. Zhang Y, Dong J, Qiao Y, He J, Wang T, Ma S. Efficacy and safety profile of antibiotic prophylaxis usage in clean and clean-contaminated plastic and reconstructive surgery: a meta-analysis of randomized controlled trials. Ann Plast Surg. 2014;72:121–30.
64. Ariyan S, Martin J, Lal A, Cheng D, Borah GL, Chung KC, et al. Antibiotic prophylaxis for preventing surgical-site infection in plastic surgery: an evidence-based consensus conference statement from the American Association of Plastic Surgeons. Plast Reconstr Surg. 2015;135:1723–39.

65. Mercer NSG. The use of preoperative swabs in cleft lip and palate repair. Br J Plast Snrg. 2002;55:176–7.
66. Moss ALH. The use of preoperative swabs in cleft lip and palate repair. Br J Plast Surg. 2002;55:533–4.
67. Chuo CB, Timmons MJ. The bacteriology of children before primary cleft lip and palate surgery. The Cleft Palat-Craniofac J. 2005;42(3):272–6.
68. Rennie AL, Treharne LJ, Richard B. Throat swabs taken on the operating table prior to cleft palate repair and their relevance to outcome: a prospective study. Cleft Palate Craniofac J. 2009 May;46(3):275–9.
69. Aznar ML, Schönmeyr B, Echaniz G, et al. Role of postoperative antimicrobials in cleft palate surgery. Plast Recon Surg. 2015;136(1):59e–66e.
70. Douglas LR, Douglass JB, Sieck JO, Smith PJ. Oral management of the patient with end-stage liver disease and the liver transplant patient. Oral Surg Oral Med Oral Pathol Oral Radiol Endod. 1998;86:55–64.
71. Guggenheimer J, Mayher D, Eghtesad B. A survey of dental care protocols among US organ transplant centers. Clin Transpl. 2005;19:15–8.
72. Lewis T, Grant RT. Observations relating to subacute infective endocarditis. BrHeart J. 1923;10:21–77.
73. Jones TD, Baumgartner L, Bellows MT, et al. Prevention of rheumatic fever and bacterial endocarditis through control of streptococcal infections. Circulation. 1955;11:317–20.
74. Wilson W, Taubert KA, Gewitz M, et al. American Heart Association. Prevention of infective endocarditis: guidelines from the American Heart Association: a guideline from the American Heart Association rheumatic fever, endocarditis and Kawasaki disease committee, council on cardiovascular disease in the young, and the council on clinical cardiology, council on cardiovascular surgery and anesthesia, and the quality of care and outcomes research interdisciplinary working group. JADA. 2008;139(suppl):3S–24S.
75. Gould FK, Elliott TSJ, Foweraker J, et al. Guidelines for the prevention of endocarditis: report of the working party of the British society for antimicrobial chemotherapy. J Antimicrob Chemother. 2006;57:1035–42.
76. Prophylaxis against infective endocarditis. National institute for health and care excellence. 2008.
77. Habib G, Hoen B, Tornos P, et al. Guidelines on the prevention, diagnosis, and treatment of infective endocarditis (new version 2009): the task force on the prevention, diagnosis, and treatment of infective endocarditis of the European society of cardiology (ESC). Endorsed by the European society of clinical microbiology and infectious diseases (ESCMID) and the international society of chemotherapy (ISC) for infection and cancer. Eur Heart J. 2009;30:2369–413.
78. Pasquali SK, He X, Mohamad Z, et al. Trends in endocarditis hospitalizations at US children's hospitals: impact of the 2007 American Heart Association antibiotic prophylaxis guidelines. Am Heart J. 2012;163:894–9.
79. Sakai Bizmark R, Chang R-KR, Tsugawa Y, et al. Impact of AHA's 2007 guideline change on incidence of infective endocarditis in infants and children. Am Heart J. 2017;189:110–9.
80. Pain terms: a list with definitions and notes on usage. Recommended by the IASP Subcommittee on taxonomy. Pain. 1979;6:249–52.
81. Feizerfan A, Sheh G. Transition from acute to chronic pain. Contin Educ Anaesth Crit Care Pain. 2015;15:98–102.
82. Luo Y, Svensson P, Jensen JD, et al. Quantitative sensory testing in patients with or without ongoing pain one year after orthognathic surgery. J Oral Facial Pain Headache. 2014;28:306–16.
83. Desjardins P. Patient pain and anxiety: the medical and psychologic challenges facing oral and maxillofacial surgery. J Oral Maxillofac Surg. 2000;58(2):1–3.
84. Pedersen A. Interrelation of complaints after removal of impacted mandibular third molars. Int J Oral Surg. 1985;14:241–4.
85. Crane M, Green P, Gordon N. Pharmacology of opioid and non-opioid analgesics. Oral Maxillofacial Surg Clin N Am. 2001;13:1–13.
86. Coulthard P, Bailey E, Patel N, Coulthard MB. Pain pathways and pre-emptive and protective analgesia for oral surgery. Oral Surg. 2013;7(2):74–80.
87. Woolf CJ, Chong MS. Preemptive analgesia treating postoperative pain by preventing the establishment of central sensitization. Anesth Analg. 1993;77:362–79.
88. Woolf CJ. Evidence for a central component of postinjury pain hypersensitivity. Nature. 1983;306:686–8.
89. Viswanath A, Oreadi D, Finkelman M, Klein G, Papageorge M. Does pre-Emptive Administration of Intravenous Ibuprofen (Caldolor) or intravenous acetaminophen(Ofirmev) reduce postoperative pain and subsequent narcotic consumption after third molar surgery? J Oral Maxillofac Surg. 2019;77(2):262–70.
90. Hutchison GL, Crofts SL, Gray IG. Preoperative piroxicam for postoperative analgesia in dental surgery. Br J Anaesth. 1990;65:500–3.
91. Ong KS, Seymour RA, Chen FG, Ho VC. Preoperative ketorolac has a preemptive effect for postoperative third molar surgical pain. Int J Oral Maxillofac Surg. 2004;33:771–6.
92. Aoki T, Yamaguchi H, Naito H, Shiiki K, Izawa K, Ota Y, Sakamoto H, Kaneko A. Premedication with cyclooxygenase-2 inhibitor meloxicam reduced postoperative pain in patients after oral surgery. Int J Oral Maxillofac Surg. 2006;35:613–7.
93. Desjardins PJ, Grossman EH, Kuss ME, Talwalker S, Dhadda S, Baum D, Hubbard RC. The injectable cyclooxygenase-2-specific inhibitor parecoxib sodium has analgesic efficacy when administered preoperatively. Anesth Analg. 2001;93:721–7.
94. Moore PA, Brar P, Smiga ER, Costello BJ. Preemptive rofecoxib and dexamethasone for prevention of pain and trismus following third molar surgery. Oral Surg Oral Med Oral Pathol Oral Radiol Endod. 2005;99:e1–7.
95. Møiniche S, Kehlet H, Dah JB. A qualitative and quantitative systematic review of preemptive analgesia for postoperative pain relief: the role of timing of analgesia. Anesthesiology. 2002;96:725–34.
96. Aznar Arasa L, Harutunian K, Figuereido R, et al. Effect of preoperative ibuprofen on pain and swelling after lower third molar removal: a randomized controlled trial. Int J Oral Maxillofac Surg. 2012;41:1005–9.
97. Evans SW, McCahon RA. Management of postoperative pain in maxillofacial surgery. Br J Oral Maxillofac Surg. 2019;57(1):4–11.
98. De Cosmo G, Congedo E, Lai C, et al. Preoperative psychologic and demographic predictors of pain perception and tramadol consumption using intravenous patient-controlled analgesia. Clin J Pain. 2008;24:399–405.
99. Coulthard P, Haywood D, Tai MA, Jackson-Leech D, Pleuvry BJ, Macfarlane TV. Treatment of postoperative pain in oral and maxillofacial surgery. Br J Oral Maxillofac Surg. 2000;38(6):588–92.
100. Mobini A, Mehra P, Chigurupathy R. Postoperative pain and opioid analgesic requirements after orthognathic surgery. J Oral Maxillofac Surg. 2018;76:2285–95.
101. Moore PA, Hersch EV. Analgesic therapy in dentistry - from a letter to the editor to an evidence-base review. Dent Clin N Am. 2019;63:35–44.
102. Fletcher MC, Spera JF. Management of acute postoperative pain after oral surgery. Dent Clin N Am. 2012;56:95–111.
103. Rudd RA, Seth P, David F, Scholl L. Increases in drug and opioid involved overdose deaths—United States, 2010-2015. Morb Mortal Wkly Rep. 2016;65:1445–52.

104. Patel N, Bailey E, Coulthard P. Opioids for pain after oral surgery. Oral Surg. 2013;7(4):196–202.
105. Moore RA, Derry S, McQuay HJ, Wiffen PJ. Single dose oral analgesics for acute postoperative pain in adults. Cochrane Database Syst Rev. 2011;9:CD008659.
106. Ceccheti MM, Negrato GV, de Melo Peres MP, et al. Analgesic and adjuvant anesthetic effect of submucosal tramadol after mandibular third molar surgery. Oral Surg Oral Med Oral Path Oral Radiol. 2014;117(3):e249–54.
107. Power I, Barratt S. Analgesic agents for the postoperative period: nonopioids. Surg Clin North Am. 1999;79:275–95.
108. Moore P, Hersh E. Celecoxib and rofecoxib, the role of COX-2 inhibitors in dental practice. J Am Dent Assoc. 2001;132: 451–6.
109. Seymour RA, Moore U, Hawkesford J, Coulthard P, Jackson-Leech D, Thomas D, Hill M, Combs ML, Renton T, McGurk M. An investigation into the efficacy of intravenous diclofenac in post-operative dental pain. Eur J Clin Pharmacol. 2000 Sep;56(6-7):447–52.
110. Derry CJ, Derry S, Moore RA, McQuay HJ. Single dose oral ibuprofen for acute postoperative pain in adults. Cochrane Database Syst Rev. 2009;3:CD010210.
111. Gyllfors P, Bochenek G, Overholt J, et al. Biochemical and clinical evidence that aspirin intolerant asthmatic subjects tolerate the cyclooxygenase 2-selective analgesic drug celecoxib. J Allergy Clin Immunol. 2003;111:1116–21.
112. Weil K, Hooper L, Afzal Z, et al. Paracetamol for pain relief after surgical removal of wisdom teeth. Cochrane Database Syst Rev. 2007;3:CD004487.
113. Laskarides C. Update on analgesic medication for adult and pediatric dental patients. Dent Clin N Am. 2016;60:347–66.
114. World Health Organization. WHO Pain Ladder. 2013. Available from URL: http://www.who.int/cancer/palliative/painladder/en/.
115. Buvanendran A, Kroin JS. Multimodal analgesia for controlling acute postoperative pain. Curr Opin Anaesthesiol. 2009;22:588–93.
116. Yong SL, Walsh T, Coulthard P. Protective analgesia for postoperative pain following third molar surgery [protocol]. Cochrane Database Syst Rev. 2010;9:CD008692.
117. Rosero EB, Joshi GP. Preemptive, preventive. Multimodal Analgesia Plast Recon Surg. 2014;134:85S–93S.
118. Rood JP, Coulthard P, Snowdon AT, Gennery BA. Safety and efficacy of levobupivacaine for postoperative pain relief after the surgical removal of impacted third molars: a comparison with lignocaine and adrenaline. Br J Oral Maxillofac Surg. 2002 Dec;40(6):491–6.
119. Chang FSC, Burrows A, Gebauer DP. Patient-controlled analgesia and length of hospital stay in orthognathic surgery: a randomized controlled trial. J Oral Maxillofac Surg. 2019;77:818–27.
120. Geha H, Nimeskern N, Beziat J. Patient-controlled analgesia in orthognathic surgery: evaluation of the relationship to anxiety and anxiolytics. Oral Surg Oral Med Oral Pathol Oral Radiol Endod. 2009;108:e33–6.
121. Hudcova J, McNicol ED, Quah CS, Lau J, Carr DB. Patient controlled opioid analgesia versus conventional opioid analgesia for postoperative pain. Cochrane Database Syst Rev. 2006;4:CD003348.
122. Peterson LJ. Postoperative patient management. In: Peterson LJ, Ellis E, Hupp JR, Tucker MR, editors. Contemporary oral and maxillofacial surgery. 3rd ed. St Louis: Mosby; 1998. p. 251.
123. Gilman AG, Rall TW, Nies AS, et al. The pharmacological basis of therapeutics (ed 8). New York, NY: Macmillan; 1990. p. 1436–52.
124. Axelrod L. Adrenal corticosteroids. In: Miller RR, Greenblatt, editors. Handbook of drug Therauv. New York. NY: Elsevier; 1979. p. 809–40.
125. Beirne OR, Hollander B. The effect of methylprednisolone on pain, trismus, and swelling after removal of third molar. Oral Surg Oral Med Oral Path. 1986;61:134–8.
126. Markiewicz MR, Brady MF, Ding EL, Dodson TB. Corticosteroids reduce postoperative morbidity after third molar surgery: a systematic review and meta-analysis. J Oral Maxillofac Surg. 2008;66(9):1881–94.
127. Alexander RE, Throndson RT. A review of perioperative corticosteroid use in dentoalveolar surgery. Oral Surg Oral Med Oral Pathol. 2000;90:406–15.
128. Montgomery MT, Hogg JP, Roberts DL, et al. The use of glucocorticosteroids to lessen the inflammatory sequelae following third molar surgery. J Oral Maxillofac Surg. 1990;48:179–87.
129. Pedersen A. Decadronphosphate in the relief of complaints after third molar surgery. Int J Oral Maxillofac Surg. 1985;14:235–40.
130. Grossi GB, Maiorana C, Garramone RA. Effect of submucosal injection of dexamethasone on postoperative discomfort after third molar surgery: a prospective study. J Oral Maxillofac Surg. 2007;65:2218–26.
131. Messer EJ, Keller JJ. The use of intraoral dexamethasone after extraction of mandibular third molar. Oral Surg Oral Med Oral Pathol. 1975;40:594–8.
132. Brucoli M, De Andreis M, Boffano BP, et al. Comparative assessment of dexamethasone administration routes for the management of postoperative symptoms following third molar surgery. J Stomatol Oral Maxillofac Surg. 2019.
133. de Almeida AC, Lemos CAA, de Moraes SLD, et al. Efficacy of corticosteroids versus placebo in impacted third molar surgery: systematic review and meta-analysis of randomized controlled trials. Int J Oral Maxillofac Surg. 2019;48:118–31.
134. Kainulainen S, Lassus P, Suominen AL, et al. More harm than benefit of perioperative dexamethasone on recovery following reconstructive head and neck cancer surgery: a prospective double-blind randomized trial. J Oral Maxillofac Surg. 2018;76:2425–32.
135. Dionne RA, Gordon SM, Rowan J, et al. Dexamethasone suppresses peripheral prostanoid levels without analgesia in a clinical model of acute inflammation. J Oral Maxillofac Surg. 2003;61:997–1003.
136. de Sousa Santos JAS, DaSilva LCF, de Santana Santos T, et al. Comparative study of tramadol combined with dexamethasone and diclofenac sodium in third-molar surgery. J Cranio-Maxillo-Facial Surg. 2012;40:694–700.
137. Matheny JL. Adrenocorticosteroids: systemic and topical therapy. In: Holroyd SV, Wynn RL, Requa-Clark B, editors. Clinical pharmacology in dental practice. 4th ed. St Louis: Mosby; 1988. p. 238–45.
138. Butler RCD, Vorono AA, Finstuen K. Dosage effects of pulsed steroid therapy on serum cortisol levels in oral and maxillofacial surgery patients. J Oral Maxillofac Surg. 1993;51:750–3.

11

# Wound Care and Closure: Tools and Techniques

Ravi Veeraraghavan

## 11.1 Wound Management

Management of soft tissue wounds needs a careful assessment of the wound, a good understanding of wound types and healing as well as adequate knowledge and skill for wound care. The various steps in wound care include cleansing and debridement, hemostasis, tetanus immunization and antibiotic medication and wound closure.

Wound closure can be accomplished in diverse ways, but suturing remains the mainstay. A wide variety of materials are available for wound suturing. One has to choose the right material and technique depending on the wound type and closure needs. Alternate techniques such as staples, tapes and adhesives are fast gaining popularity.

Wounds are treated by

1. Cleansing and debridement,
2. Haemostasis,
3. Tetanus immunisation,
4. Wound dressings,
5. Wound closure,
6. Antibiotic medication.

## 11.2 Wound Closure

Artificial closure of the wounds is required if significant connective tissue is exposed. Wound closure leads to faster wound healing with reduced complications. Even though suturing is the mainstay of wound closure, other alternatives are fast gaining popularity.

R. Veeraraghavan (✉)
Department of Oral and Maxillofacial Surgery, Amrita School of Dentistry, Ernakulam, India

### 11.2.1 Purposes of Wound Closure

Before going into the intricacies of material selection and techniques of wound closure, one needs to be clear about the actual need for artificially closing a wound. The main indication for wound closure is significant exposure of connective tissue. In general, there are five reasons behind the concept of wound closure.

1. *Healing by Primary Intention*
   This is the most important purpose of wound closure. The open wounds, which are likely to heal by secondary intention, are made to heal in a 'more' primary manner by the intervention of wound closure. This hastens the healing process and also reduces scar formation, with resultant advantages in aesthetic and functional facets.
2. *Coverage of Deep Tissues*
   When the epithelium is breached and connective tissue is bared, it exposes the inner tissues to mechanical and biological threats. This threat becomes even more serious when deeper structures such as the viscera or bone is exposed.
3. *Prevent Contamination*
   An open wound is under constant attack by the pathogenic microorganisms, more so in the oral cavity. Such relentless contamination is likely to lead to a full-blown infection and/or delayed healing. Sooner the wound is closed, the lesser the risk of major contamination.
4. *Haemostasis*
   This is not one of the primary purposes of wound closure. But sutures may help in impeding blood loss by preventing mechanical disturbance to the clot.
5. *Prevention of Dead Space*
   If only the superficial cutaneous sutures are placed over a deep wound, a dead space can result beneath the surface. This condition usually leads to wound breakdown and/or wound infection. Dead space is prevented by closing the deep tissues in multiple layers.

## 11.3 Wound Suturing

Suturing is the process of wound closure by holding the edges of the wound together using a thread. This thread, called a 'suture', is used to approximate the wound edges together and to hold them in position till the tissue healing is sufficiently advanced to maintain themselves in the corrected anatomic position and alignment to each other. The surgeon uses a 'suture needle' to pass the thread through the tissues on either side of the wound so as to hold the separated edges in the proper position.

### 11.3.1 Suturing Instruments

Apart from the suture thread and needle, some instruments are used to perform the suturing process. Commonly used instruments include a needle holder, a tissue holding forceps and a pair of scissors.

#### 11.3.1.1 Needle Holder

The needle holder (needle driver) is the primary instrument used for suturing. Similar to a haemostat, it is used to grasp and manipulate the suture needle to which the thread is attached. A needle holder has three parts—a pair of beaks, a joint ('pivot') and a pair of handles with rings. Many designs are available, examples being Webster, Halsey and Mayo-Hegar. Most designs have a serrated or cross-hatching pattern of teeth for the beaks. This helps to grip the needle securely without damaging it. A locking mechanism similar to haemostats is present to lock the needle grasp.

The classical way to hold the instrument is to engage the handle-rings with the thumb and the fourth finger. The middle finger is used for support and the index finger is used to direct or orient the instrument in the required direction. Alternatively, while suturing on tough tissues, one may be 'palmed', i.e. may be held against the palm with fingers around. While palming the needle holder, some surgeons still rest the fourth finger lightly in the handle-ring.

#### 11.3.1.2 Tissue Holding Forceps

The pickup forceps are used to delicately handle and manipulate the wound edge which is being sutured. The fine-toothed Adson forceps is the workhorse for most interior and cutaneous wound closures. The forceps is held in the non-dominant hand and is used to grasp, lift and evert the wound edge so that the surface is made more amenable to a perpendicular needle entry. Fine skin hooks may also be used for the same purpose.

#### 11.3.1.3 Suture Cutting Scissors

The suture cutting scissors is used to cut the suture thread tags after the knot is tied. It is also used to cut the thread during suture removal.

These scissors should be differentiated from scissors used for cutting tissue. Many of them have specifically designed blades and tips, which are uniquely shaped to lift and grasp up the handing tags or the tied suture thread away from the tissue and to cut it safely without injuring the tissues. Short and long versions are available. The tip may be straight or curved and may have a sharp slot for the thread to be cut. Some manufacturers have incorporated a cutting component in the needle holder itself, using which the surgeon can cut the suture tag without switching instruments.

### 11.3.2 Suture Needles

The suture needles help to pass the suture threads through tissues. In ancient days, needles were made of natural materials such as bones, ivory, horns, wood or thorns. In fact, eyed needles from as early as 30,000 AD have been unearthed. Later, metals such as silver, copper and aluminium bronze were used. The modern needles are diligently shaped and contoured as per use and are smooth and strong so that they withstand the stresses of suturing and least traumatic to tissues at the same time.

The suture needle has three parts: the tip, the body and the suture attachment. Made of stainless steel or carbon steel, they are thin, smooth and sharp, designed to pass through tissues with ease (Fig. 11.1).

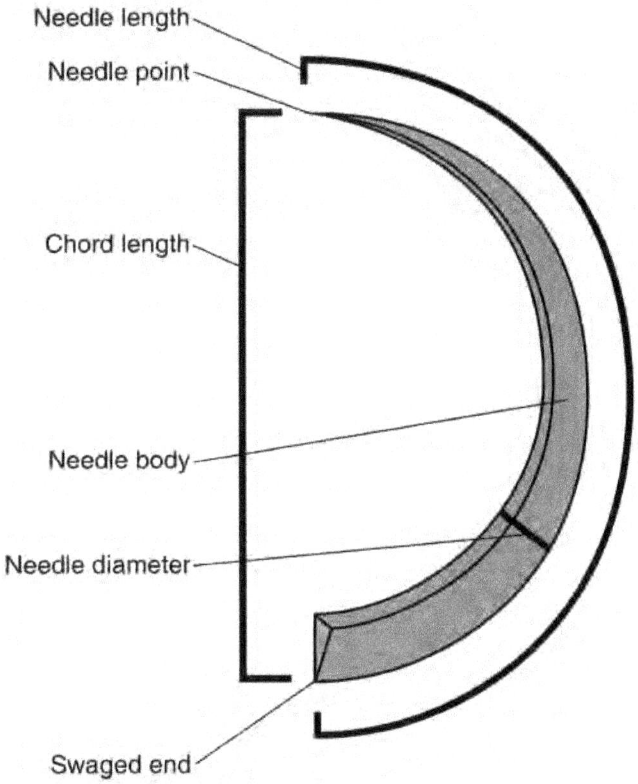



**Fig. 11.1** Parts of suture needle

**Fig. 11.2** Needle shapes/ curvature

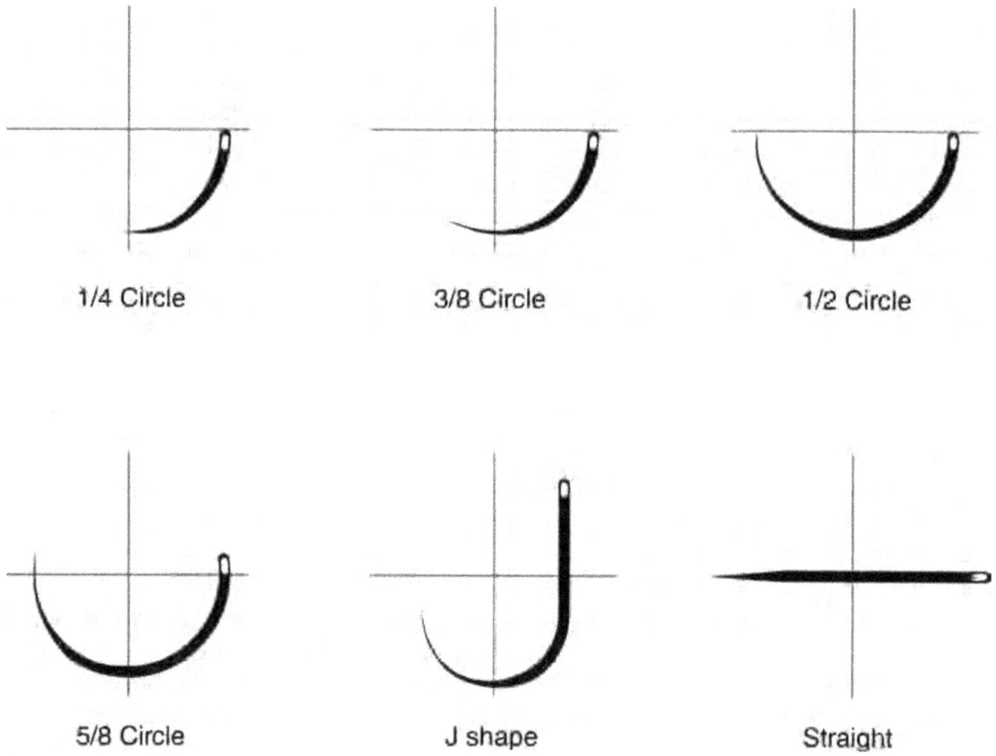




### 11.3.2.1 Needle Shape

The suture needles are usually curved as an arc of a circle. Straight needles, though available, have very limited practical applications. The curvature is described as the span of the arc, in terms of ¼, $^3/_8$, ½ and $^5/_8$ of a circle. Most of the regular suturing in oral and maxillofacial surgery is done with half circle needles. A smaller arc such as $^3/_8$ can be used for suturing flat skin surfaces. Longer arc, i.e. $^5/_8$ circle, needles are used in narrow tunnelled surgical fields such as in cleft palate or inside the nose (Fig. 11.2).

The cross section and the tip of the needles can be widely varied. Depending on these aspects, the suture needles can be.

1. Round bodied,
2. Conventional cutting (Fig. 11.3) or
3. Reverse cutting.

Round bodied needles are generally used to suture viscera and other internal structures such as muscle and fascia. It can also be effective on non-keratinised mucosa. The tip of the round-bodied needle can be blunt or sharp. The blunt tip needle is specifically used in the inner abdominal wall and in friable tissues. The sharp tip is used for most other purposes. But even the sharp tip is hard to pass across the skin and keratinised mucosa. The shape of the 'cutting' needle overcomes this problem. In the cutting needles, the needle cross section is a triangle, with the inner curve side being pointed and the outer convex side flat. This shape enables the needle to 'cut' through the dense tissues to make the needle passage easier. But the cutting design presented a new problem. Even under minimum tension, the needle behaved like a knife, and the sharp edge often tended to lacerate the tissue resulting in a 'cut-through' of the wound edge. This was solved by the reverse-cutting design, wherein the inner curve is flat and the outer curve is pointed. This helps to retain the cutting nature while avoiding the risk of wound edge laceration. In oral and maxillofacial surgery, the tissues encountered may be keratinised (skin, gingiva and palate) or non-keratinised (buccal mucosa, floor of mouth and lips). Mostly, reverse-cutting needles are now being used since they are well-suited to pass through all oral tissues without causing inadvertent tears.

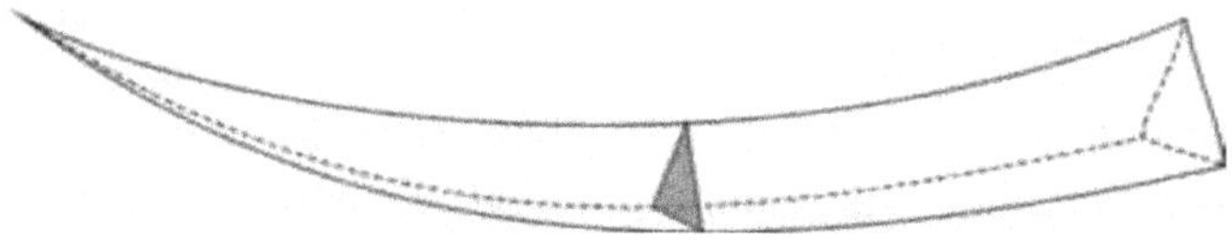



**Fig. 11.3** Needle cross section of a conventional cutting needle

### 11.3.2.2 Needle Size

The suture needle size generally depends on the size of the suture. In general, smaller the suture size, smaller the needle. It is important to recognise the various dimensions of a needle.

The 'needle length' refers to the end-to-end measurement along the curve of the needle. The straight line distance from the tip to the other end is called 'chord length'. The chord length determines the bite-width of the needle in the tissues. The bite-depth into the tissue is defined by the 'chord diameter' which is perpendicular from the chord length to the centre of the needle body. Needle diameter and needle radius are dimensions which refer to the cross-sectional thickness and not to the needle curve.

#### 11.3.2.3 Eyed vs Swaged Needles

The eye of the needle is a small hole at one end for attaching the suture thread. This necessitates an increase in the needle thickness at the attachment end, increasing the risk of potential tissue trauma. The suture is passed through the eye, and may then be tucked or tied for better retention. Both tucking and tying further increases the tissue drag and causes additional trauma. The attached suture now follows the needle through the tissues. The eyed needles are cheaper and can be reused after resterilisation.

Modern suture needles do not have an eye. Instead, the suture thread is sealed inside the needle for a permanent attachment. This mechanism, called 'swaging', reduces the tissue trauma significantly as the needle diameter is not increased for thread attachment. Further, only a single thread strand passes through the tissue at all times. So these needles are often called 'atraumatic needles'. The swaged needle with thread is available as a sterile pack, and cannot be reused.

## 11.4 Suture Thread

Many different types of suture threads are available for use. Each type has its specific benefits and indications for application (Table 11.1).

A basic classification divides them into 'natural' and 'synthetic'. Suture materials sourced from natural sources include catgut, steel and silk. Synthetic plastic materials such as nylon, polypropylene and polymers of glycolic acid, lactic acid, etc., have become popular in recent decades.

Suture materials can also be classified as absorbable and non-absorbable. Absorbable sutures hold the tissues together till they have healed sufficiently to withstand normal stress, and are then absorbed by the tissues where they are embedded. Non-absorbable sutures, on the other hand, are not absorbed, and they should be removed after the initial stabilisation of the wound edges has occurred. In reality, most or all natural materials will get absorbed by the body in due course of time. Thus, for clinical practice, a suture is considered non-absorbable if it retains its tensile strength in tissues for more than 60 days.

**Table 11.1** Suture material classification

| Basis of classification | Types |
|---|---|
| Source | Natural, synthetic |
| Absorbability | Absorbable, non-absorbable |
| Thread size | 3, 2, 1, 0, 1–0, 2–0, 3–0..........................11–0 |
| Filament type | Monofilament, multifilament (braided) |

According to the filament type, the sutures may be monofilament or multifilament. A monofilament suture is essentially a single strand of fibre. This simple structure enables these sutures to pass through tissues with least resistance. Though this makes it the material of choice in delicate tissues such as the vascular tissues, there are some notable drawbacks. The handling and knot-tying are generally more taxing, and the knot has less friction to keep its position. In addition, the cut edges tend to be stiff leading to probable irritation of movable and delicate regions like the tongue and buccal mucosa.

The multifilament sutures are made of multiple fibre strands, which are either coated or braided together to make one fine thread. The process of braiding bestows a higher tensile strength as well as better pliability and flexibility. This improves the handling characteristics and the ease of knot-tying. They also better resist the tendency of the knot to untie itself. The cut edges are usually smooth and soft, and are not irritating to oral tissues. The disadvantages of multifilament sutures include the higher risk of harbouring pathogens in its structure and the tendency to 'wick' the oral fluids into deeper tissues through the suture track. This, in turn, can lead to occurrence to unaesthetic suture tracks visible on the skin.

### 11.4.1 Suture Thread Size

The suture thread is available in different thicknesses. The thickness is usually mentioned as 'number of zeroes'. This system follows the U.S. Pharmacopeia, and has gained wide acceptance. The most commonly used thread size for intraoral use is mentioned as 3–0 or 000 size. Sutures are available from size 6 to 11–0 (Table 11.2).

**Attributes of an Ideal Suture Material**

1. Sterile or sterilisable,
2. Good handling characteristics,
3. Ensure a secure knot,
4. Adequate tensile strength,
5. Retention of strength during the healing phase,
6. Rapid absorption after healing.
7. Stay inert in tissues without causing antigenicity or other adverse tissue reaction.

**Table 11.2** Suture sizes—U.S. Pharmacopeia designation and equivalent metric measurements

| USP designation | 11–0 | 10–0 | 9–0 | 8–0 | 7–0 | 6–0 | 5–0 | 4–0 | 3–0 | 2–0 | 0 | 1 | 2 | 3 |
|---|---|---|---|---|---|---|---|---|---|---|---|---|---|---|
| Diameter (mm) | 0.01 | 0.02 | 0.03 | 0.04 | 0.05 | 0.07 | 0.1 | 0.15 | 0.2 | 0.3 | 0.35 | 0.4 | 0.5 | 0.6 |

It is beyond the purview of this chapter to go into the details of all the types of suture materials available in the market, chemical structure, method of resorption, qualities, indications, advantages, etc. Details of few suture materials widely used in oral and maxillofacial surgery are given below.

## 11.4.2 Natural Absorbable Sutures (Absorbed by Proteolysis)

The absorbability characteristics of many natural materials had been recognised for millennia. All absorbable natural suture materials contain predominantly collagen. Over the years, they have progressively fallen out of favour due to the risk of antigenicity and adverse tissue reaction [1].

### 11.4.2.1 Catgut

Catgut has been the most popular material in this group. Its use has been prevalent at least from the time of Galen of Pergamon (200 AD). This material is made of tissue taken from the submucosal layer of sheep intestine or from the serosal (adventitial) layer of the cattle small intestine intima. The collagen strands are twisted together and the resultant thread is precision-ground to form a monofilament. Catgut has long been a popular fibre to make string instruments and tennis racquets. For many centuries, catgut (surgical gut) had been the only absorbable suture material available. The absorption is by proteolytic biodegradation brought about by proteolytic enzymes.

Performance-wise, catgut has good flexibility but relatively poor tensile strength, poor knot stability and high tissue reactivity. Full tensile strength remains only for 7 days.

### 11.4.2.2 Chromic Catgut

It has been found that many poor characteristics of catgut can be overcome by impregnating the suture material with chromic salts. This modified product, called chromic catgut, has higher tensile strength and delayed absorption time. Chromic catgut retains its maximum tensile strength for about 2 weeks. It also has reduced tissue reaction as compared to plain gut.

Manufacturers package catgut sutures soaked in the disinfectant isopropyl alcohol solution to retain the flexibility and to increase shelf life. This necessitates rinsing of the suture in sterile saline to remove the irritant alcohol before use. Some manufacturers use a glycerine coating on chromic catgut to do away with the alcohol in packaging. Glycerine-coated chromic gut is smoother and thicker and has better handling characteristics.

## 11.4.3 Natural Non-absorbable Sutures

These are the oldest suture materials known to mankind. People tended to use any threaded material known to them for holding the wound edges together. Non-absorbable natural materials include cotton, linen, steel and silk.

### 11.4.3.1 Cotton and Linen

Cotton and linen sutures primarily contain cellulose polymer. Both the materials get absorbed in due course, but are considered non-absorbable because of delayed absorption time. Cotton is sourced from the hair of the cotton seed while linen is made from flax. The fibres are twisted to form a suture. It has good tensile strength, but there is moderate tissue reaction. Handling is average but knot-holding is good. Linen has the advantage that it gains tensile strength when wet.

Cotton and linen have largely fallen out of favour because of adverse tissue reactions and the high 'wicking' effect which causes seepage of fluids into the suture track.

### 11.4.3.2 Silk

Silk has been a well-known textile material from fourth millennium BC. It is produced by the silkworm larvae to form the cocoon. Natural silk is a protein fibre, the main components being fibroin and sericin. Fibroin forms the basic structure and contributes to the tensile strength. Sericin is a gum layer which holds the strands together. The silkworm larvae are cultivated and once they start pupating, the cocoons are dissolved in boiling water to extract the individual fibres which are fed into the spinning reel. To make it suitable as a medical product, the sericin protein component is later removed by a degumming process.

Silk is the most widely used natural non-absorbable suture material. Surgical silk is made from the larvae of the silkworm *Bombyx Mori*. The silk suture consists of a group of strands braided around a core and has a wax or silicon coating. It is usually dyed black in colour for better visibility.

The most impressive property of the silk suture is the ease of handling. It is extremely pliable and smooth and has good knot-holding capability. But the tensile strength is pretty low. The other drawbacks include high levels of tissue friction, capillary action and tissue inflammatory response. The wax coating helps to counteract all these negative attributes.

Silk is now not considered an appropriate material for cutaneous suturing, except on specific sites such as eyelids and lips. It is very often used for ligating blood vessels and for hitching drains. It is the most popular material used in dentistry. Its soft and pliable nature makes it suitable for use in oral mucosa which is mobile and wet.

### 11.4.4 Synthetic Non-absorbable Sutures

#### 11.4.4.1 Polyamide/Nylon (Ethilon, Dermalon)

Nylon belongs to the first generation of commercially successful synthetic thermoplastic polymers, having started production in 1927. It is made of repeated units linked by aliphatic or aromatic amide links (polyamide). It has been a very versatile material and has been used as fabric, fibres, films, coatings and moulded shapes for wide applications in diverse fields.

Nylon surgical sutures were introduced in 1940. Monofilament nylon sutures are very popular for cutaneous suturing. The main advantages are their high tensile strength, exceptional elasticity and low tissue reaction. The elasticity helps the material to accommodate tissue swelling and maintain wound edge apposition. The nylon sutures are dyed black in colour.

The biggest shortcoming of this material is its shape memory, which negatively affects its knot-tying and knot-holding properties. Often, one needs 3–4 knots to hold a stitch in place. Also, the monofilament may be stiff. Multifilament nylon sutures are available with increased pliability and handling features. Addition of fluid (alcohol) in the package reduces the shape memory and improves pliability.

#### 11.4.4.2 Polypropylene (Prolene, Surgipro)

Polypropylene is another thermoplastic polymer used as a non-absorbable suture material. It is produced by chain-growth polymerisation of the monomer propylene. It is pigmented blue to enhance visibility, hence the name polypropylene blue.

Similar to nylon, polypropylene has a very high tensile strength, excellent elasticity and minimal tissue reaction. It can extend up to 30% without breakage, making it highly suitable for suturing cutaneous wounds. The shape memory is also similar to nylon and can contribute to knot slippage. This feature, though, is advantageous in subcuticular suturing since it slides out smoothly during suture removal.

The excellent mechanical properties and inert nature have made polypropylene the material of choice in stressful sites. It is widely used in the management of hernia and vaginal prolapse, often in the form of a mesh in addition to sutures.

#### 11.4.4.3 Polyester (Ethibond, Surgidac, Dacron)

Polyester is a general term used for any organic polymer which has an ester functional group in the main chain. More specifically, the term is used for the material polyethylene terephthalate. It is a type of petroleum-based plastic, made by mixing ethylene glycol and terephthalic acid. Because of its durability, cleanability, anti-wrinkle and quick-drying characteristics, it swiftly made a name in the textile industry as a reliable material.

Polyester is a non-absorbable, braided, surgical suture with high tensile strength and low tissue reactivity. The braided nature adds to enhanced handling, knot-tying and retentivity. Thus, it combines the positive features generally attributed to monofilaments and multifilaments. It is thus the suture of choice in cardiovascular surgery, prosthetic implants and facelifts.

Polyester braided sutures are usually dyed green in colour. They may be coated or uncoated. The uncoated variant has a rough surface which produces drag in the tissues. The coating is made of PTFE or polybutylate.

#### 11.4.4.4 Polybutester (Novafil, Vascufil)

Polybutester is a relatively new thermoplastic material with unique stress-strain properties. It is a copolymer comprised of polybutylene terephthalate and poly teramethylene ether glycol, and is coated with polytribolate. The polybutester monofilament sutures are designed to have high strength, elasticity and pliability. The flexibility and lack of memory allow it to be handled with ease resulting in a high knot security. The unique features have made this a popular material for abdominal wound closure.

The elasticity of polybutester is phenomenal. It can stretch 50% of its length at initial loads. It has a biphasic expansion curve wherein it expands well in response to initial stress and maintains pressure without cutting the tissue, and at the same time withstanding creep by not undergoing permanent deformation even under constant pressure.

#### 11.4.4.5 Polytetrafluroethylene (Gore-Tex, Cytoplast, Coreflon, Teflon)

Polytetrafluroethylene (PTFE) is a synthetic material which has found extensive application globally. It is a fluoropolymer of tetrafluoroethylene (-$CF_2$-$CF_2$-), made by free-radical polymerisation of monomer units. PTFE is a strong, tough, waxy, non-flammable material popular for its non-stick properties.

PTFE suture is considered as the ideal material for oral surgeries, especially for dental implant surgeries. It is inert, non-absorbable and monofilament in nature. The strong fluoro-carbon bond is thought to be the reason for its inertness. Unlike other synthetic monofilament sutures, PTFE is smooth, supple and soft. The cut ends cause no irritation to delicate oral tissues. It has no shape memory. It is well tolerated in the oral cavity and has excellent handling, knot-tying and knot-holding abilities. Thus, it has most of the positive attributes of braided sutures, at the same time avoiding the risk of bacterial contamination by wicking effect.

#### 11.4.4.6 Stainless Steel

Surgical stainless steel non-absorbable surgical suture is composed of 316 L austenitic stainless steel. It can be monofilamentous or multifilamentous. The obvious advantages of stainless steel sutures are strength and low tissue reaction. Its drawbacks include very poor flexibility that makes it highly demanding in suturing skills. Incorrect technique can cause an excessive pull or tear on the tissues resulting in necrosis of wound edges. Barbs at the end can cause glove punctures and trauma to adjacent tissues.

Stainless steel suture is used in sternal closure and in orthopaedic procedures involving cartilage and tendon repair. It is also sparingly used for abdominal wound closure and hernia repair.

### 11.4.5 Synthetic Absorbable Sutures (Absorbed by Hydrolysis)

Till polyglycolic acid sutures were introduced in the 1970s, all absorbable sutures were natural. The synthetic absorbable sutures are all polymers based on glycolic acid, l-lactic acid, paradioxanone, trimethylene carbonate and e-caprolactone [2]. They are sterilised either by ethylene oxide gas or by gamma radiation. These polymers have definite advantages over chromic catgut in clinical use. They are much stronger, evoke minimal tissue reaction, stay longer before absorption and leave no reactive changes after they are resorbed. They are absorbed typically by hydrolysis reaction which breaks the polymer chains. The hydrolysis end products are $CO_2$, $H_2O$ and the monomer.

#### 11.4.5.1 Polyglycolic Acid (Dexon, PolySyn, PGA)

Polyglycolic acid suture, introduced in the early 1970s, was the first absorbable synthetic suture material. It is braided homopolymer of glycolic acid. The uncoated version is beige in colour while the polycaprolate-coated product may be undyed or dyed green, violet or bicoloured. When compared to catgut, the tensile strength and knot security are excellent. It retains 65% of its tensile strength after 2 weeks, by which time catgut would have lost all its strength.

The polylycolic acid soon became very popular but fell out of favour later as better products were developed in due course of time.

#### 11.4.5.2 Polyglactin 910 (Vicryl, Polysorb)

Polyglactin 910 is a synthetic heteropolymer consisting of 90% glycolic acid and 10% lactic acid. Introduced in 1974, this is a multifilamentous, braided suture with a lubricant coating of polyglactin 370 (30:70 ratio) and calcium stearate. The final product is usually dyed violet in colour, but an undyed beige version is also available. Polyglactin 910 is among the most popular absorbable sutures used for surgical wound closure today.

The main advantages of polyglactin over polyglycolic acid include consistently higher residual tensile strength and faster absorption. The absorption happens between 40 and 70 days. The coating ensures smooth passage. Since the coating is made of similar material, the risk of flaking is very low. Calcium stearate used in the coating is an absorbable organic lubricant. The shelf life of polyglactin is as high as 5 years.

As the material became very popular and widely used, manufacturers began to bring out modified products providing specific benefits. One of them is a monofilament version which does not require a coating. Another one is an 'antibacterial suture' with embedded triclosan, which is said to be very effective in preventing surgical site infections. Yet another useful modification is 'rapidly absorbing polyglactin' (Vicryl Rapide/Velosorb Fast). By treating the coating with γ-radiation, it is made to lose strength by second week and is fully absorbed by sixth week. This variant is widely used in oral surgery, where faster resorption is desired.

#### 11.4.5.3 Polydioxanone (PDS, PDO)

Polydioxanone was the first monofilament suture available of large size (larger than 3–0). It is a polyester product and is synthesised through the ring opening of the monomer paradioxanone (1, 4-dioxan 2-one). As a monofilament suture, it has much less drag through the tissues than polyglactin or polyglycolic acid. Since it retains its tensile strength over a long span of time (80% strength at 2 weeks and 60% after 6 weeks), it is considered a better alternative to polyglactin for suturing of fascia.

A modification called PDS II is chemically similar but is annealed above melting temperature to soften the external surface, imparting improved flexibility to the final product.

#### 11.4.5.4 Poliglecaprone 25 (Monocryl/Biosyn/Petcryl Mono/Monoglyde)

Often seen as the monofilament alternative to polyglactin, poliglecaprone is a segmented block polymer consisting of 75% glycolide and 25% ε-caprolactone. It is available as an undyed or a violet dyed version. The key feature that differentiates poliglecaprone from other monofilament sutures is the high level of pliability and handling properties. This is achieved through the formation of an interim soft polymer chain 'pre-polymer' which is high in caprolactone. In the ensuing stages of manufacturing, more glycolide is added to supplement hard segments to the pre-polymer. In this way, we get a final product with high tensile strength without compromising on the pliability.

The tensile strength of the undyed poliglecaprone suture degrades to 50% in 1 week and 30% in the second week. The dyed version retains 70% strength after 1 week. Complete absorption by hydrolysis happens in about 100 days.

#### 11.4.5.5 Polyglyconate (Maxon)

This copolymer has a molar ratio of 64% glycolic acid and 36% trimethylene carbonate. It is an uncoated monofilament which may be undyed or dyed dark green. Polyglyconate has good handling properties. But its main advantage is the retention of tensile strength over a long time span. It retains at least 50% of its strength 4 weeks after implantation, making this an excellent choice in situations where long-term retention is needed. The slow absorption makes it relatively unsuitable for subcuticular sutures, since the dyed suture may be visible under the surface.

#### 11.4.5.6 Glycomer 631 (Biosyn)

It is a synthetic absorbable coated monofilament polyester suture. It is a tri-block copolymer and contains glycolide (60%), trimethylene carbonate (26%) and p-dioxanone (14%). It may be undyed or dyed violet. It has high flexibility, low memory and minimal tissue reactivity.

It passes through the tissues easily but has poor knot-holding capability. Degradation and absorption are similar to polyglactin. Full absorption is complete in around 100 days.

#### 11.4.5.7 Polyglytone 6211 (Caprosyn)

Polyglytone 6211 is the only suture available with four different monomers in its core structure. It is a polyester copolymer of glycolide, caprolactone, trimethylene carbonate and lactide in the ratio 6:2:1:1. It is a monofilament, uncoated, absorbable suture which is undyed or dyed violet.

Polyglytone 6211 is a suture for the short-term approximation of tissues. Because of its quick disintegration, it offers an inert alternative to catgut that can evoke inflammatory response. Its strength decreases to 50–60% at 5 days and to 20–30% at 10 days post-implantation.

## 11.5 Knot-Tying

The suture knot-tying can be accomplished by using an instrument (usually the needle holder) or using hands. Three main techniques are described.

### 11.5.1 Two-Handed Tie

The two-handed tie is cumbersome and is not routinely used. The suture is tied together by holding one tag in each hand and intertwining them.

### 11.5.2 One-Handed Tie

The one-handed tie is the most popular hand-tie method. It is quicker and can be accomplished in a smaller space. One end of the suture thread tag ('the long end') is held with thumb and forefinger of the dominant hand. The other side tag ('the short end') is placed a bit distal to the first tag, running in the same direction. The middle finger is folded and is used to guide the short end around the long end, and then the two tags are pulled away.

### 11.5.3 Instrument Tie

Instrument tie is the most popular technique for tying a suture knot. The long end is wrapped around the needle holder. Then the needle holder beaks are opened to grasp the short end, which is then pulled to form a tie. One such tie is called a 'throw'.

## 11.6 Suture Knots

The suture thread tags are intertwined to form a knot. The knot should be firm and tight, and should not lie on the wound/incision line. It is important that the knot stays tight and maintains strength during the healing phase. Knot slippage or breakage before healing can be detrimental to the wound. In general, knot security is higher for braided and uncoated sutures because of higher friction coefficient.

The knots placed for the surgical suturing are of simple design. Those employed commonly are the square knot, surgeon's knot and granny's knot. These three variants are very similar to each other and differ from each other only in minor aspects.

### 11.6.1 Square Knot/Reef Knot

A square knot is among the simplest of the knot designs. It involves a simple intertwining of the two threads. This 'half-hitch' knot (one 'throw' around the instrument) need to be complemented with an additional similar throw to make it secure. Preferably the second hitch should be in the opposite direction, i.e. if the first throw is in clockwise direction, the second one should be in anticlockwise orientation.

The classical square knot formed by a clockwise and a counterclockwise hitch can be further complimented by more similar hitches in alternatively changing directions.

### 11.6.2 Surgeon's Knot

A surgeon's knot is a minor modification of the square knot in which the initial intertwining is doubled. This is accomplished by doubling the first throw, by doing two turns of the thread around the instrument. This is followed by a regular second throw in the opposite direction.

### 11.6.3 Granny's Knot

In the granny's knot, two initial throws are placed in the same direction, followed by a third throw in the opposite direction.

**Principles of Wound Suturing**

Regardless of the specific technique, some basic principles are to be followed while performing a suturing procedure. It is to be remembered that these are only general principles, and can be modified or rejected in specific situations depending on the clinical context.

1. The suture needle is to be held with the needle holder about ¾th of the distance from the needle tip.
2. The selected suture size should be the smallest possible which will hold the wound edges securely.
3. The needle tip should enter the tissue perpendicular to the tissue surface.
4. The needle penetrations should be at equal distances from the wound edge on both sides of the wound. The actual distance depends on the suture/needle size but is generally agreed to be 2–3 mm.
5. The passage of the needle through the tissues should follow the curvature of the needle.
6. When one side of the wound is fixed to the underlying tissues, one should first engage the mobile wound edge.
7. When one side of the wound is thicker than the other, the thinner wound edge should be engaged first.
8. When one side is deeper and the other more superficial, the deeper side should be engaged first.
9. The depth of needle penetration should be more than the distance from wound edge to needle penetration point. This will ensure eversion of wound edges.
10. The sutures should ensure proper tissue approximation of wound edges at the same time avoiding excessive tension on the tissues. Excessive tissue tension can lead to blanching, tear and necrosis. In case the edges are not approximating passively, the flaps may be undermined to achieve better mobilisation so that a tension-free closure can be achieved.
11. The knot should lie on one side of the wound, and not over the wound edges.
12. The spacing between the individual sutures depends on the type of tissue and the size of sutures. Generally placed 3–4 mm apart, they should be closer together at areas of underlying muscular activity and when the sutures are smaller in size.

## 11.7 Specific Suturing techniques [3] (Video 11.1)

There are quite a large number of techniques available to stitch a wound. Only the commonly used methods are mentioned.

**Factors to Be Considered on Specific Material and Technique**

1. Type of tissue,
2. Type of wound,
3. Time available,
4. Aesthetic requirements,
5. Functional needs,
6. Likely tension on the wounds.
7. Expected time for tissue healing.

### 11.7.1 Simple Interrupted Suture

A simple interrupted suture ('simple loop') is the most common method to suture a wound. This is the simplest design of wound closure. The suture passes once through each side of the wound in a simple loop and is then tied in a knot above the surface. Multiple such ties are made over the length of the wound, resulting in several independent sutures collectively securing the tissue edges together. The same technique is frequently employed for internal suturing of tissue layers also [4].

The needle penetrates the surface 2–3 mms away from the wound edge on one side and proceeds into the subcutaneous tissue. The curve of the needle is then used to pass it through to the subcutaneous tissue on the opposite side. The needle then exits through the surface. The initial and final tags, now outside of the tissues, are then tied in a knot. The configuration inside the tissue is thus in the form of a loop. If the wound sides are of unequal depth, then the needle should travel deeper in the lower side while staying superficial on the higher side. This will help to correct the depth disparity and ensure proper surface levelling.

This technique is easy to learn and employ. This suture provides good tensile strength and carries minimal risk of wound oedema or impaired circulation. Several adjustments to the design are possible with this method depending on the wound characteristics. Since there is a series of multiple sutures, even if one suture fails, the others may provide sufficient strength to keep the wound edges together (Fig. 11.4).

The major drawback of this method of suturing is the high possibility of 'rail-road track' shaped scars caused due to the ingrowth of epithelium into the suture tracks. There is also a tendency to cause 'wound inversion' (depression of the surface at the wound site) due to tissue contracture during healing. The inversion can be prevented by making the suture configuration 'flask-shaped' inside the tissues, by making the needle travel farther laterally away from the wound within the tissues. When compared to continuous suturing techniques, the interrupted method is more time-consuming as it requires many more knots need to be tied.

### 11.7.2 Simple Buried Suture

The buried suture is a modification of the simple interrupted suture and is reserved for stitching the inner (deeper) tissue layers. The only difference is that the knot ends up in the tissues deeper to the suture loop, i.e. away from the surface. In essence, this is a simple interrupted suture in the reverse orientation.

The wound edge is first reflected using fine forceps or hooks. The needle is then inserted into the underside of the dermis on one side. The needle then proceeds along its curvature to exit in the wound edge more superficial to the initial bite. The needle then pierces the dermis wound edge (near the surface) on the opposite side, proceeds in a path mirroring its motion in the first side and comes out at a deeper point which corresponds to the first bite. Though the tie is done outside, the knot gets buried deep inside the tissues as it is tightened (Fig. 11.5).

This technique is extremely useful in suturing the inner tissue layers before the surface closure. As the knot is buried deep, it does not interfere with the closure of superficial layers. This aspect is extremely useful while closing cutaneous facial wounds.

Two major drawbacks have been observed with this suture. One is a skin dimpling which typically happens if the suture arc inadvertently involves the epidermis. Another problem is the tendency for wound inversion to occur. Small modifications such a set-back dermal buried suture or a vertical mattress buried suture can be employed to overcome this

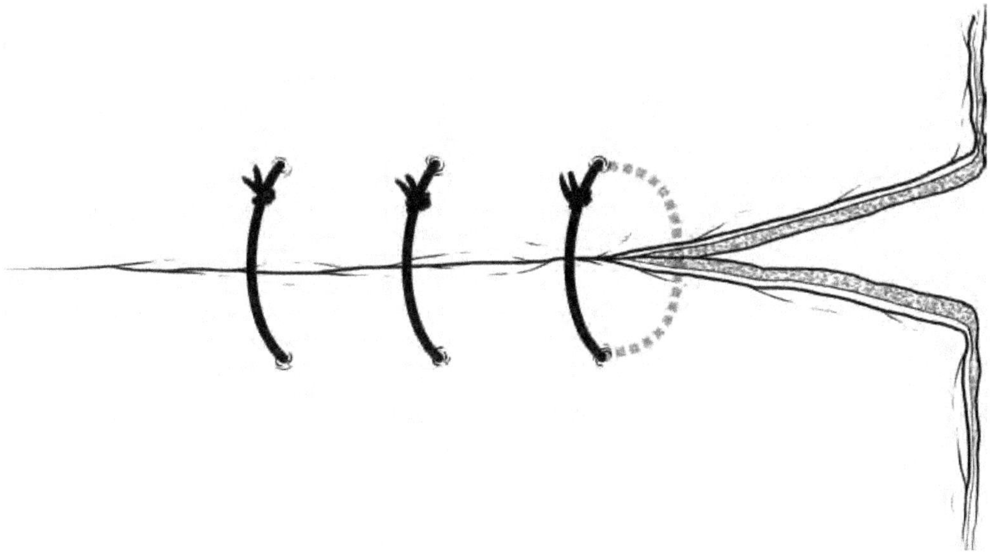

**Fig. 11.4** Simple interrupted suture technique

**Fig. 11.5** Buried suture

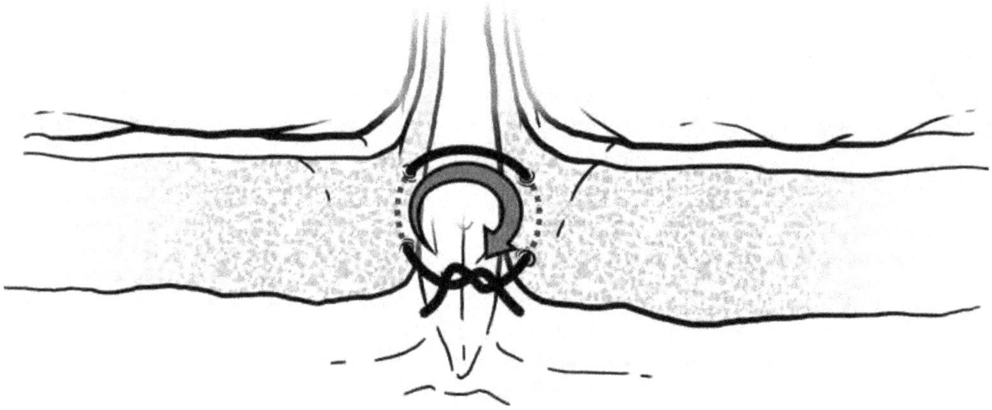



**Fig. 11.6** Vertical mattress suture

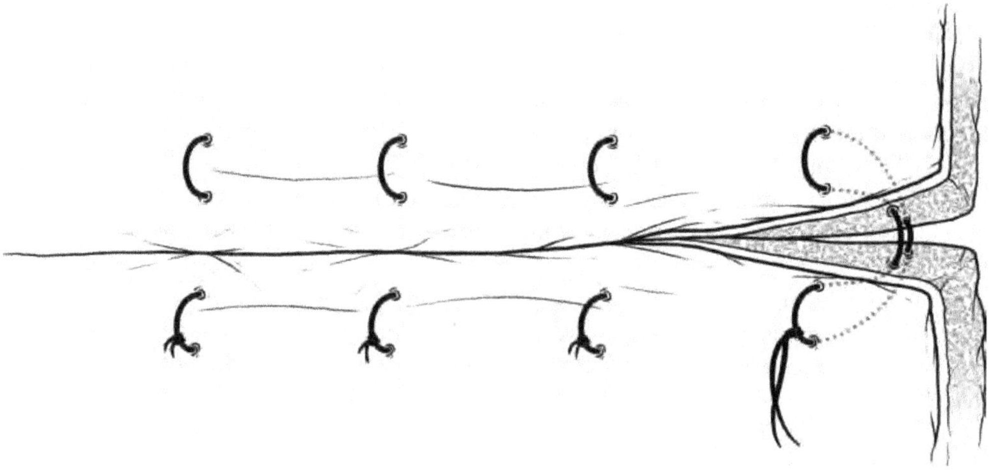



problem. These modifications attempt to pass the bridging suture segments to be deeper, thus resulting in wound eversion.

### 11.7.3 Vertical Mattress Suture

The vertical mattress suture is in part similar to simple interrupted sutures but includes an additional suture bridge close to the wound edge. Also known as Donati Suture, or 'far-far, near-near' suture, this is the most frequently used suturing technique to obtain wound eversion [5]. This suture design is very popular in abdominal and limb surgeries.

The needle is first penetrated far from the wound edge (about 6 mm), and then proceeds through the deeper tissue to the opposite side and emerges out at an equal distance from the edge. The needle is then reinserted at a point closer (2–3 mm) to the wound edge on the second side itself. It is then rotated superficially through the tissues and is exited on the other side at a corresponding near point. This results in a double bridging of the wound, one deep in the tissues and another superficial and nearer to the wound edge. Thus, both tags of the thread are now on one side of the wound. They are tied together gently (Fig. 11.6).

The primary advantage of this suture is the resultant wound eversion. This eversion is expected to compensate for the anticipated contracture occurring along the wound margin. As the suture is bridging the wound twice, the binding strength is more. Elimination of dead space is another obvious advantage. The suture thread does not pass the wound edge on the surface, minimising the chance of track marks.

On the flip side, fine wound edge approximation is almost never achieved with this suture. Excessive tightening could lead to over-constriction and sometimes exposure of the raw area. This may necessitate placement of additional interrupted sutures for better results.

The vertical mattress concept can be used in a buried suture situation also by ensuring that the more superficial suture thread passed back to the first side in a path parallel to the first, deeper suture bridge. This will result in a better wound eversion.

### 11.7.4 Simple Continuous Suture

Simple continuous suture ('running loop', 'standard running suture') is a good method for rapid closure of small wounds. It gives an even distribution of tension all along the wound span. It combines many benefits of the simple interrupted sutures with the additional advantage of a quicker finish.

The technique is very simple. The first part follows the same process as a simple interrupted suture. The first knot becomes the anchoring knot for the ensuing running line. The tags are not cut and the longer tag (with the needle) is used for making the remaining loops. The needle is inserted back into the tissues a few millimetres away from the first piercing. Then the needle (followed by the thread) passes through the tissues in a path parallel to the first loop. Once it comes out of the second loop, it is not tied. Instead, the loop is tightened and the thread crosses over obliquely across the wound and enters the tissue surface again, a few millimetres away from the second piercing. This process continues over and over until one reaches the other end of the wound. As the last loop goes through the tissues, the thread is only partially pulled through, leaving some loose thread on the opposite side. The suture is then tied to this loose thread for the final knot. Thus, the suture material runs across the wound in repetitive loops, and there are only two knots—one at either end (Fig. 11.7).

The obvious advantages of this technique are the quickness of suture placement and the ease of avoiding many knots. Also, if the tissue wells up in one site, the remaining part of the suture can provide some compensatory slack.

The principal drawback is that the integrity of the entire suture line is vested in just two knots. Any breakage to the suture at any point leads to the entire line getting untied. Since the loops are in continuous succession, fine-tuning of design for each loop is not possible. Also, since the tension is the same across all loops, the areas of the wound with greater tension, usually the central part, may tend to gape.

### 11.7.5 Locking Continuous Suture

This is a variation of the simple continuous suture technique used for surface wounds. Each loop of the continuous suture is 'locked' on itself before making the next loop. This is the most popular continuous suturing technique especially for closing wounds over long spans. As with other superficial continuous sutures, this method is frequently used as a surface layer after the internal tissue layers have been closed.

Similar to the simple continuous technique, the first loop is passed and the knot tied. After the second loop has gone through the tissues and exited, the suture is not immediately tightened. The needle and the leading thread it is made to pass through the earlier loop. After making this 'lock', the suture is tightened and is then passed into the tissues for the third loop. The assistant should maintain this tension until the next loop is passed. This process is repeated for the entire line of succeeding loops (Fig. 11.8).

The locking helps to align the tissues in a proper anatomic orientation perpendicular to the wound. There is an added haemostatic effect due to the tension on tissues. Uniform degree of tension is maintained across all the loops. At the same time, the running locks partially detach the tension on the individual loops from one another. Thus, to an extent, individual control of tension depending on the site can be obtained.

This technique inherits the main disadvantage of the simple continuous sutures of being dependent on only two knots, and the risk of complete loss of suture integrity in case of breakage at any point. The locks, if they are too tight, may cause vascular compromise of underlying tissues.

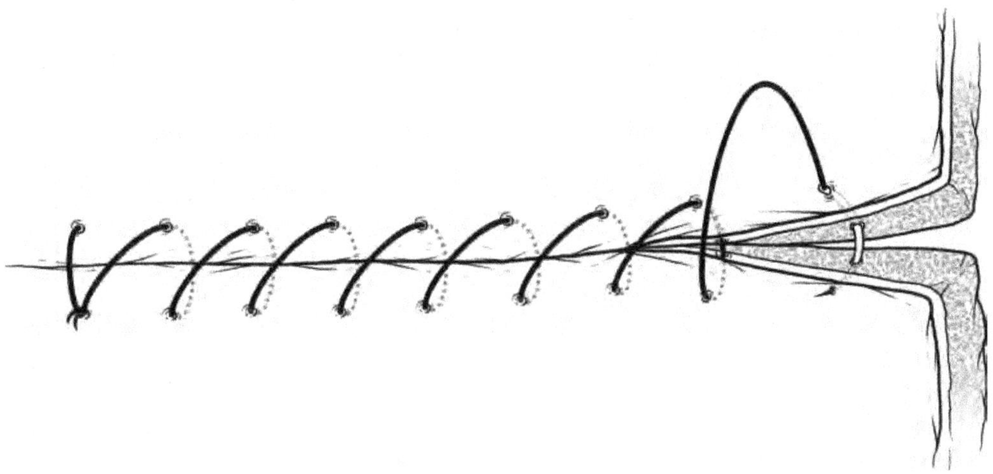

**Fig. 11.7** Simple continuous suture

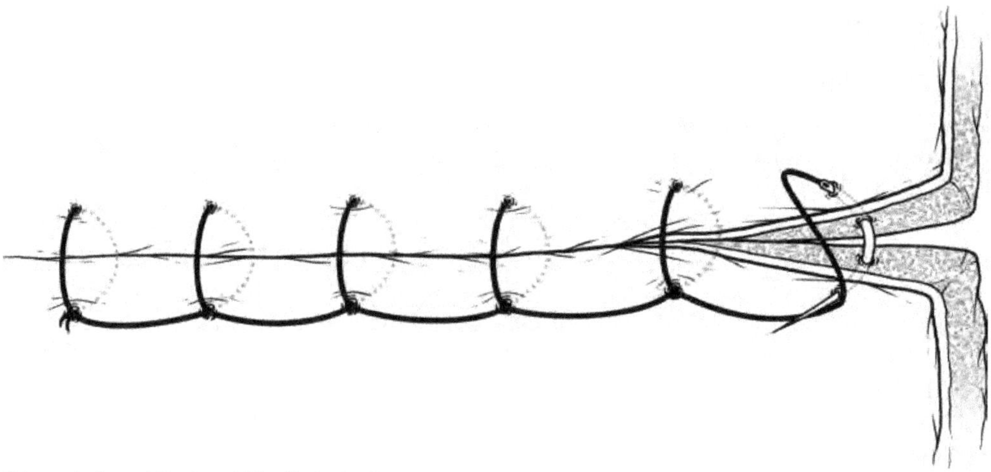



**Fig. 11.8** Locking continuous suture

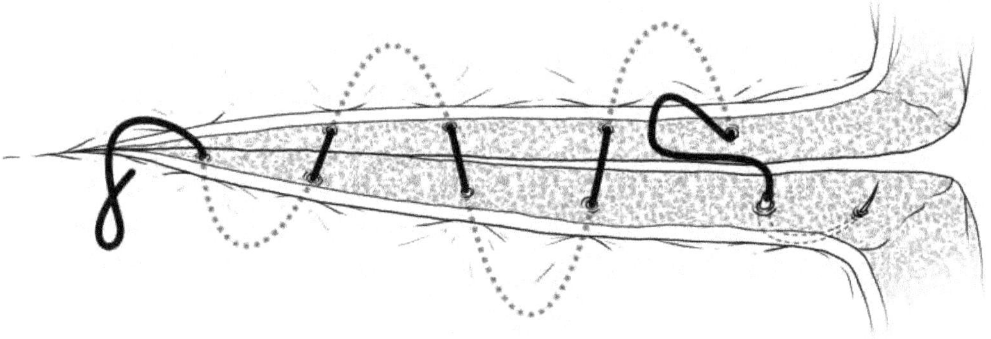



**Fig. 11.9** Subcuticular suture

## 11.7.6 Subcuticular Suture

This is a mostly buried, continuous, epidermal wound closure which is used for surface closure. The suture ends exit a few mms away from the wound corner. The subcuticular suture is employed only after the deeper structures and dermis have been secured well with absorbable sutures. It is popular as an aesthetic suture for face [6].

The suture may be absorbable or non-absorbable, and is usually thin (size 5–0 or 6–0). The needle insertion is at one end of the wound, 2–5 mm away from the apex. It is passed along the curve into the wound, where it exits in the interior, close to the apex. Then the needle is inserted again into the dermis on any one side of the wound edge walls. Thereafter, it passes horizontally parallel to the surface, and following the needle curve to come out into the wound interior a small distance away. The same step is then repeated on the other side of the wound. This process is repeated till one reaches the other end of the wound, wherein the needle is made to pierce the far end apex and to come out in the surface. This last step is a mirror image of the initial steps. Then each of the suture tags on both sides is tied separately on to itself. Alternatively, the tags may be secured with adhesive strips, surgical tape or tissue glue (Figs. 11.9 and 11.10).

The biggest advantage of this technique is the much decreased risk of scars. The close approximation achieved in the dermis region makes the need for a further surface suturing unnecessary. The tension is aligned centrally across the wound and is evenly distributed all along the length of the suture. Also, this technique is highly suitable in cases where the suture material is required to stay in place for a long period of time.

On the negative side, the subcuticular suture takes longer time to perform. Leaving a large quantity of foreign material in situ can increase the risk of foreign body reaction and infection. If non-absorbable material is used, there is a minor risk of long and thin suture track following removal. If absorbable material is used, an undyed suture should be chosen to prevent cutaneous visibility. Incorrect technique can leave small segments of exposed raw area, which need to be addressed with additional surface sutures.

### 11.7.7 Purse-String Suture

This is essentially a modification of the simple continuous suture, and is designed to reduce the size of a two-dimensional surface defect. It is not a cosmetically superior technique and is rarely used in the face. The purse-string effect causes a puckering in the surrounding skin tissue. But this is an effective method to reduce wound area. It may also be used to achieve haemostasis.

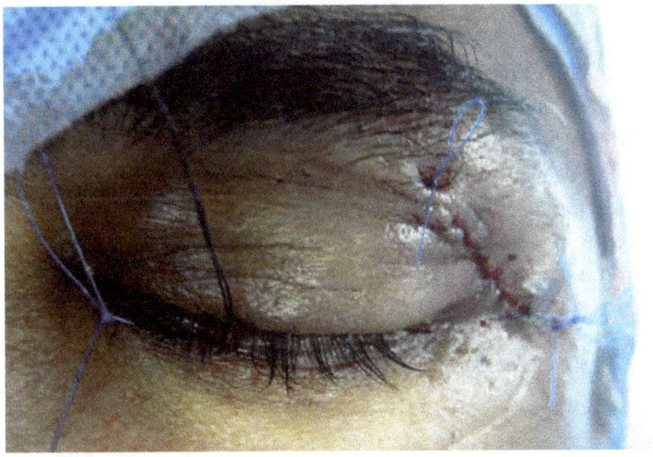



**Fig. 11.10** Subcuticular suture at the subciliary incision site and at the pre-existing lateral orbital laceration in a case of zygomatic complex fracture fixation

At first, the wound edges of the defect need to be freshened and underlined. The needle and thread is passed along the edge of the defect in a course running parallel to the wound edge. Thereafter, it continues in a series of loops running along the edge of the surface wound along its entire circumference. As the thread completes the full distance and reaches near the initial needle entry, it is pulled taut, leading to complete or partial closure of the wound. Then the tags are tied together.

### 11.7.8 Three-Point Suture

Also known as 'tip stitch' or 'half-buried horizontal mattress suture', this technique is used for managing a situation where three ends of the tissue have to be sutured together. In maxillofacial surgery, this situation is encountered while repairing V-shaped lacerations and while closing flaps with sharp corners (such as the triangular flap at the vermilion border for cleft lip repair)

This suture is placed only after the flaps are brought into position using buried dermal sutures. The surface suture thread is used, that is, 6–0 for face and 3–0 for scalp. The needle is first inserted into one side of the non-flap side of the wound. It follows the needle curve to exit in the inner aspect of the wound. The next tissue insertion is into the superficial dermis of the flap tip. Then the needle passes horizontally and comes out through the dermis on the other side of the flap tip. After releasing from the flap tip, it re-enters the dermis of the non-flap side on the other side and comes out through the skin at a point corresponding to the initial entry. The tags are then knotted together (Figs. 11.11 and 11.12).

**Fig. 11.11** Three-point suture technique

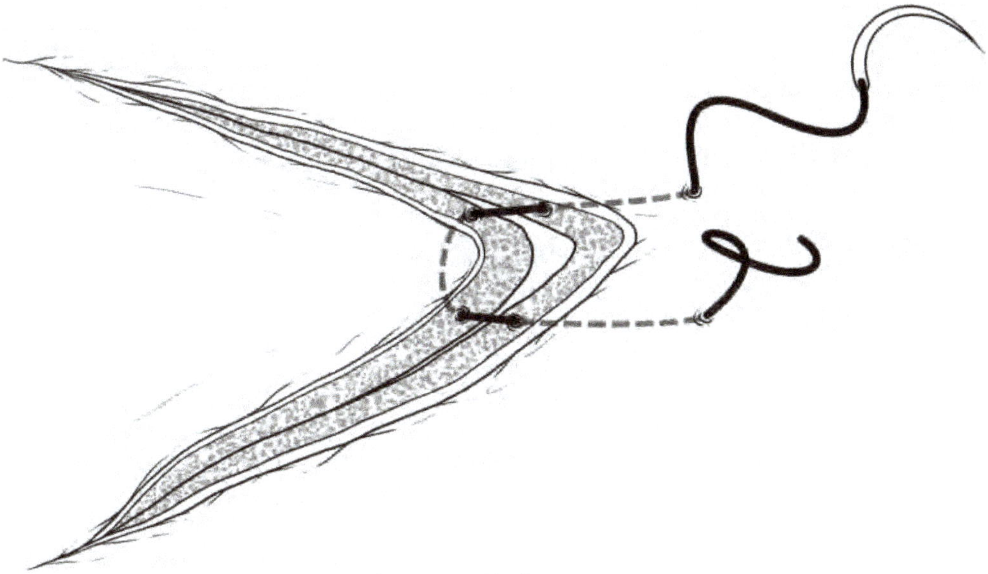

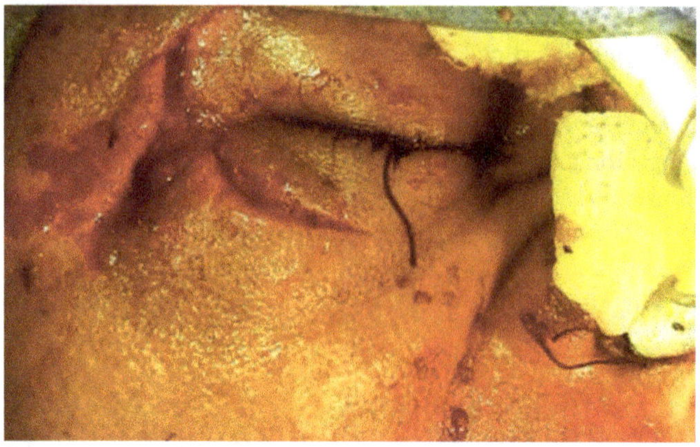



**Fig. 11.12** A laceration that needs three-point suturing

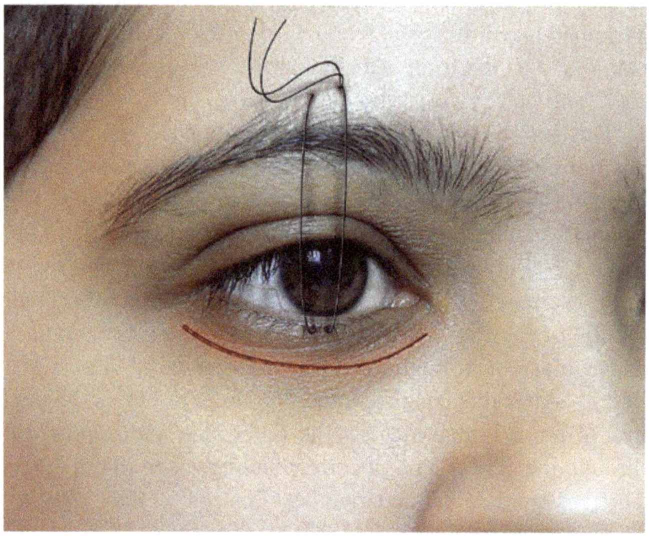



**Fig. 11.13** Frost suture

### 11.7.9 Frost Suture

The Frost suture is a temporary eyelid suspension suture, used to ensure proper lower eyelid placement during the post-operative period [7].

After the closure of the lower eyelid incision, a needle bite is taken on the tarsal plate or just inferior to it. Then a second bite is taken just above the eyebrow, ensuring the anatomic position and alignment of the lower lid. These tags are then tied or secured with tapes or tissue glue (Fig. 11.13).

These sutures may be removed on third post-operative day, but need to be kept longer if there has been significant trauma to the tissues.

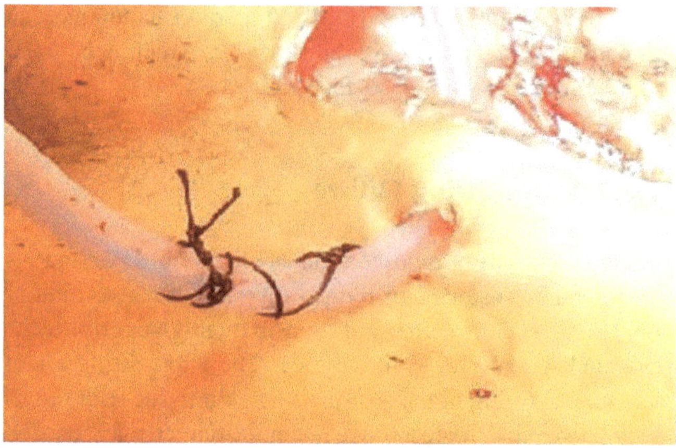



**Fig. 11.14** Drain anchoring suture

### 11.7.10 Drain Anchoring Suture

Different types of drains are used in surgery, such as corrugated rubber drain, the suction drain, intercostal drain, etc. After the drain has been inserted, it needs to be securely fixed to the body to prevent displacement.

The most common means to secure drains is the Roman Garter method, which uses silk sutures. A strong bite is first taken on the skin near the drain entry site. After making a knot, the two suture tags go around the drain tube in a series of windings. A knot may be tied after each 2 or 3 turns around the tube. The large number of windings around the tube increases the friction, holding the tube in position without dislodgement (Fig. 11.14).

Other techniques which have been described include the use of nylon suture, safety pin, drain clip, adhesives and Tie-lok.

## 11.8 Dentoalveolar Suturing

The tissues and the surgical environment in the dentoalveolar region are different from other parts of the body. Consequently, the wound closure requirements also differ. Wound closure in dentoalveolar surgery involves suturing in situations such as

1. Suturing of buccal and/or lingual flaps back to its place after dentoalveolar surgery around teeth or implant accessories.
2. Wound closure after tooth extraction.
3. Flap closure in edentulous ridge.

In most cases, the needle passage is through keratinised mucosa with little or no subcutaneous tissue, obviating the need for multilayered closure. The presence of teeth or artificial crown on one side of the flap forces the surgeon to innovate on the basic suture design. Another difference is when the extraction wound is closed—the wound is usually closed only at the edges and is largely left open in the middle. Also, the suture site will have to endure itself in a challenging environment with the presence of saliva, food materials and a very dynamic milieu where tongue movements and masticatory forces abound [8].

If marginal gingiva is not involved in the flap (as in a semilunar flap), the wound closure models are usually not different from the general cutaneous designs which were discussed in the previous section.

### 11.8.1 Simple Interrupted Suture (Interdental Suture)

As in any case of wound closure, the simple interrupted suture is the mainstay in closing dentoalveolar flaps [9]. In general, it involves suturing the detached interdental papillae together. The needle passes from the buccal aspect of the buccal flap, emerges on the inside of the flap and then passes between the tooth roots to enter the inner aspect of the lingual flap. As it pierces the lingual flap and emerges through the mucosa, the needle is turned back and is taken back via the interdental region to the buccal side. The two suture tags are then tied together. Thus, the knot remains on the buccal side and is accessible for removal.

If only one flap (usually buccal) has been raised, the needle can still pass through the attached lingual flap and the suture design stays the same. In post-extraction wounds also, the procedure is the same, and the tooth socket space is not totally closed.

### 11.8.2 Interrupted Reversing Suture

In this modified interrupted suture, the direction of the needle is reversed for engaging the lingual papilla. Once it passes through the buccal papilla and reaches the lingual side, the needle orientation is reversed and it is made to enter the lingual papilla from outside (lingual side). The needle exits the flap on the inside, passed across to the buccal side and is then tied. Thus, both the papillae are engaged in an 'outside-to-inside' orientation, ending in a figure-of-eight formation in the vertical plane (Fig. 11.15).

This technique is especially useful in cases where both buccal and lingual flaps are raised during surgery, such as in periodontal surgeries.

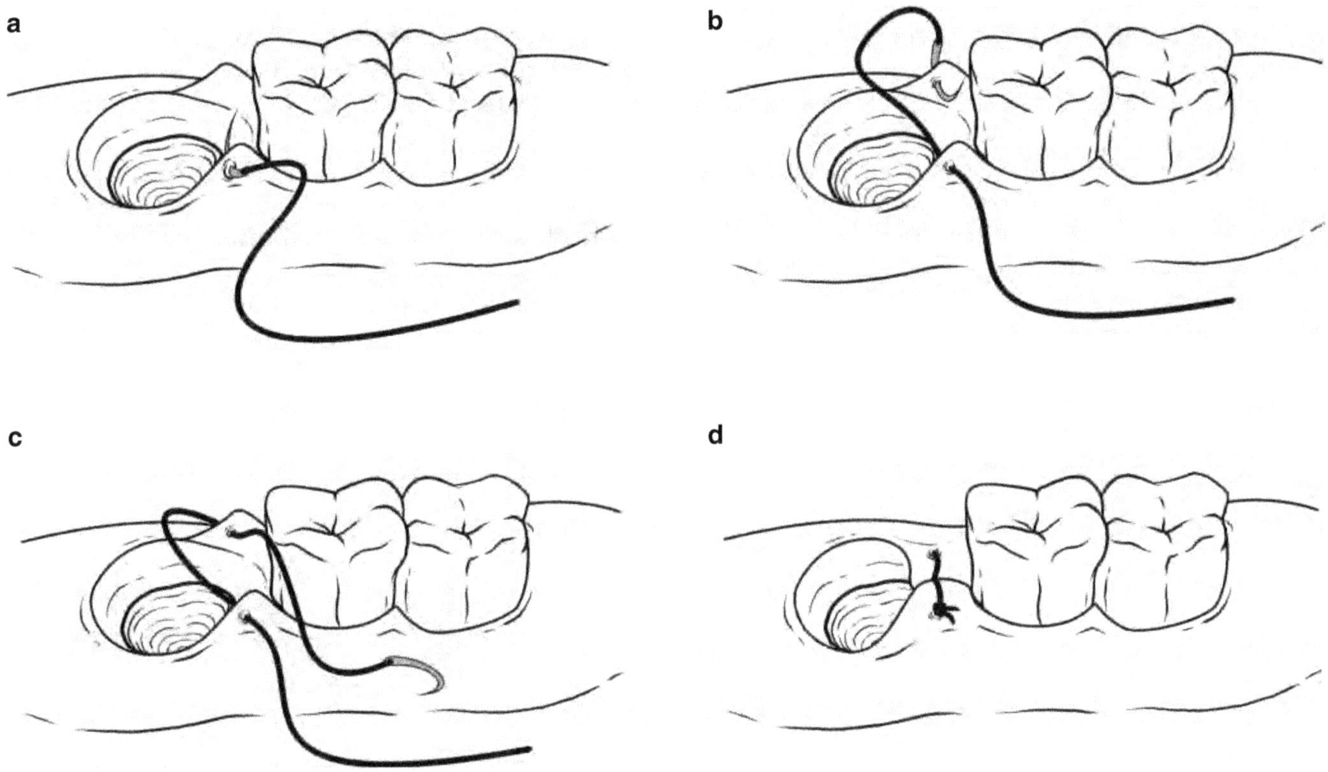




**Fig. 11.15** Interrupted reversing interdental suture

### 11.8.3 Vertical Mattress Suture

Vertical mattress technique in dentoalveolar surgery is a modification of the papilla-attaching simple interrupted technique. After the initial passage of the needle through the buccal and lingual papillae, the needle is turned back and picks a small bite at the tip of the lingual papilla before passing back to the buccal side. Then it again pierces the tip of buccal papilla before knot-tying.

While this technique helps in pressing the papilla into the interdental space, it is not a popular technique because of the difficulty in getting a solid bite at the papilla tip without 'cutting through'. Obviously, one needs to use an atraumatic needle with a small thread (4–0 or smaller) for this purpose.

### 11.8.4 Horizontal Mattress Suture

This is a two-dimensional suturing technique where the suture thread is spread in a horizontal fashion in the tissues. It is not very popular for general cutaneous suturing but is especially useful in dentoalveolar surgery.

When closing flaps in edentulous areas, the needle first passes through both flaps. Then it is reinserted into the flap on the same side, a little distance away from the earlier exit point. The reinserted needle now passes through both flaps and emerges out a similar distance away from the initial entry point. Both the thread tags, now on the same side, are tied together (Fig. 11.16).

In dentulous areas, this technique sutures two adjacent papillae together, eventually tying four papillae segments around a tooth in a horizontal square fashion. To close extraction wounds, only the papillae are approximated and the tooth socket space is not closed completely.

The advantage of this technique is that a single horizontal mattress suture serves like two separate interrupted sutures, thus helping to reduce the number of sutures. It compresses the wound from four corners and helps in haemostasis. It also results in some degree of wound eversion.

### 11.8.5 Horizontal Mattress Modification: Dental Anchor Suture

In this modification, the suture does not pass through the lingual soft tissues. After passing through the buccal papilla, the suture passes through the interdental region into the lingual side. Without engaging the lingual papilla, it goes around the tooth and comes back to the buccal side via the interdental space on the other side. Then it engages the buccal papilla before being tied. In this way, it secures the papilla to the bone using the tooth as its 'anchor'.

This technique can also be used in a reversing fashion, where only the papilla on the lingual side is engaged and the buccal side papillae are not pierced.

### 11.8.6 Horizontal Mattress Modification: Mattress Sling Suture

This technique attempts to combine the benefits of vertical mattress suture with those of horizontal mattress suture. The basic technique goes similar to the horizontal mattress but the final tag re-enters the buccal papilla at the tip and traverses a reverse path around the tooth to exit near the initial entry. In this way, it ensures the engagement of both buccal papillae in a vertical mattress fashion.

### 11.8.7 Horizontal Mattress Modification: Figure-of-Eight Suture (Cruciate Mattress Suture/Cross Suture)

The figure-of-eight suture is the most popular modification of the horizontal mattress technique. This is used mostly in closure of extraction wounds, and never in the presence of teeth at the wound site.

The needle first penetrates the buccal papilla on one side and then the lingual papilla. Then the thread crosses across the edentulous site, and the needle is reversed in orientation to pierce the buccal papilla of the other side from outside

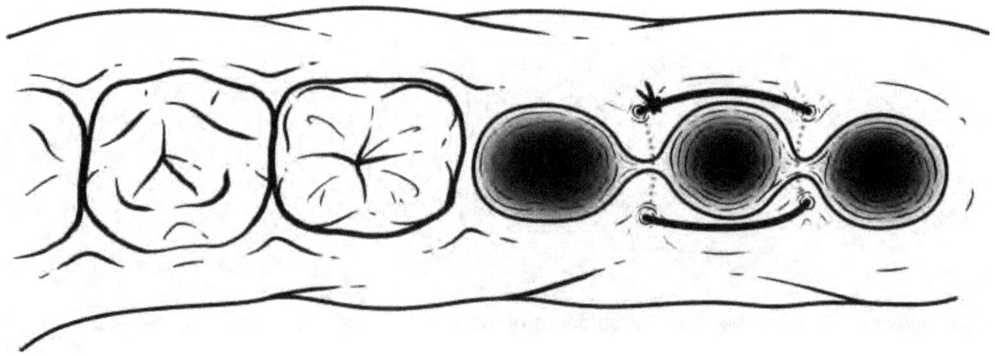

**Fig. 11.16** Horizontal mattress suture (extraction wound)

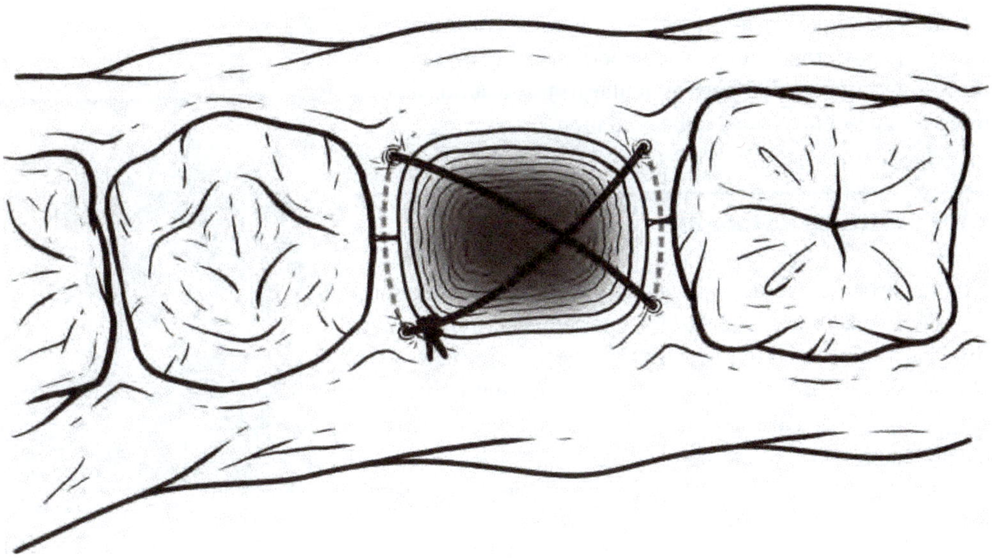


**Fig. 11.17** Figure-of-eight suture

(buccal side) to pass through the lingual papilla and exit on lingual side. Then the thread passes across the site to be tied with the initial tag. The suture thus ends with the appearance of suture material crossing the wound site in a 'cross' shape (Fig. 11.17).

Many surgeons consider the figure-of-eight suture to be the most comprehensive way to suture a single tooth extraction site. This method ensures an even tension on the tissues from four corners, effectively constricting the wound. There is a positive effect on haemostasis also, due to the tension on the flap and due to its presence a mechanical barrier to clot loss.

## 11.8.8 Simple Continuous Suture

The continuous sutures are almost exclusively used for edentulous situations including post-extraction closure. After making a conventional interrupted suture knot, the longer tag is not cut and is instead used to make a series of 'running loops' approximating the succeeding pair of papillae one after the other. Gentle tension must be maintained on the thread to keep the loops tight while the needle passes through the next tissue. Knots are not tied for each loop but is done only at the other end of the long wound. Some surgeons prefer to tie a knot after 3 or 4 running loops. In the end, the part of the suture passing through the inner tissues are perpendicular to the wound, and the superficial, exposed parts lie across the wound in an oblique fashion.

The continuous sutures save time and effort while closing wounds of long span. It also ensures an even distribution of tension across the wound. The obvious disadvantage is the fact that if one loop or part of the suture is compromised (by untying, cutting through or loosening), the entire suture line gets loosened.

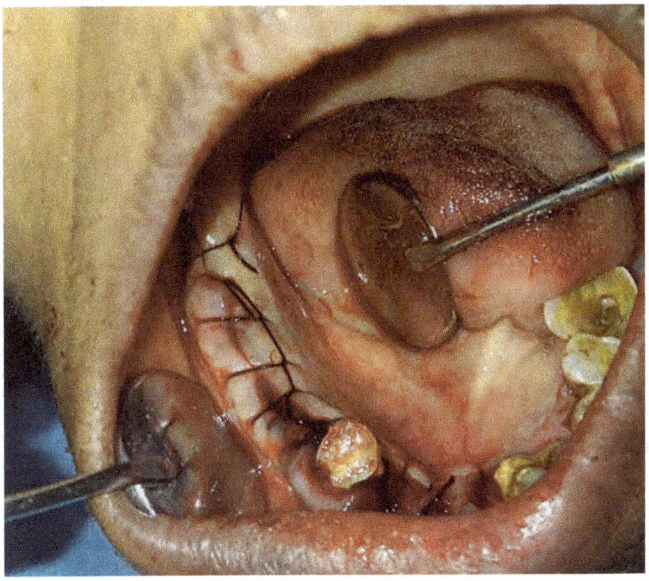


**Fig. 11.18** Continuous locking suture (dentoalveolar)

## 11.8.9 Continuous Locking Suture

The continuous locking suture is a continuous suture in which a 'lock' is incorporated by passing the thread under the previous loop before it is pulled through the tissue. It is important to keep maintaining the tension on the previous loops as the needle makes the next pass through the tissue (Fig. 11.18).

This technique ensures a better orientation of the sutures with respect to the wound. The superficial, exposed parts of the suture are oriented perpendicular to the wound, leading to better anatomic wound approximation.

## 11.9 Suture Removal

Non-absorbable sutures on skin and mucosa should be removed after the wound surface has achieved initial stability. The timing of suture removal is very important. They should remain in tissue long enough to prevent dehiscence and scar spread. On the other hand, early removal reduces tissue reaction and suture marks.

Sutures on facial skin and in oral cavity are usually removed in 5–7 days. The recommended interval is 3–5 days for eyelids, 7 days for neck and 7–10 days for scalp. Those on trunk and limbs should remain in place for 10–14 days.

The suture line is cleansed with antiseptic. The knot is grasped and is pulled away mildly from the surface and to one side of the wound. An uncontaminated segment of the thread is exposed on the other side by this pull. The thread is cut at this segment near to the surface. Then the suture is pulled out, making sure that no contaminated (exposed) part is ragged through the tissues.

In the case of a continuous suture, every single loop should be cut and pulled out separately. A subcuticular suture is removed by cutting the knot off at any one end, and then pulling the suture out gently from the other end. It is important to make sure that the suture does not break within the tissues.

## 11.10 Other Wound Closure Methods

### 11.10.1 Staples

The use of specialised staples for wound closure was popularized in 1900s by the Hungarian surgeon Hümér Hültl, known as the 'father of surgical stapling'. Compared to suturing, surgical stapling is a quicker method to close the skin in large wounds, and the inflammatory response is relatively less. Staples provide good wound edge eversion without strangulation of the tissue. It is an excellent method to employ in cases which require quick wound closure and where aesthesis is not a major concern [10] (Fig. 11.19).

Though titanium staples were initially used, almost all of the contemporary hardware is stainless steel. However, titanium retains the advantages of being biocompatible and MRI-compatible. Bioresorbable staples, based on polyglycolic acid, are also available. The stapler devise itself may be of stainless steel (reusable) or plastic (disposable), into which the disposable staple cartridges can be loaded.

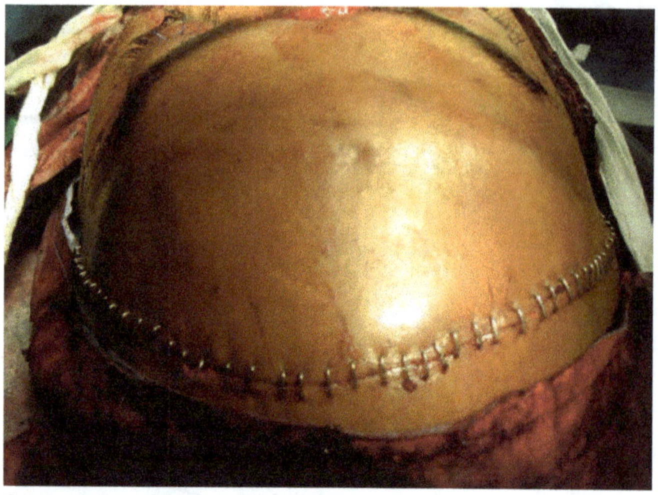



**Fig. 11.19** Stapled scalp incision in a coronal approach

In maxillofacial surgery, staples are frequently used to close scalp wounds and neck incisions, following the closure of internal layers with conventional sutures. Staples are also popular in reconstructive surgery to secure skin grafts and to close the flap donor sites. They are not generally used to close facial wounds, since there is a tendency to produce 'rail-road track' scars. Skin staples are removed after 7-10 days with a specialized staple remover device.

### 11.10.2 Tapes

Different types of surgical adhesive tapes are used to effect wound closure, to reduce tension on sutured wounds and to reinforce wound site after suture removal.

The indications of this method for wound closure per se are limited. Tapes can be used to close superficial lacerations where tissue tension is minimal. They are also employed in the closure of superficial layer after buried dermal sutures have been employed for wound edge approximation and tension reduction. A major indication is its use an additional reinforcement and protection over sutured wounds. The advantages of using tapes for wound closure are.

(a) They are rapid and easy to perform.
(b) The tape application is painless (patient anxiety and discomfort are minimal).
(c) Residual suture track scars are avoided.
(d) There is no need for a review visit to remove the tape.
(e) Tapes, being non-invasive, are less prone to infection than other methods.
(f) They are suitable for thin, fragile skin of the elderly and infants.

On the other hand, there are significant limitations to the use of tapes to close wounds. The most obvious contraindication is an area under significant tension. Tapes are difficult to apply on to highly convex surfaces, irregular wounds and in areas of tissue laxity. They do not attach well to wet surfaces (e.g. oral mucosa). They may get detached easily in hairy areas and those which tend to sweat.

These tapes are typically made of synthetic reinforced material with a hypoallergenic adhesive and are made porous to make them 'breathable' for skin. Some products are made elastic to account for oedema tension while some have incorporated antibiotic to reduce the incidence of surgical site infection. Modifications of tape-based wound closure include incorporation of a zip-lock mechanism and a clip attachment, both techniques designed to pull the wound edges together for better approximation.

### 11.10.3 Adhesives

The use of tissue adhesives is an efficient way to close wounds in select cases. Just like surgical tapes, tissue adhesives can be used to approximate wounds that do not require deep-layer closure and do not have significant tension on the edges [11].

All currently available tissue adhesives are chemically cyanoacrylates (esters of cyanoacrylic acid). These compounds were discovered by Ardis in 1949 and were first used in surgery by Coover in 1959. These are chemically similar to methacrylates, the only difference being the methyl ($CH_3$) group substituted with cyano/nitrile (CN) group. The water present on the skin or mucosal surface activates the acryl groups in the resin to rapidly polymerise and form long, strong chains. Three types of tissue adhesives are currently available for clinical use—2-octyl cyanoacrylate, N-butyl-2-cyanoacrylate and isoamyl 2-cyanoacrylate. The adhesion involves two mechanisms—mechanical interlocking into the surface irregularities and chemical covalent bonding with the nucleophilic amine groups on skin surfaces.

Tissue adhesives are mainly used to treat superficial skin tears (that do not extend past the dermis) and for surface closure after the deeper layers are secured with sutures. Other indications include stabilisation of bone fragments during plating, sealing of CSF leaks and sinus perforations, attaching grafts, achieving peripheral nerve reanastomosis and closure of dentoalveolar flaps [12]. They are also widely used to achieve haemostasis at surgical sites and as a biologic cover on ulcers. The relative contraindications include wounds over or near joints and wounds under significant static or dynamic skin tension. Also animal bite wounds, crushed wounds and wounds in high friction areas and those with cross mucocutaneous borders are not considered suitable for a closure using adhesives.

The procedure for using the tissue adhesives for surface closure involves thorough cleaning and haemostasis. Though moisture is a prerequisite for adhesion, the presence of excessive water or blood at the site is detrimental to a good result. The surface is dried before applying the adhesive in at least three to four thin layers along the length of the wound's surface. It is advisable to extend it approximately 5–10 mm from each side of the wound. The edges of the wound are held together for at least 1 minute as the adhesive dries.

The main advantages of tissue adhesives over other wound closure methods are the rapidity and painless application [13]. In addition, the suture track scars are avoided, leading to a much better cosmetic result. The risk of suture site infection is also found to be less. The material sloughs off in 5–10 days, as the skin sheds.

The obvious disadvantage is that it cannot be used in areas of tension. Additionally, there is a minor risk of toxicity and foreign body reactions. If the clinician's gloved fingers, gauze or plastic instruments contact the tissue adhesive during application, these materials may adhere to the patient's skin.

## 11.11 Conclusion

Wound care primarily involves measures to ensure that the wound heals quickly without going through adverse situations such as infections. Along with mechanical debridement, antibiotic medication and dressings, the various wound closure methods form the foundation of wound care practices. Depending on the patient needs and the wound types, one should choose from a wide variety of materials and techniques to implement effective wound closure.

## References

1. Buckley MJ, Keller JC. Emerging biomaterials and tissue engineering. Oral Maxillofac Surg Clin North Am. 2002 Feb;14(1):ix.
2. Herford AS, Haug RH. Emerging biomaterials and techniques in tissue regeneration. Oral Maxillofac Surg Clin N Am. 2017;29(1):1–120.
3. Kandor J. Atlas of suturing techniques. Approaches to surgical wound, laceration, and cosmetic repair. New York: McGraw-Hill; 2016.
4. Hupp JR. Guide to suturing. Section 2. J Oral Maxfac Surg. Aug 2015;73(Suppl 1):9–35.
5. Kudur MH, Pai SB, Sripathi H, Prabhu S. *Sutures* and *suturing* techniques in skin closure. Indian J Dermatol Venereol Leprol. 2009;75(4):425–34.
6. Gusman DN. Suture materials and techniques. In: Lower extremity soft tissue and cutaneous plastic surgery, vol. 1. Nottingham: Saunders; 2012. p. 77–100.

7. Connolly KL, Albertini JG, Miller CJ, Ozog DM. The suspension (frost) suture: experience and applications. Dermatol Surg. 2015 Mar;41(3):406–10.
8. Koshak HH. Dental suturing materials and techniques. Glob J Otolaryngol. 2017;12(2):1–11. GJO.MS.ID.555833
9. Griffin TJ, Hur Y, Bu J. Basic suture techniques for oral mucosa. Clin Adv Periodontics. 2011, Nov;1(3):221–32.
10. Iavazzo C, Gkegkes ID, Vouloumanou EK, Mamais I, Peppas G, Fallagas ME. Sutures versus staples for the management of surgical wounds: a meta-analysis of randomized controlled trials. Am Surg. Sept 2011;77(9):1206–21.
11. Tuptis A, Salma I. Fibrin sealant in maxillofacial surgery (literature review). https://www.rsu.lv/en/scientific-papers/fibrin-sealant-maxillofacial-surgery-literature-review. 2015.
12. Kaderi MA, Menaka KB, Metgud RM, Gharat MR, Naik PS, Ajmani JM, et al. In-vitro evaluation of antibacterial potential of cyanoacrylate tissue for intra-oral wound closure. J Dent Mater Tech. Sep 2017;6(4):163–9.
13. Oladega AA, James O, Adeyemo WL. Cyanoacrylate tissue adhesive or silk suture for closure of surgical wound following removal of an impacted mandibular third molar: a randomized controlled study. J Craniomaxillofac Surg. 2019 Jan;47(1):93–98.

# 12

# Providing Postoperative Care to Patients

J. Naveen Kumar and Poornima Ravi

Postoperative care of the patient encompasses the time from the completion of the surgical procedure to the complete return of the patient to the normal physiological state. This is divided into three phases. Phase I is early recovery and takes place in the postanesthesia care unit (PACU). Phase II is intermediate recovery, and takes place in the ward. Phase III is late recovery that occurs after discharge.

## 12.1 Assessment of the Patient After Surgery

### 12.1.1 Assessment of the Patient Immediately After Surgery

Postoperative care of the patient begins immediately after the surgical procedure has been completed, even before the anesthesia is reversed. The first step is clearing the airway of blood and debris. Maxillomandibular fixation and occlusal splints, if placed earlier need to removed [1]. The next step is the removal of the throat pack.

#### 12.1.1.1 Care of the Airway

The decision to extubate or not must be made in conjunction with the anesthetist. Cases in which there is a high risk of airway edema will require the ET tube to be retained [1]. These include:

- Space infections compressing on the airway, e.g. Ludwig's angina.
- Severe facial trauma where there is likelihood of blood ooze, edema, or tongue fall back.
- Prolonged surgery, e.g. Free flap reconstructions.

In other cases, the patient may be extubated on the table. Awake extubation is usually preferred for head and neck surgery. The patient may be extubated when the following criteria are met [1]:

- No bleed from surgical site or secretion in the oropharynx.
- Patient is able to follow verbal commands.
- Patient is able to sustain head lift for at least 5 seconds.
- Patient is breathing on his own, with respiratory rate less than 24/min, tidal volume greater than 5 ml/kg, and Spo2 > 90%.

Once the extubation is done, an oropharyngeal airway can be inserted to prevent clenching of teeth and the tongue from falling back, which can cause obstruction. Alternatively, a nasopharyngeal airway can be used in case the surgeon deems oral cavity unfit for manipulation using the former. This must remain in place until the patient is conscious and obeys commands.

Some patients, such as those who have undergone extensive face and neck resection, may have required a tracheostomy prior to surgery. The tube must be secured after surgery by taping the stay sutures to the neck or chest. Tracheostomy care in the postoperative period is critical; a blocked or dislodged tube can have disastrous consequences [2].

1. The tube must be checked at frequent intervals.
2. The tube stoma must be covered with a humidifying bib, or a moist gauze.

J. N. Kumar (✉)
Oral and Maxillofacial Surgery, Sri Ramachandra Institute of Higher Education and Research, Chennai, India
e-mail: naveenkumarj@sriramachandra.edu.in

P. Ravi
Department of Oral and Maxillofacial Surgery, SRM Dental College, Ramapuram, Chennai, Tamil Nadu, India

3. The tube must be suctioned regularly to prevent clogging due to secretions. The suction catheter must be inserted to half of its length, which will correspond to the carina (Patients usually cough when this point is reached). Suction is then applied while simultaneously withdrawing the catheter.
4. To break up secretions, small quantities of sterile water can be syringed in and suctioned immediately.

#### 12.1.1.2 Need for Ventilation in the PACU

In some instances, ventilation may be required even after anesthetic recovery. Some examples include:

1. Patients who have history of COPD.
2. Severe trauma or infection.

While monitoring the patient who is on a ventilator, it is important to be aware of the various modes that the ventilator operates on [3]. These have been summarized in Table 12.1. Patients who have been on the ventilator for long periods of time need to be weaned off slowly. OMF surgeons frequently come across such patients in neurosurgical ward having concomitant traumatic brain injuries and craniomaxillofacial fractures. This may be done by setting the ventilator in CPAP mode (Continuous Positive Airway Pressure). This allows the patient to breathe, with the ventilator taking over if the patient is unable to do so.

#### 12.1.1.3 Monitoring in the PACU

Once the patient has been shifted to the recovery room, the cardiac monitor and pulse oximeter must be attached for proper monitoring. The following parameters must be monitored continuously:

- *Oxygen Saturation:* Hypoxia can occur in the postoperative period and the patient must be kept on oxygen for 1–2 h (2–6 L/min) to prevent this. Oxygen may be delivered using a face mask or through nasal prongs.
- *Pulse, blood pressure:* Increase in these parameters may indicate pain. Serious complications (Infarction, Malignant hyperthermia) may produce a drastic change in these parameters and must be recognized.
- *ECG waveform:* To monitor cardiac status.
- *Postanesthesia tremors/shivering:* This can occur on the table during recovery from anesthesia. It can occur if the patient is hypothermic, and is commonly associated with the use of halogenated anesthetics. Management consists of rewarming the patient. Tramadol and meperidine may be used to stop uncontrollable shivering [4].

The suction apparatus must be kept handy to evacuate blood ooze or secretions that may hamper the airway. It is advisable to avoid Maxillomandibular fixation (MMF) in the immediate postoperative period; if required, this may be done after 24 h.

Detailed surgical notes must also be recorded, along with the number and type of implants that were used. Postoperative instructions must also be documented in detail. A list of notes to be completed by the surgeon before leaving the operation theater complex is summarized in Table 12.2.

#### 12.1.1.4 Briefing the Patient and Family

Immediately after the surgery, the surgeon must interact with the patient's immediate caregivers, giving them the details of the procedure, and any anticipated complications.

#### 12.1.1.5 Discharge from PACU to Ward

This is done when the patient has regained consciousness, with adequate respiratory function and stable vitals. Decisions can be made based on a standard scoring system, such as the Aldrete scoring system [5]. The scoring system which was originally proposed in 1970, underwent modifications in 1995 and 1999. The various factors considered

**Table 12.1** Ventilator modes and settings

| Ventilator mode | Type of setting | Description/indications |
|---|---|---|
| Volume control | Continuous mandatory ventilation (CMV) | Patients with respiratory muscle weakness or LV dysfunction<br>If patient breathes rapidly, may cause hyperinflation and respiratory alkalosis |
| | Synchronous intermittent mandatory ventilation (SIMV) | Patient breathes partially on their own; meant for patients who breathe rapidly on CMV<br>Mandatory breaths are synchronized with spontaneous breathing |
| Pressure control | Pressure controlled ventilation (PCV) | Patients with neuromuscular disease but normal lungs who can control volume. |
| | Pressure support ventilation | Used during weaning, patient determines respiratory volume and frequency, but the ventilator provided continuous positive airway pressure (CPAP) |

**Table 12.2** Checklist for completion before leaving the theater complex

| Checklist to complete before leaving the OT |
|---|
| Surgical notes |
| Details of implants and hardware used |
| Postoperative instructions to be followed by nursing staff |
| Postoperative fluid management instructions |
| Postoperative medication dose and schedule |
| Biopsy requisition form |
| Requisition form for aspirates/swabs and others |
| Investigation requisition form |

**Table 12.3** Subjective assessment of the patient

| Subjective parameters evaluated | Assessment made |
|---|---|
| Pain (use visual analog scale- VAS/ faces scale) | Whether the pain medication is adequate or whether it needs to be increased or discontinued (see Sect. 12.2.2.1) |
| Nausea/vomiting | If the patient has experienced this, assess the need for antiemetics, and insertion of nasogastric tube to decompress the stomach. (Sect. 12.2.5.5) |
| Mobility | The patient must be encouraged to sit up and walk by the first postoperative day. (Section IID) |
| Function- e.g. swallowing, speech, nerve function | It is important to evaluate branches of the facial nerve and trigeminal nerve that may have been at risk of damage during surgery |
| Passing urine/stools/ flatulence | Inability to pass urine may indicate inadequate fluid therapy, and may lead to acute renal failure. (see Sect. 12.2.5.6)<br>Inability to pass stools may be a sign of paralytic ileus; may occur after iliac crest harvest |

are patient activity, respiration, circulation, consciousness, $O_2$ saturation, pain, surgical site bleeding, and nausea/vomiting. Patients scoring greater than 9 on this scale can be moved to the ward for the next phase of care. Readers are advised to refer the article for getting a detailed idea of the scoring table.

### 12.1.2 Comprehensive Assessment of the Patient in the Ward

This is done according to the SOAP format [6]. SOAP is an acronym for Subjective, Objective, Assessment, and Plan. In Subjective evaluation, the patient must be asked if they have any complaints. Specific complaints are recorded. In Objective evaluation, a thorough evaluation of the patient is done by the physician. This includes evaluation of the vital signs, fluid intake and output, as well as an assessment of the surgical site. Helpful information may be obtained from the TPR chart, input/output chart, and nurses' notes. Based on the subjective and objective evaluation, the patient's current status is assessed (Tables 12.3 and 12.4). This is used to formulate a plan.

#### 12.1.2.1 Postoperative Investigations

Sometimes investigations may be required in the postoperative period, either to check the health status of the patient or to confirm the diagnosis of certain complications. A list of investigations that may be ordered and the indications for the same are summarized in Table 12.5.

**Table 12.4** Objective assessment of patient

| Objective parameters evaluated | Assessment made |
|---|---|
| *Vital signs* | |
| Temperature<br>Pulse<br>Blood pressure<br>Respiratory rate | Is postoperative fever present? If so, it must be worked up (Sect. 12.2.5.2)<br>Changes in pulse and blood pressure have several causes (Sect. 12.2.5.3)<br>If abnormal, evaluate whether the patient has respiratory distress (Sect. 12.2.5.4) |
| *Fluid input/output* | Is the input adequate? (Sect. 12.2.1)<br>Is urinary output adequate? This helps assess renal function(Sect. 12.2.5.6) |
| *Surgical site evaluation* | The wound must be inspected, and assessed for healing. (Sect. 12.3) |

**Table 12.5** Postoperative investigations

| Investigation | Indications |
|---|---|
| Hemoglobin | If there has been extensive blood loss during surgery, to determine the need for blood transfusion. |
| Serum electrolytes | Suspicion of electrolyte imbalances (seizures, palpitations, muscle cramps) |
| WBC TC/DC | Suspicion of spreading infection |
| Chest x-ray | Suspicion of atelectasis/aspiration pneumonia |
| OPG/other facial radiographs | To check the accuracy of reduction and status of plating. |

## 12.2 Formulating a Plan of Care Based on Assessment

### 12.2.1 Fluid Therapy in the Postoperative Period

The patient is usually 'nil per mouth' for a few hours prior to surgery and after surgery. Apart from this, there is a loss of blood and body fluids in any surgery, which requires replacement. It is therefore essential to infuse intravenous fluids during this period [7, 8]. This is done for two purposes.

**Replacement** Any fluid deficit that has occurred must be replaced by infusion. This could have occurred during either of the following periods:

- Preoperative period: This could be due to
  - NPO status.
  - Blood or fluid losses that may have occurred due to trauma, burns, etc.
- Intraoperative period: Surgical blood loss of greater than 500 ml or 7 ml/kg requires replacement.

**Maintenance** This is to maintain the ongoing fluid requirements, till the patient resumes oral intake of fluids. Maintenance fluids are essential to maintain proper pH and electrolyte balance and for adequate organ perfusion.

#### 12.2.1.1 Types of Fluids Used

There are three types of fluids than can be used—crystalloids, colloids, blood and blood products. The preference of one type of fluid over another has several controversies, and there are no clear-cut guidelines available [9]. A few indications for each fluid type are given below.

**Crystalloids**

Crystalloids are balanced salt solutions with or without the addition of a buffering agent. When infused into the bloodstream, crystalloids tend to leave the capillaries and enter the extravascular fluid compartment. Crystalloid infusion will increase fluid in the extravascular tissues and does little to expand the circulating blood volume. In maxillofacial surgery, crystalloids are favored as maintenance fluids during the postoperative period.

**Colloids**

Colloids are protein-containing solutions. Since these proteins have a large molecular size, under ordinary circumstances, these are prevented from crossing the capillary endothelial cells and going into the extravascular space. Therefore, they tend to expand vascular volume alone. Colloids are mostly used in the intraoperative period if there has been significant blood loss and the plasma volume needs to be expanded. It is not common to use colloids in the postoperative setting.

Commonly used iv fluids are listed in Table 12.6.

**Table 12.6** Commonly used postoperative IV fluids

| IV Fluid | Composition (in meq/l) | Indications | Risks |
|---|---|---|---|
| *Crystalloids* | | | |
| Lactated Ringers (RL) | Na –130; Cl –109; K –4; Ca –3; Lactate –28 | Fluid of choice in postoperative maintenance | Lactic acidosis if liver function is poor |
| Dextrose Normal Saline (DNS) | Na –154; Cl –154; Dextrose –50 g | Alternative to RL | Hyperchloremic acidosis |
| Normal Saline (NS) | Na –154; Cl –154 | Alternative to DNS in diabetics | Hyperchloremic acidosis |
| 5% Dextrose (D5W) | Dextrose 50 g | Replacing free water deficit | Hyperglycemia in diabetics |
| *Colloids* | | | |
| Hetastarch | 6% hydroxyethyl starch | Plasma volume expansion | Nephrotoxicity, coagulopathy |

#### 12.2.1.2 Strategy for Estimating Fluid Requirement

1. The input-output chart must be verified before determining the fluid requirement. This will help to estimate fluid excess (positive balance), or deficits (negative balance) and plan requirements.
2. Calculate the Estimated Fluid Requirement (EFR) for each hour:
   This is done using Holliday and Segar's formula (The 4-2-1 rule) [10].
   - First 10 kg: 4 cc/kg.
   - Next 10 kg: 2 cc/kg.
   - Above 20 kg: 1 cc/kg.

   E.g. a 60 kg adult will require $(4 \times 10) + (2 \times 10) + (1 \times 40) = 40 + 20 + 40 = 100$ ml/h.
3. Calculate the total Estimated Fluid Deficit: This depends on the number of hours from the last oral intake to the next oral intake. For example, if the patient has not had oral intake for 12 h:
   EFD = EFR × no. of NPO hours = $100 \times 12 = 1200$ ml.
4. Estimate the surgical blood loss. If crystalloids are used to replace this blood loss, for a particular volume of blood, three times the volume of crystalloids are used for replacement. If colloids are used, the same volume is sufficient.
5. Estimate the amount of fluids that have already been infused during anesthesia.
6. Total postsurgical fluid requirement:
   EFD+(blood loss × 3)−fluids replaced during surgery.
   In the above scenario, if 300 ml of blood was lost, and one liter of fluid was infused during surgery, then:

   Total postsurgical fluid requirement:
   $1200 + (300 \times 3) - 1000 = 1200 + 900 - 1000 = 1100$ ml.

#### 12.2.1.3 Liberal Versus Restrictive Fluid Therapy

In recent years, the above method of estimating fluid requirements has been criticized, as it tends to overestimate the amount of fluids needed by a patient [11]. Excessive fluid infusion may cause fluid shift into the extravascular compartment, which in turn can result in overload complications such as renal injury, acute respiratory distress syndrome, etc. On the other hand, liberal fluid infusion can reduce postoperative complications such as nausea, vomiting, and drowsiness.

For major systemic surgeries, the current trend is either to follow a 'restrictive' approach or a goal-directed therapy. Goal-directed therapy measures hemodynamic parameters such as stroke volume, and fluids are given accordingly. While this has been found useful in major surgeries, particularly abdominal surgeries, there is no evidence on its effectiveness in postoperative recovery for maxillofacial surgery. A liberal approach may be preferred for most kinds of

**Table 12.7** Risks vs. benefits of blood transfusion

| Risks of blood transfusion | Benefits of blood transfusion |
|---|---|
| Transmission of infections that cannot be identified by screening (cytomegalovirus, Epstein-Barr virus, B-19 parovirus, dengue, chikungunya, HHV-8, malarial parasite)<br>Transfusion reactions | Better functional status<br>Lower morbidity and mortality (for levels below 7.0 mg/dl) |

**Table 12.8** Indications for postoperative blood transfusion

| Postoperative hemoglobin level | Risk factors/compensatory mechanisms present | Transfusion requirement |
|---|---|---|
| <6 g/dl | | Required |
| 6–8 g/dl | No risk factors | Not required |
| | Presence of risk factors (coronary artery disease, heart failure, cerebrovascular disease/limited mechanisms of compensation) | Required |
| | Presence of symptoms indicative of hypoxia (physiological transfusion triggers: Tachycardia, hypotension, electrocardiographic signs of ischemia, lactic acidosis, etc.) | Required |
| 8–10 g/dl | Presence of symptoms indicative of hypoxia (physiological transfusion triggers: Tachycardia, hypotension, electrocardiographic signs of ischemia, lactic acidosis, etc.) | Required |
| | Absence of above symptoms | Not required |
| >10 g/dl | | Not required |

maxillofacial surgery, which generally fall under low or intermediate risk procedures. Nevertheless, as long as postoperative fluids are being administered, the patient must be monitored for signs of overhydration such as peripheral edema, dyspnea, high blood pressure, and a bounding pulse. If any of these are present, the current fluid regimen must be reassessed [12].

#### 12.2.1.4 Transfusion of Blood and Blood Products

Postoperative blood transfusion is rarely required in routine maxillofacial surgery. It has been stated that the risks of blood transfusion outweigh the benefits [13] (See Table 12.7), and currently a restrictive approach to blood transfusion is favored.

If there has been extensive blood loss during surgery, or preexisting anemia, the postoperative hemoglobin must be assessed, and the decision to transfuse is based on this level [14]. This is described in Table 12.8.

### 12.2.2 Postoperative Medication

The maxillofacial surgeon must be aware of the type and dosage of medication that is required in the immediate postoperative period. Pain control and prophylaxis against infection are the most important factors to be kept in mind while prescribing medication.

#### 12.2.2.1 Pain Control

Pain control is an important goal after every surgical procedure as it can not only affect the patients' attitude, but it can also impair oxygenation and thereby delay wound healing. The pain must be assessed subjectively, by asking the patient to rate their pain on a standard scale (e.g. Visual Analogue scale or Faces pain scale). If the patient is in pain, pain medication must be increased or changed.

Preemptive analgesia is an evolving, controversial technique that involves the administration of analgesics prior to the onset of noxious stimuli. This is believed to limit the sensitization of the nervous system, thereby reducing the need for postoperative analgesia [15]. One effective preemptive technique is the infiltration of a long-acting local anesthetic, such as bupivacaine, into the incision site before closure. This provides effective pain relief throughout the postoperative period.

In the postoperative period, various classes of analgesics may be used [16]. Some of the commonly used analgesics are summarized in Table 12.9.

The best method of choosing the appropriate analgesic is using the WHO analgesic ladder (Fig. 12.1). If the pain is not well controlled, the patient can move to the next step of the ladder. Once the pain is controlled, patients must be weaned by moving down the ladder [17]. This step ladder approach is just a broad lattice and has its own share of controversies and modifications. Readers are encouraged to read appropriate references for getting a broader picture of the analgesic ladder and a detailed discussion is beyond the scope of this chapter.

**Patient-controlled Analgesia** Postoperative patients often require immediate pain relief at varied intervals. PCA allows the use of iv pumps which, when the patient presses a button, allows a bolus dose of analgesic to be delivered for immediate relief [18]. This allows analgesics to be tailored to the patients' requirements and also records the amount of opioid being administered per day.

#### 12.2.2.2 Anti-inflammatory Drugs

The role of corticosteroids in postoperative care is controversial. Corticosteroids are potent anti-inflammatory agents and are often used after surgery. It has been established that corticosteroids reduce pain and inflammation [19]. There is also evidence that single doses of steroids can reduce postoperative nausea and vomiting, and improve fatigue after surgery. However, the benefit of extended doses of steroids seems controversial and comes with the risk of impaired wound healing, infectious complications, and hyperglycemia. It is

**Table 12.9** Analgesics commonly used for postoperative pain control

| Drug | Classification | Dosage and frequency | Precautions and adverse effects |
|---|---|---|---|
| Diclofenac | NSAIDS (aryl acetic acid derivatives) | 75 mg bd adults<br>1.5 mg/kg bd children | Has been linked to adverse cardiovascular events—Avoid in patients with heart disease<br>Gastric ulceration and bleeding may worsen<br>Nephrotoxic; avoid in patients prone to kidney disease |
| Aceclofenac | | 100 mg bd adults<br>Safety not established in children | Less than diclofenac, mild GI symptoms have been reported |
| Ketorolac | NSAIDS | 20–30 mg q6hr<br>0.5 mg/kg q6hr | GI symptoms, hypertension reported in few patients |
| Acetaminophen (paracetamol) | NSAIDS (Para-amino phenol derivative) | 0.5–1 g tds adults<br>10–15 mg/kg children | Hepatotoxicity |
| Tramadol | Synthetic opioid | 50 mg bd or sos<br>Safety not established in children. | May worsen nausea and vomiting. Like all opioids, respiratory depression is higher. |
| Morphine | Natural opioid | 0.2–0.8 mg/kg bd | Respiratory depression, nausea, vomiting, constipation. Not suitable in immediate postop as consciousness cannot be evaluated |

therefore recommended that steroids be used only till the first postoperative day. Dexamethasone 8 mg is generally used twice a day. For single day dosing, taper is not generally required.

Enzymatic anti-inflammatory medication is also used to reduce postoperative edema [20]. These include serratiopeptidase (10 mg tds) or trypsin:chymotrypsin (chymoral, 100,000 IU). However, its efficacy is based mostly on anecdotal reports and there is hardly any scientific evidence to back its use.

#### 12.2.2.3 Antibiotic Prophylaxis

The use of antibiotic prophylaxis (for wound infections) in maxillofacial surgery is a controversial area. Literature evidence is insufficient to ascertain whether prophylaxis is required or not, and the duration of prophylaxis has no definite guidelines. Based on recent systematic reviews, Table 12.10 sums up current recommendations [21, 22].

Preferred antibiotics for prophylaxis include:

Amoxicillin-Clavulanate 1.2 mg IV bd.
Amoxicillin 500 mg per oral tds (OR) Cefotaxime 1 g IV bd with Metronidazole 500 mg IV tds.
Prophylaxis must be started 30–90 min before the surgical procedure. The postoperative regimen has no clear guidelines, but must continue for at least 24 h after the procedure. After this, the wound must be monitored for infection, and therapeutic antibiotics may be instituted only if required. This section is covered in more detail in Chap. 10, of this book

#### 12.2.2.4 Medication to Prevent Postoperative Gastritis and Vomiting

Preoperative and intraoperative fasting, as well as drugs used in the postoperative period, can induce gastric irritation in the surgical patient. To counter this, drugs that reduce the acidity of gastric secretions may be used. Ranitidine, a H2 blocker, may be used in a dose of 50 mg bd. An alternative drug is Pantoprazole, which may be used in a dose of 40 mg once a day.

Prevention of postoperative nausea and vomiting is an important factor in postoperative care. One of the important drugs used for the management of PONV is Ondansetron, which is given in a dose of 4 mg [23]. This is usually a rescue medication and is not given on a routine basis.

#### 12.2.2.5 Drugs for Thromboprophylaxis

Patients undergoing prolonged surgery or hospitalization may be at increased risk of developing thromboembolic events, namely deep vein thrombosis and pulmonary embolism. Additional risk factors include smoking, pregnancy, oral contraceptives, and malignancy. These patients must be placed on thromboprophylactic drugs. In indicated cases, TED (thromboembolic deterrent) stockings have to be used in the postoperative patients. The guidelines are summarized in Table 12.11 [24].

#### 12.2.2.6 Other Drugs That May be Required Based on the Patients' Medical History

If the patient has other medical comorbidities, medication that was being taken prior to the procedure may need to be continued or modified. It is best to confer with the patients' physician to determine the dosage and kind of drugs needed. These have been summarized in Table 12.12.

### 12.2.3 Nutritional Status in the Postoperative Period

Maxillofacial surgical procedures provide a unique challenge to the nutritional status in the postoperative period. Pain and edema in the oral region often prevent the patient

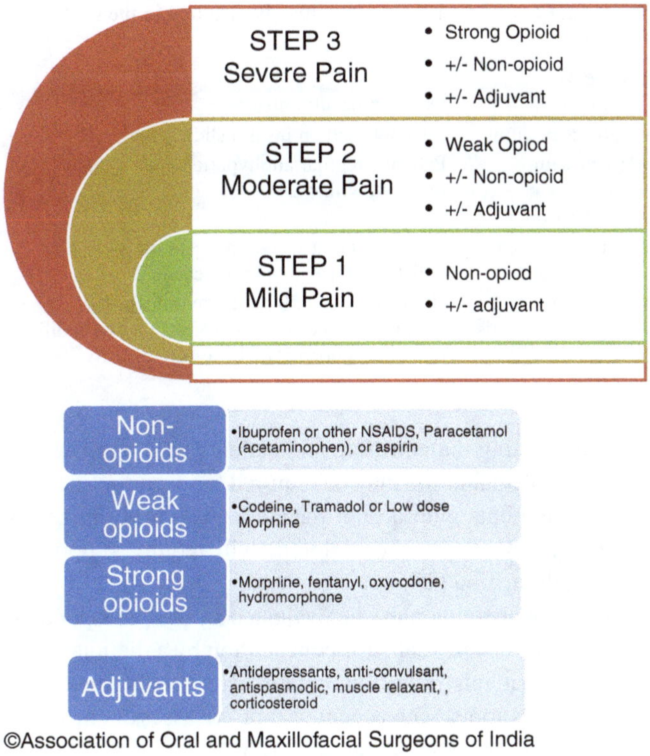


**Fig. 12.1** WHO analgesic ladder

**Table 12.10** Recommendations for antibiotic prophylaxis

| Type of surgery | Recommendation for antibiotic prophylaxis |
|---|---|
| Orthognathic surgery | Strongly recommended |
| Trauma—compound fractures | Recommended |
| Resections involving oral and cervical region | Recommended |
| Reconstruction | Weak evidence; physician judgment |
| Cleft surgery | Weak evidence; physician judgment |
| Minor oral surgery | Weak evidence; physician judgment |

from taking food comfortably, and there is a tendency to eat less or not at all. In patients with intermaxillary fixation, there is an inability to open the mouth and chew food. In certain kinds of surgery, such as reconstructive flaps involving the oral region, the patient is asked to avoid taking food by mouth at all to prevent the possibility of infection and flap failure in the postoperative period.

It is important, however, that the nutritional status is maintained. Inadequate nutrition has been shown to increase morbidity and mortality and can delay wound healing. It also increases the patient's susceptibility to infection. In the young, healthy adult patient, nutritional support may not be required, as the body compensates for decreased intake by increased glycogenolysis, gluconeogenesis, lipolysis, and amino acid oxidation. However, in young children, patients

**Table 12.11** Thromboprophylaxis guidelines

| Risk level | Criteria | Thromboprophylaxis required |
|---|---|---|
| Low | Minor surgery, age < 40 yrs., no additional risk factors | Early and persistent mobilization |
| Moderate | Minor surgery in age 40–60 yrs., with risk factors<br>Major surgery <40 yrs., no risk factors<br>Patients with medical illnesses or burns, with one risk factor<br>Neurosurgical patient with one risk factor | Low molecular weight heparin, <3400 units per day OR intermittent pneumatic compression devices |
| High | Minor surgery >60 years<br>Major surgery >40 years with risk factors<br>Patients with malignancy<br>Patients with medical illness or burns with two or more risk factors<br>Neurosurgical patient with two or more risk factors<br>Trauma patients with one or more risk factors | Low molecular weight heparin, >3400 units per day OR intermittent pneumatic compression devices |
| Highest | Patients with multiple risk factors, pelvic and lower extremity trauma or surgery, head injuries | Low molecular weight heparin, >3400 units per day AND intermittent pneumatic compression devices |

**Table 12.12** Additional drugs that may be required in the postoperative period

| Medical comorbidity | Drugs to be administered |
|---|---|
| Diabetes mellitus | Insulin based on insulin sliding scale |
| Patient with chronic hypertension | Patient's regular antihypertensive regimen to be restarted within 24 h |
| Patient on anticoagulants | Low molecular weight heparin for 24 h, after which warfarin should be resumed |
| Patient on long-term steroids | Hydrocortisone 50 mg three times a day, (equivalent to dexamethasone 2 mg) in addition to patient's normal dose, for up to 72 h |

with preexisting malnutrition, and patients with wasting diseases, supplementation may be required for even routine procedures. Patients who do not have adequate oral intake for 7–14 days (3–10 days in children) will require support to avoid malnutrition [25].

Nutritional status must be evaluated in the postoperative patient. This usually calls for consultation by a dietician. For long-term patients, nutritional status can also be measured using certain tools. The accepted tool for assessment is the subjective global assessment scale [26].

In patients on intermaxillary fixation, the classic use of the nasogastric tube must be discouraged. Patients may be educated on taking food through the retromolar region, using a feeding tube. NG tubes may be reserved for cases in whom oral feeds are contraindicated to avoid infection. Nutritionally complete formulas (e.g. Ensure) are available for enteral feeds. The patient may be started on 50 ml formula every 4 h, and this may be gradually increased in 50 ml increments until the desired target is achieved. After each feed, the tube must be flushed with 30 ml water to prevent blockage.

In cases of extensive neck surgery, where swallowing may be impaired, percutaneous gastrostomy (PEG) or jejunostomy tubes may be placed. For these tubes, infusion feeds (at the rate of 20 ml/h, increased in 20 ml increments every 4 h) may be given.

Total parenteral nutrition is usually not preferred because it has been linked to higher rates of infectious complications as compared to enteral nutrition. Patients who have complete block of the gastrointestinal system or those who cannot tolerate or retain enteral feeds are candidates for TPN. Dextrose solutions are preferred, with a dose of 10–20 g/kg/day of glucose. This is used in conjunction with amino acid solutions (0.5–3.5 g/kg/day) and lipid emulsions (50 ml/hr) [25].

### 12.2.4 Postoperative Mobilization of the Maxillofacial Surgery Patient

After the surgical procedure, early mobilization is recommended for all patients. Early mobilization is believed to enhance recovery by reducing the incidence of postoperative complications. It reduces secretions in the lungs, accelerates peristalsis, and improves venous blood flow to the extremities, thereby preventing thrombophlebitis and deep vein thrombosis [27]. Immobilization increases the risk of complications such as DVT and pressure sores. It can also lead to urinary retention.

For most maxillofacial procedures, the patient may be allowed to sit up with legs dangling 6 h after surgery. The patient may be mobilized within 24 h, and it is recommended that they ambulate every 4–6 h (during waking hours) till discharge. Caution must be employed in patients who have had grafts or flaps taken from the fibula. While the early mobilization protocol must be followed, protected weight bearing may be employed.

For patients who require prolonged bed rest, the use of alternating pressure mattresses or gel mattress overlays must be considered to prevent pressure sores.

Chest physiotherapy forms an important component of postoperative care. The in-hospital patient is prone to increased lung secretions and infections, which may be cleared using chest physiotherapy.

### 12.2.5 Management of Complications in the Postoperative Period

#### 12.2.5.1 Sudden Airway Obstruction

Maxillofacial surgery and surgery to the neck carry a risk of edema and hematoma developing in the postoperative period that can compress on the airway. The airway must be monitored closely, both in the immediate postoperative period and during the stay in the ward.

If the patient presents with hypoxia and airway obstruction, the head tilt-chin lift-jaw thrust maneuver must be employed. The airway must be checked manually and cleared of obstruction such as vomitus or blood. If the airway obstruction is at or above the oropharynx, insert an airway (such as Guedel's) to keep the passage patent. If there is a hematoma compressing the airway, surgical sutures must be removed to allow a release of pressure. In extreme cases, emergency airway procedures such as cricothyroidotomy may need to be performed.

#### 12.2.5.2 Fever in the Postoperative Period

Fever is defined as a rise in body temperature above 38 °C (100.4 °F). Postoperative fever represents a diagnostic challenge for most surgeons. Although most cases of fever are self-limiting, some can be serious and need urgent intervention. The timing of postoperative fever often gives a clue as to its diagnosis and management [28, 29].

**Immediate Fever (During Surgery or Within the First 24 h).**

Fever in the immediate postoperative period is most likely to be an inflammatory response to surgery. The surgical procedure causes *release of pyrogenic cytokines*, which stimulate the anterior hypothalamus to release prostaglandins, causing a rise in body temperature. The extent of fever depends on the amount of tissue trauma, but usually resolves in 24 h. Laboratory and diagnostic workup is not warranted for this kind of fever.

Occasionally, immediate fever can occur due to more serious reasons, and it is important to identify these. *Malignant hyperthermia* is a rare, life-threatening disorder that can manifest in susceptible individuals when they are exposed to inhalational anesthetics, or succinylcholine. There is an immediate rise in body temperature during or up to 1 h after surgery. It may be recognized by an immediate rise in $ETCO_2$, tachypnea, tachycardia, and muscle rigidity. Prompt intervention is required to avoid muscle lysis and organ system failure. Treatment involves immediate intravenous Dantrolene sodium (2.5 mg/kg), repeated every 5 min till reversal occurs, or till the maximum dose is reached (10 mg/kg).

If the fever occurs during or immediately *after a blood transfusion*, it is a sign of transfusion reaction. Transfusion of incompatible (mismatched) blood can cause a severe hemolytic reaction, which, in addition to fever, can present with dyspnea, fever, and myoglobinuria. In such cases, the transfusion must be discontinued immediately. Sometimes, febrile reactions can also occur with compatible blood, due to reaction of recipient antibodies with antigens in the transfused blood. This fever will be accompanied by headache, nausea, and vomiting. Slowing the transfusion may suffice, but it must be stopped if the reactions become severe.

*Adverse drug reactions* can rarely cause fever. This is usually a diagnosis of exclusion, and if suspected, all drugs must be discontinued one at a time to identify the offender. If replacement is necessary, a chemically unrelated drug must be used.

### Early Postoperative Fever (24–48 h After Surgery)

A serious cause of postoperative fever in this time period is *deep vein thromboembolism*. This must be suspected if the patient has known risk factors, such as a history of smoking, malignant disease, prolonged surgery, advanced age, or prolonged immobility after surgery. Diagnosis is made by ultrasound or impedence plethysmography. If present, prompt systemic anticoagulation must be started to avoid fatal pulmonary embolism. The use of Homan's sign (Pain in the calf on forced dorsiflexion of the foot) is no longer recommended because of the risk of dislodging the thrombus into circulation. A suspected PE may be confirmed with a ventilation-perfusion (V/Q) scan of the lungs.

*Thrombophlebitis* can also cause a rise in body temperature. Any iv line in place for more than 24 h can cause phlebitis. This presents with pain, erythema, and edema at the affected site. The iv line must be removed and replaced, and anti-inflammatory drugs may be given. A topical ointment containing heparin and benzyl nicotinate (thrombophob) may be applied locally.

*Atelectasis* was once thought to be a cause of fever, but it is now believed that fever and atelectasis are unrelated, though they can coexist. *Aspiration pneumonia* is more likely to be a respiratory cause of fever, but it presents 3–5 days after surgery.

### Delayed Postoperative Fever (After 48 h)

*Surgical site wound infections* can result in fever 3–5 days after surgery. The surgical site must be examined for pain, swelling, and pus discharge if fever occurs during this period. If an infection is present, it must be managed as detailed in the following sections.

*Aspiration pneumonia* can occur if the gastric fluid is aspirated into the lungs, owing to a depressed cough reflex after surgery. The risk increases in patients on maxillomandibular fixation.

### Fever Beyond Fifth Postoperative Day

Fever beyond the fifth postoperative day is usually a sign of systemic infection and needs a diagnostic workup. The most common infections that can occur are *urinary tract infection* and *upper respiratory tract infection*.

Indwelling urinary catheters are the main source of UTIs. Women are at greater risk because they have a shorter urethra; however, both genders can develop UTI if the catheter is in place for more than 72 h. Concomitant signs such as burning sensation on passing urine may be present. Urine will appear cloudy. Diagnosis is best confirmed by urine culture; empirical antibiotics may be started in the meantime.

Respiratory tract infections can range from sinusitis to hospital-acquired pneumonia. In Hospital Acquired Pneumonia (HAP), chest auscultation may reveal crackles or rales, and diagnosis is made by chest x-rays. Treatment is by empirical antibiotics.

A rare infection that can occur beyond the fifth day is *necrotizing soft tissue infection*. Although this is more common after colorectal surgery, cervical necrotizing infection has been reported after maxillofacial surgery as well [30]. Diagnosis may be made by detecting subcutaneous 'gas' on x-rays or CT imaging. Treatment involves the use of broad spectrum antibiotics and fluid resuscitation.

With all systemic infections, blood culture must be done to rule out sepsis. It is also important to monitor the patient's vitals closely to ensure that the patient does not go into septic shock.

> It may be of interest to know that in the literature there is a mnemonic of 6 W's, with regard to causes of postoperative fever. The W's being *Waves* (ECG changes, MI), *Wind* (atelectasis, pneumonia), *Water* (UTI), *Wound* (surgical site infection), *Walking* (Venous thromboembolism), *Wonder* drugs(drug-related fever).

The workup for postoperative fever is shown in Fig. 12.2.

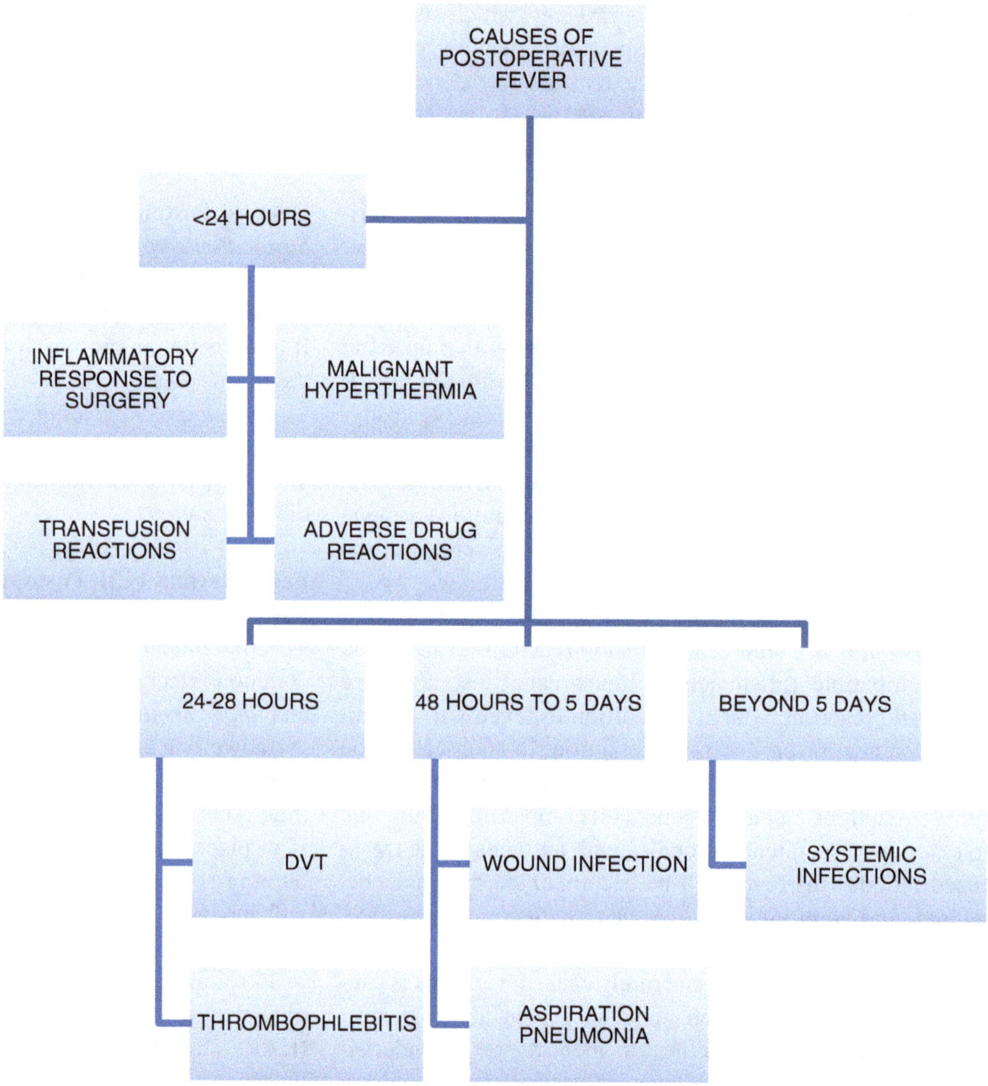


**Fig. 12.2** Postoperative fever workup

#### 12.2.5.3 Changes in Pulse and Blood Pressure

Any gross deviation from the normal vital signs must be looked into. Changes in pulse (tachycardia or bradycardia) are usually associated with changes in the other vital signs as well, and these must therefore be evaluated first.

Hypotension in the postoperative period can occur due to several causes [6] (Fig. 12.3). Hypotension is usually the result of reduced plasma volume; this may be due to inadequate fluid resuscitation, or ongoing blood loss. Excessive usage of opioid analgesics may also cause a fall in blood pressure. A myocardial infarction and blood sepsis may also present with hypotension. Hypotension with tachycardia can be a sign of developing shock; which must be treated immediately with a fluid challenge (rapid bolus of fluid). Regardless of the cause, hypotension must be managed by increasing fluid input and supplemented by high-flow oxygen to improve the perfusion.

Raised blood pressure usually occurs in patients who have had preexisting hypertension. If the patient has a history of ischemic heart disease or cerebrovascular disease, it must be managed with appropriate medication, to reduce the risk of developing myocardial infarction or stroke postoperatively. Sometimes, hypertension may occur in healthy adults with no history. In these cases, it could reflect pain and anxiety, or distension of the bowel and/or bladder. Excessive fluid resuscitation may also result in hypertension [6].

#### 12.2.5.4 Changes in Respiration

Increase in respiratory rate (tachypnea) is usually a sign of respiratory distress, and may be accompanied by decreased

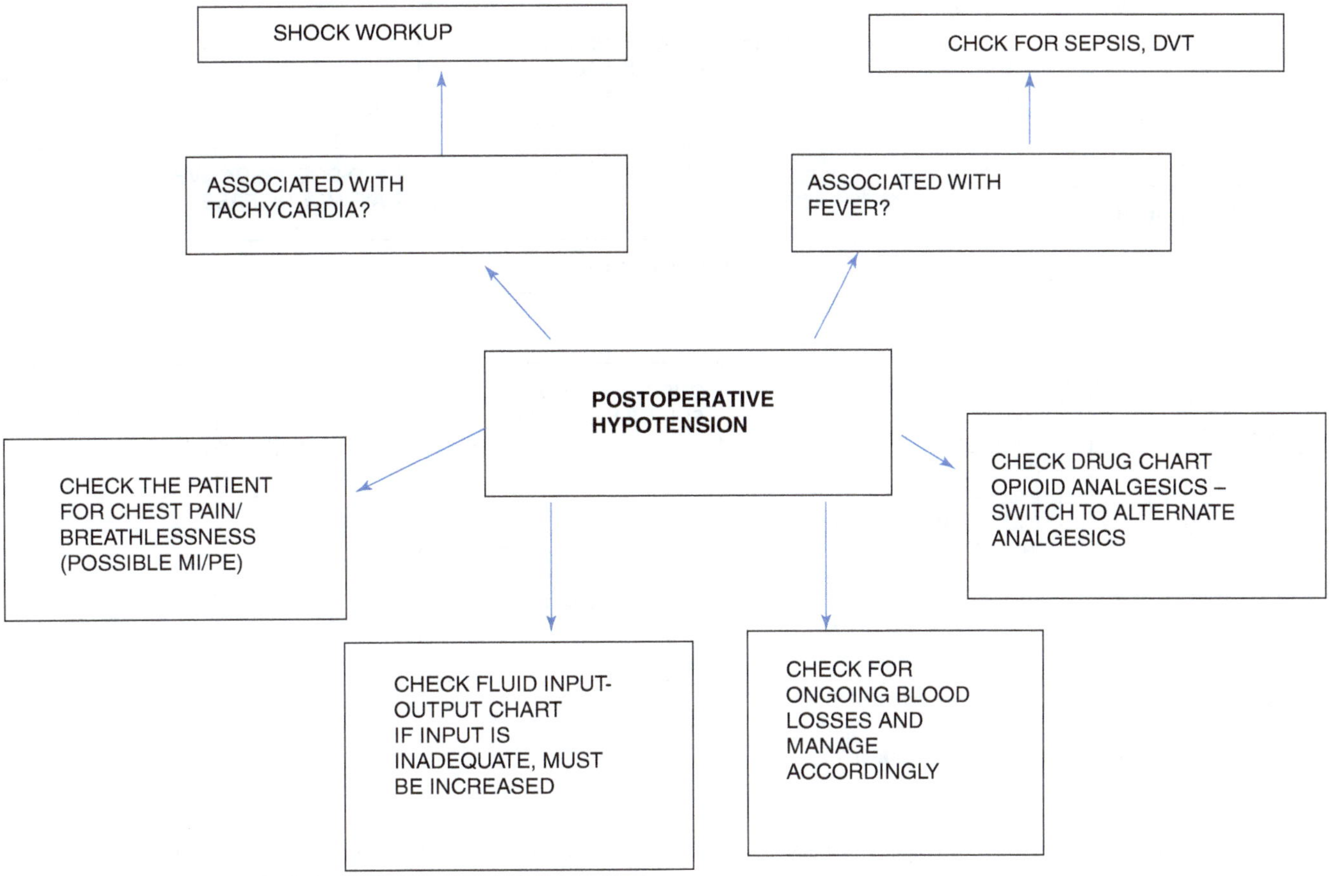




**Fig. 12.3** Postoperative hypotension workup

oxygen saturation, and use of accessory muscles of respiration [6]. Sudden acute shortness of breath may be a sign of pulmonary embolism. Gradual onset that occurs within 2–5 days of surgery is commonly due to atelectasis. Atelectasis is the collapse of a small segment of the lung and commonly occurs after general anesthesia. Atelectasis after maxillofacial surgery may be obstructive in nature, occurring secondary to epistaxis or mucus secretion. Another reason for the slow onset of respiratory distress is Acute Respiratory Distress Syndrome (ARDS), which can occur secondary to hypovolemia, sepsis, or trauma. Respiratory infection and cardiac causes such as myocardial infarction or cardiac failure can also alter respiratory rate. The various causes are illustrated in Fig. 12.4.

If a person experiences shortness of breath, high-flow oxygen must be started, and a chest x-ray and EKG must be taken. Laboratory tests including cardiac enzymes and arterial blood gases must be performed to ascertain the cause. If sputum is present, it must be sent for culture and gram staining.

#### 12.2.5.5 Postoperative Nausea and Vomiting

This is a common complication that occurs due to activation of the nucleus tractus solitarius and vomiting center by inhalational anesthetics. Patients who undergo maxillofacial surgery, particularly orthognathic surgical procedures, are at increased risk of developing postoperative nausea and vomiting, due to accumulation of blood in the throat. It can affect 20–80% of all patients, the risk being higher in young patients, females in the first 8 days of their menstrual cycle, and obese patients [23]. This complication is best managed symptomatically using antiemetics such as ondansetron and metoclopramide.

#### 12.2.5.6 Oliguria and Acute Renal Failure

The normal urine output is 1 ml/kg/h in infants, 0.5 ml/kg/h in children, and at least 400 ml/day in adults. Any drop below this level is referred to as oliguria and this must be addressed to prevent acute kidney injury (AKI). AKI is diagnosed as oliguria, along with serum creatinine levels 1.5 times above baseline [6]. The various causes of postoperative oliguria and management are outlined in Table 12.13.

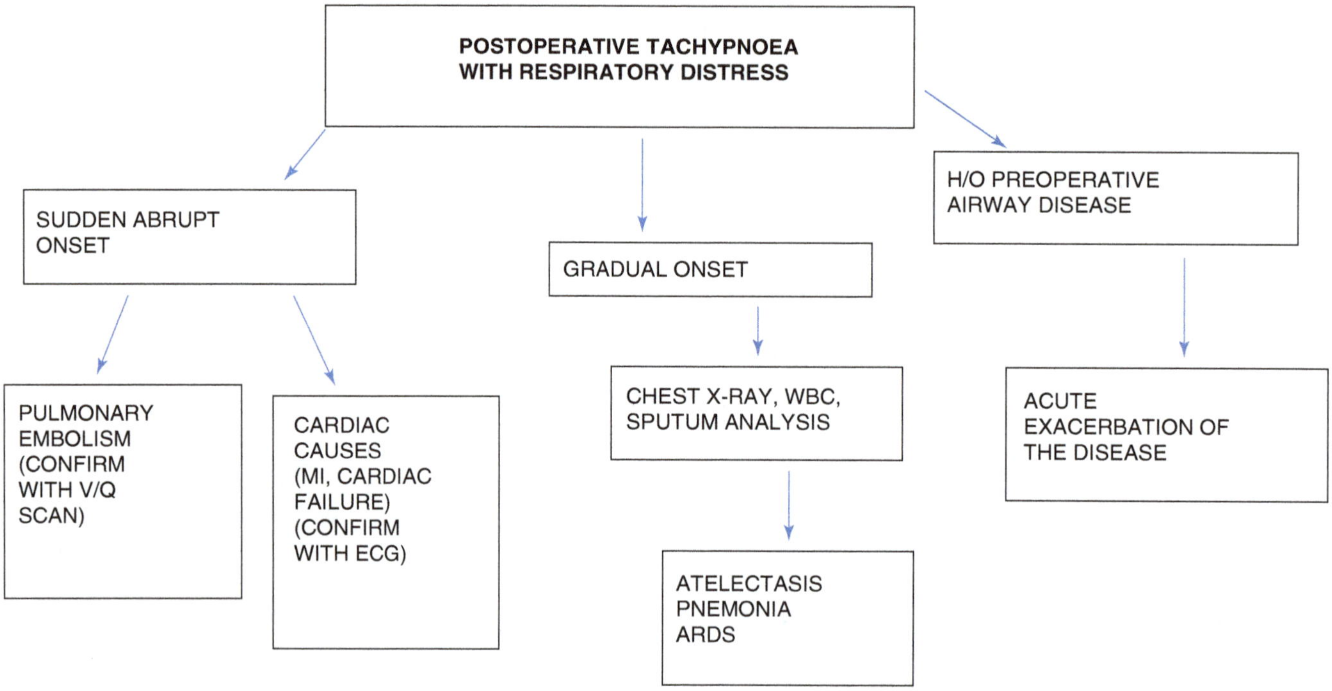




**Fig. 12.4** Postoperative respiratory distress workup

**Table 12.13** Types of postoperative oliguria and management

| Type of oliguria/ AKI | Cause | Management |
|---|---|---|
| Prerenal | Hypovolemia | Fluid challenge of 250 ml iv fluid over 1 h |
| | Hypotension | Address the cause of hypotension |
| Renal | Nephrotoxic drugs: NSAIDS, aminoglycosides, steroids | Discontinue the offending drug |
| | Sepsis | Aggressive treatment with broad spectrum antibiotics and fluid resuscitation |
| Post-renal | Blocked Foley's catheter<br>Blocked ureter | Relieve obstruction |

## 12.3 Care of the Surgical Wound Site

### 12.3.1 Immediate Care in the Operating Room

Care of the surgical wound site begins even before closure of the wound has been completed. It may be necessary to place drains or catheters within the wound.

**Surgical Drains**

A drain is a device that is intended to evacuate fluids and air from the surgical wound site. By evacuating accumulated pus, blood, and serous fluid, they help prevent infection of the surgical site. By evacuating air, they help eliminate dead spaces, which results in faster wound healing.

The various kinds of drains are summarized in Table 12.14. Drains may be classified as:

- Active drains: These work under negative pressure and actively remove fluids and air from the surgical site.
- Passive drains: They drain fluids passively, and are dependent on gravity. Passive drains may be open or closed.

Technique of inserting a surgical drain:

- The drain must be inserted before the last layer of sutures is placed.
- The drain tube has a needle at one end and perforations at the other end.
- The needle is inserted from the deeper edge of the surgical wound, and pulled out through the skin surface, about 2 cm away from the wound margin. The end with the perforations must remain within the surgical site.
- The exit of the needle must be in a dependent area, lower than the incision line.
- The needle is cut off from the tube and discarded safely.
- The drain tube is secured with sutures to the skin surface.
- The bulb or container is deflated completely, to ensure negative pressure, and is then attached to the exit end of the tube.
- Dressing with betadine gauze is done around and over the drain tube.

**Table 12.14** Types of drains

<table>
<tr><th>Type of drain</th><th></th><th>Example</th><th>Indications for use</th><th>Image</th></tr>
<tr><td>Active</td><td></td><td>Jackson-Pratt drain</td><td>Inserted into the surgical site to drain blood and serous fluid; to eliminate dead spaces</td><td>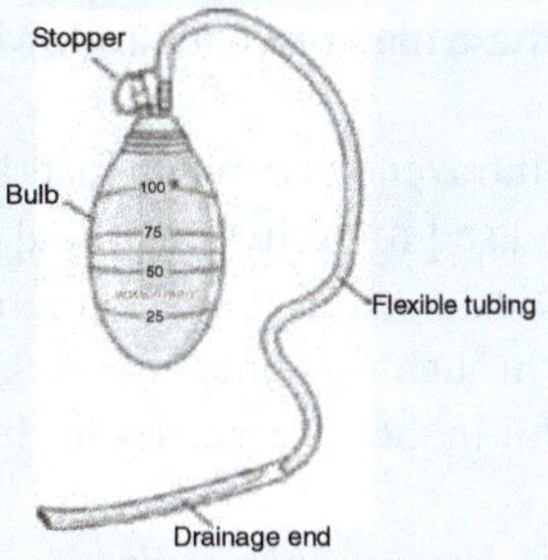
</td></tr>
<tr><td></td><td></td><td>Hemovac</td><td></td><td>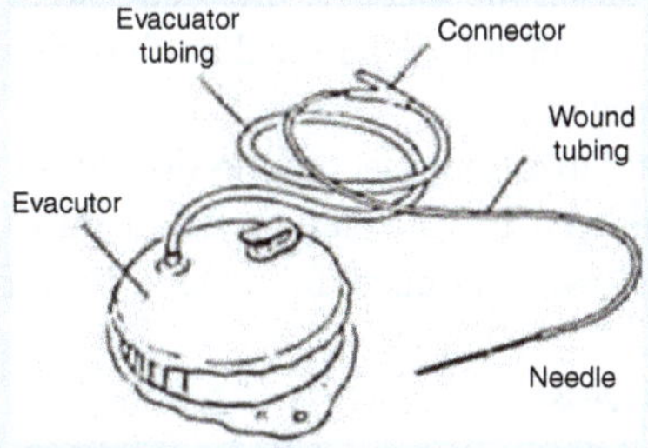
</td></tr>
<tr><td>Passive</td><td>Open</td><td>Corrugated rubber drain</td><td>To drain pus from infected abscesses and anatomical spaces</td><td>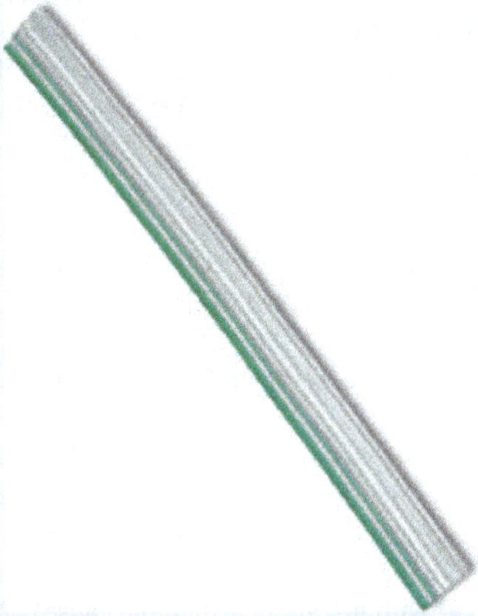</td></tr>
<tr><td></td><td></td><td>Penrose drain</td><td></td><td>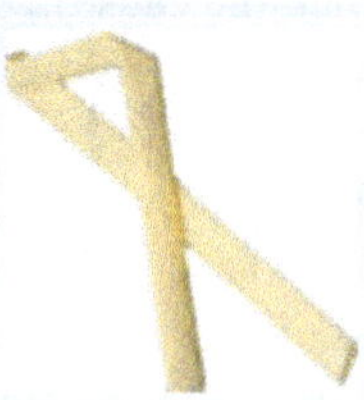</td></tr>
<tr><td></td><td>Closed</td><td>Nasogastric tube, Foley's catheter</td><td>To drain body secretions (gastric fluid, urine)</td><td>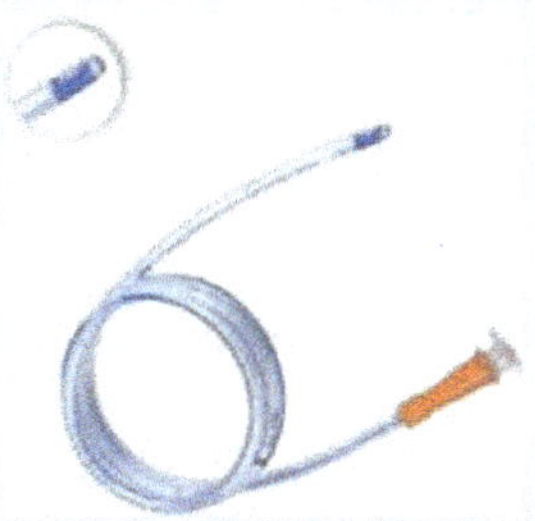</td></tr>
</table>

**Surgical Site Catheters**

Catheters may be inserted directly into the surgical site beneath the skin sutures. These may serve the following purposes:

- Analgesia: An intravenous cannula inserted into the surgical site may be used for delivering local analgesia. Long-acting anesthetics, such as ropivacaine and bupivacaine, are delivered through this into the surgical site. This is especially useful in the iliac crest after harvest of autogenous bone.
- Local antibiotic therapy: Infected spaces or osteomyelitic bone may benefit from local antibiotics that are delivered via catheters.
- Marsupialization: Decompression of a cystic lesion may be followed by catheter insertion into the cystic cavity. This allows continued drainage of fluid from the cyst.

**Wound Dressing**

Once complete suturing of the wound has been completed, appropriate dressing of the wound site must be carried out. Various types of dressing material are available [31]. These are detailed in the Chap. 11 on soft tissue injuries and management.

### 12.3.2 General Guidelines for Postoperative Wound Care [32]

- Aim to leave the wound undisturbed for at least 48 h after surgery.
- Premature removal of the wound dressing may, however, be required in certain situations. These include:
- Excess exudate or blood soaking through the dressing.
- Suspicion that the wound site is infected (e.g. Postoperative fever with no other attributable cause).
- The dressing is no longer serving its purpose (e.g. Falling off).
- If the wound dressing is being changed, check if there is excess exudate or devitalized tissue that may delay wound healing. If these are present, the wound must be cleansed. This is done by gentle irrigation of saline (for the first 48 h) or clean tap water (after 48 h) using a syringe. The wound must never be swabbed with gauze, as this can delay healing.

**Postoperative Care of Drains and Catheters**

- The drain must be monitored every 4 h and more frequently if the discharge from the wound is excessive.
- The drain container must be evacuated at least once every day.
- Once the drain fluid collection goes below 25–50 ml/day, the drain may be removed.

Surgical site catheters must be removed by the third postoperative day.

### 12.3.3 Surgical Site Complications

**Postoperative Bleeding, Hematoma, and Seroma**

Bleeding after surgery is classified as primary (occurs during or immediately after the surgical procedure), reactionary (occurs after few hours, possibly due to slipped ligatures), and secondary (occurs after few days, commonly due to infection). Active, ongoing bleeding is referred to as hemorrhage.

Hematoma refers to a clotted collection of blood below the tissues, which occurs due to damage to vessel walls. Most hematomas are self-limiting. Larger hematomas can be treated with ice packs or compression dressings. Analgesics may be given if the swelling is painful. Hematomas in the submandibular and neck region, or other regions which can potentially compress the airway, must be drained surgically.

Seromas are collections of serous fluid that generally develop 5–7 days after surgery. They are more common in extensive surgeries, particularly in neck dissection, where lymph nodes have been removed. Small seromas resolve over time. If the seroma is large and painful, the fluid may be aspirated and a pressure dressing can be applied.

**Infected Wound**

As maxillofacial procedures are clean-contaminated surgeries, they carry a higher risk of developing infection as compared to clean surgeries. Signs and symptoms of an infected wound include:

- Unexplained fever 3–5 days after surgery.
- Localized pain at the wound site.
- Erythema around the wound.
- Wound dehiscence, with pus discharge from the wound.

If the wound appears infected, a few sutures must be removed and pus must be drained out. A swab must be sent for culture and sensitivity testing, and the patient must be started on empirical antibiotics. The patient must be monitored closely for signs of systemic infection. The infected wound can be treated by local debridement and antibiotic irrigation.

**Wound Dehiscence**

This generally occurs as a result of one of the above complications, most commonly subacute infection. Sometimes, however, it may simply be the result of excessive wound tension due to inadequate tissue undermining. If the wound is uninfected less than 24 h postoperatively, re-suturing may be attempted. Otherwise, the wound is best left to heal by secondary intention. Resistant wound dehiscence may lead to orocutaneous communications and may become difficult to handle. The decision to either allow these to granulate or surgically provide a cover depends on individual scenarios.

## 12.4 Postoperative Care for Specific Types of Surgeries

While the general rules apply to all kinds of surgeries, there may be extra measures which are required in each specific surgery type. These are outlined below [2].

**Postoperative Care for the Trauma Patient**

- In the immediate postoperative period, the airway must be monitored. This may get compromised due to bleeding or edema.
- For fractures of the zygoma and orbit, monitoring for retrobulbar hemorrhage is important. This can be diagnosed by the three Ps—pain (in the orbit), proptosis, and pupillary defects [33]. The postoperative care team is generally required to check papillary reflexes on an hourly basis for the first 6 h which can be relaxed to once in 2 h for the next 6 h. Any impending sign of diminishing vision or pupillary inactivity is brought to the notice of the consultant and steps initiated accordingly.
- Assess and document paresthesia along any nerves involved in the fractured segment. This includes the inferior alveolar nerve for mandibular fractures and infraorbital nerve for zygomaticomaxillary complex fractures.
- The accuracy of reduced fractures must be checked on the first postoperative day using radiographs. For fractures involving the dentoalveolar segments, occlusion may be used as a guide.

**Postoperative Care for Orthognathic Surgery Patients**

- As with trauma patients, airway compromise due to bleeding and edema must be monitored.
- Considerable facial swelling is common. Ice packs and systemic steroids can help reduce swelling.
- Occlusion must be checked on the first postoperative day, and elastics must be placed if required. Class II elastics are placed from the upper anterior teeth to lower posterior teeth. Class III elastics are placed from lower anteriors to upper posterior teeth.

**Postoperative Care for Oncology and Reconstruction Patients**

- These patients usually undergo extensive surgery that lasts for hours, and will therefore need intensive monitoring in the postoperative period. Tracheostomy care may be required (See Sect. 12.1.1).
- Most of these patients will be unable to feed properly till wound healing is complete. Ryle's tube or PEG insertion must be done on the day of surgery or the first postoperative day.
- Patients must be on DVT prophylaxis. The malignancy, prolonged surgery, and in-hospital stay increase the risk of the patient developing DVT.

**Flap Monitoring**

- Reconstructed flaps must be monitored for vitality. If the blood supply to the flap is lost due to thrombi, it may be salvageable within the first 48 h. Periodic monitoring ensures prompt surgical intervention if the need arises.
- Flaps may be monitored using a handheld Doppler. Capillary refill may be assessed for flaps which are not buried. The needle prick test is simple, but must be done only to confirm congestion or loss of vitality.
- Flaps must be monitored hourly for the first 24 h, and 4 hourly for the next 48 h.

## 12.5 Postoperative Complications Specific to each Type of Surgery

Table 12.15 lists the complications that may be encountered with each specific surgery.

## 12.6 Criteria for Discharging the Patient

Prolonged hospital stay increases the patient's risk of developing nosocomial infections. Therefore, the patients must be discharged as soon as feasible. Criteria for discharge are as follows:

- Patient is hemodynamically stable, and all vitals are stable.
- Patient can take nutrition independently or with the aid of a caregiver.
- Wounds are healing well with no signs of infection.

Discharge summary: This is a record given to the patient, detailing the diagnosis, procedure performed, and any implants that were used. Instructions and medications to be taken must also be noted.

Follow-up appointments must be made for review. In case facial and neck incisions were placed, an appointment for suture removal must be given.

**Table 12.15** Specific postoperative complications

| Type of surgery | Complication | Management |
|---|---|---|
| Trauma | Malunion/nonunion | Reopen, remove cause of malunion, induce bleeding, use of graft |
| | Ptosis, diplopia, enophthalmos (orbital and ZMC repair) | Secondary surgical correction |
| | Persistent paresthesia | Palliative |
| TMJ surgery/ condylar fractures | Frey's syndrome (gustatory sweating) | Botox injection, surgical intervention |
| | Sialocele, salivary fistula | Debride the fistula lining and keep the area clean till healing occurs. |
| | Facial nerve palsy | Temporary—Palliative care<br>Permanent—Facial nerve reanimation |
| Orthognathic surgery | Condylar malpositioning leading to anterior open bite (BSSO) | Re-surgery, removal of plates, repositioning the condyle and re-fixation |
| | Inferior alveolar nerve paresthesia | Palliative management |
| | Alar base widening (maxillary surgery) | Alar cinching |
| | Nasal septal deviation | Septoplasty |
| | Aseptic necrosis of segment | Removal and reconstruction |
| | Malocclusion | Orthodontic treatment |
| Neck dissections | Chyle leak | Chyle duct repair |
| | Shoulder syndrome (spinal accessory nerve damage) | Physiotherapy |
| | Paresthesia of sensory nerves, e.g. greater auricular, lingual nerves | Palliative |
| | Carotid blowout | Surgical emergency, immediate repair needed. |

## 12.7 Conclusion

Postoperative care requires a thorough understanding of the patient, the procedure they have undergone, and the expected outcome. Surgeons must realize that more often it may be the first experience for a patient in going under the knife and lying at the ICU or ward. Hence, a perfect coherence of scientific and psychological views is required of the surgical team at all levels. The chapter emphasizes the need for comprehensive management of the maxillofacial patient at the ward after their procedure. The reader is expected to understand that outcome depends, but not ends at operating room or ward/ICU.

## References


1. Ogle O. Postoperative care of oral and maxillofacial surgery patients. Oral Maxillofac Surg Clin North Am. 2006;18(1):49–58.
2. Cascarini L, Schilling C, Gurney B, Brennan P. Oxford handbook of oral and maxillofacial surgery. Oxford: Oxford University Press; 2018 August 2.
3. Chatburn RL, Primiano JF. A new system for understanding modes of mechanical ventilation. Respir Care. 2001 Jun;46(6):604–21.
4. Buggy DJ, Crossley AW. Thermoregulation, mild perioperative hypothermia and post-anaesthetic shivering. Br J Anaesth. 2000 May 1;84(5):615–28.
5. Aldrete JA. The post anaesthesia recovery score revisited [letter]. J Clin Anesth. 1995;7:89–91.
6. Williams N, O'Connell PR, editors. Bailey & love's short practice of surgery. 26th ed. Boca Raton, FL: CRC Press; 2013 Feb 18.
7. Alfonsi P. Postanaesthetic shivering. Epidemiology, pathophysiology and approaches to prevention and management. Minerva Anestesiol. 2003;69:438–41.
8. Giannakopoulos H, Albakoff J. Fluid and electrolyte management and blood product usage. Oral Maxillofac Surg Clin North Am. 2006;18:7–17.
9. Kayilioglu SI, Dinc T, Sozen I, Bostanoglu A, Cete M, Coskun F. Postoperative fluid management. World J Crit Care Med. 2015;4(3):192–201.
10. Chesney RW. The maintenance need for water in parenteral fluid therapy, by Malcolm A. Holliday, MD, and William E. Segar, MD, Pediatrics, 1957; 19: 823–832. Pediatrics. 1998 Jul 1;102(Supplement 1):229–30.
11. Doherty M, Buggy D. Intraoperative fluids: how much is too much? Br J Anaesth. 2012;109(1):69–79.
12. Della Rocca G, Vetrugno L, Tripi G, Deana C, Barbariol F, Pompei L. Liberal or restricted fluid administration: are we ready for a proposal of a restricted intraoperative approach? BMC Anesthesiol. 2014;14(1):62.
13. Chao J. Transfuse or not to transfuse: for postop anemia. Am J Clin Med. 2011;8(1):11–4.
14. Liumbruno GL, Bennardello F, Lattanzio A, Piccoli P, Rosetti G. Recommendations for the transfusion management of patients in the peri-operative period. III. The post-operative period. Blood Transfus. 2011;9:320–35.
15. Ong CK, Lirk P, Seymour RA, Jenkins BJ. The efficacy of preemptive analgesia for acute postoperative pain management: a meta-analysis. Anesth Analg. 2005 Mar 1;100(3):757–73.
16. Coulthard P, Haywood D, Tai M, Jackson-Leech D, Pleuvry B, Macfarlane T. Treatment of postoperative pain in oral and maxillofacial surgery. Br J Oral Maxillofac Surg. 2000;38(6):588–92.
17. Vargas-Schaffer G. Is the WHO analgesic ladder still valid? Twenty-four years of experience. Can Fam Physician. 2010 Jun 1;56(6):514–7.
18. Grass JA. Patient-controlled analgesia. Anesth Analg. 2005 Nov 1;101(5S):S44–61.
19. Fleischli J, Adams W. Use of postoperative steroids to reduce pain and inflammation. J Foot Ankle Surg. 1999;38(3):232–7.
20. Bhagat S, Agarwal M, Roy V. Serratiopeptidase: a systematic review of the existing evidence. Int J Surg. 2013;11(3):209–17.
21. Escobar JIS, de Velasco AAF. Antibiotic prophylaxis in Oral and maxillofacial surgery. Med Oral Patol Oral Cir Bucal. 2006;11:E292–6.

22. Kreutzer K, Storck K, Weitz J. Current evidence regarding prophylactic antibiotics in head and neck and maxillofacial surgery. Biomed Res Int. 2014;2014:1–7.
23. Dobbeleir M, De Coster J, Coucke W, Politis C. Postoperative nausea and vomiting after oral and maxillofacial surgery: a prospective study. Int J Oral Maxillofac Surg. 2018;47(6):721–5.
24. Lachiewicz PF. Comparison of ACCP and AAOS guidelines for VTE prophylaxis after total hip and total knee arthroplasty. Orthopedics (Online). 2009 Dec 1;32(12):74.
25. Fang J, Chirag D, Dym H. Nutritional aspects of care. Oral Maxillofac Surg Clin North Am. 2006;18(1):115–30.
26. da Silva FJ, Daniel de Mello P, Daniel de Mello E. Subjective global assessment of nutritional status – a systematic review of the literature. Clin Nutr. 2015;34(5):785–92.
27. Dolgun E, Giersbergen M, Aslan A, Altınbaş Y. The investigation of mobilization times of patients after surgery. Asian Pac J Health Sci. 2017;4(1):71–5.
28. Ansari R. Fever work-up and management in postsurgical oral and maxillofacial surgery patients. Oral Maxillofac Surg Clin North Am. 2006;18(1):73–9.
29. Jadwani S, Bansod S, Chug A, Misra B. Management of postoperative fever in oral and maxillofacial surgery patients. Asian J Oral Maxillofac Surg. 2010;22(1):2–6.
30. Tung-Yiu W, Jehn-Shyun H, Ching-Hung C, Hung-An C. Cervical necrotizing fasciitis of odontogenic origin: a report of 11 cases. J Oral Maxillofac Surg. 2000;58(12):1347–52.
31. Ovington LG. Advances in wound dressings. Clin Dermatol. 2007 Jan 1;25(1):33–8.
32. Yao K, Bae L, Yew WP. Postoperative wound management. Aust Fam Physician. 2013;42(12):867–70.
33. Bater MC, Ramchandani PL, Brennan PA. Post-traumatic eye observations. Br J Oral Maxillofac Surg. 2005 Oct 1;43(5):410–6.

# Permissions

All chapters in this book were first published by Springer; hereby published with permission under the Creative Commons Attribution License or equivalent. Every chapter published in this book has been scrutinized by our experts. Their significance has been extensively debated. The topics covered herein carry significant information for a comprehensive understanding. They may even be implemented as practical applications or may be referred to as a beginning point for further studies.

The contributors of this book come from diverse backgrounds, making this book a truly international effort. We would like to thank all the contributing authors for lending their expertise to make the book truly unique. They have played a crucial role in the development of this book. Without their invaluable contributions this book wouldn't have been possible. They have made vital efforts to compile up to date information on the varied aspects of this subject to make this book a valuable addition to the collection of many professionals and students.

This book was conceptualized with the vision of imparting up-to-date and integrated information in this field. To ensure the same, a matchless editorial board was set up. Every individual on the board went through rigorous rounds of assessment to prove their worth. After which they invested a large part of their time researching and compiling the most relevant data for our readers.

The editorial board has been involved in producing this book since its inception. They have spent rigorous hours researching and exploring the diverse topics which have resulted in the successful publishing of this book. They have passed on their knowledge of decades through this book. To expedite this challenging task, the publisher supported the team at every step. A small team of assistant editors was also appointed to further simplify the editing procedure and attain best results for the readers.

Apart from the editorial board, the designing team has also invested a significant amount of their time in understanding the subject and creating the most relevant covers. They scrutinized every image to scout for the most suitable representation of the subject and create an appropriate cover for the book.

The publishing team has been an ardent support to the editorial, designing and production team. Their endless efforts to recruit the best for this project, has resulted in the accomplishment of this book. They are a veteran in the field of academics and their pool of knowledge is as vast as their experience in printing. Their expertise and guidance has proved useful at every step. Their uncompromising quality standards have made this book an exceptional effort. Their encouragement from time to time has been an inspiration for everyone.

The publisher and the editorial board hope that this book will prove to be a valuable piece of knowledge for students, practitioners and scholars across the globe.

# Index


**A**

Acute Asthma, 49, 56
Acute Kidney Injury, 39, 43, 47, 241
Acute Renal Failure, 43, 47, 233, 241
Airway Anatomy, 17
Airway Management, 17, 77, 85, 90, 93, 96, 98, 108, 113
Airway Problems, 106
Ambulatory Anesthesia, 11, 78, 83, 85, 90
Analgesic Ladder, 203, 235, 237, 246
Aneroid Manometer, 99
Anesthesia, 10-12, 15, 18-20, 22-23, 25-27, 33-34, 38-39, 48, 55, 58, 60-68, 70-80, 83-92, 114, 132, 171-172, 187, 192, 201, 204, 208, 231-232, 234, 241
Anesthesia Training, 78, 85
Anti-inflammatory Drugs, 202-203, 239
Articaine, 37, 39, 60-62, 75-76
Asthmatic Attack, 48-49, 56

**B**

Benzodiazepines, 18, 34-35, 78, 89

**C**

Carotid Artery, 103-104
Chemotherapy, 5-6, 13, 44-45, 47, 93, 200, 208
Chromic Catgut, 214, 216
Continuous Locking Suture, 227
Controlled Hypotension, 96, 103-105, 111
Conventional Laryngoscopy, 110

**D**

Dental Chair, 33, 52, 174
Dental Vibe, 73, 76
Dentistry, 3-4, 7, 10, 46-47, 60, 76, 90-91, 144, 208, 210, 215

**E**

Elective Tracheostomy, 105
Epilepsy, 11, 32-33, 46, 54-57, 202

**F**

Facial Injuries, 109-110, 196
Fibre Optic Bronchoscopy, 97, 99, 110

**G**

Glossopharyngeal Nerve Block, 71-73, 76
Greater Auricular Nerve Block, 71-73

**H**

Haemostasis, 32, 103, 105, 210, 223, 226-227, 229
Hematoma, 17, 37, 66, 68-70, 145, 238, 244
Horizontal Mattress Suture, 223, 226
Hypertension, 18, 20, 23, 25-27, 33, 36, 40, 43, 46, 56, 92, 111, 206, 236, 238, 240
Hypotensive Drugs, 104

**I**

Imaging Investigation, 117-119, 137
Intermaxillary Fixation, 33, 189, 237-238

**K**

Knot-tying, 213, 215-217, 226

**L**

Larynx, 17, 109, 127
Lidocaine, 37, 42, 60-63, 75, 90
Local Anesthetic Agents, 60-61

**M**

Mandibular Nerve Block, 61, 63-65, 67, 71-72, 76
Mask Ventilation, 17, 93, 106, 109-110, 113
Maxillary Tuberosity, 67, 71
Maxillofacial Considerations, 33-34
Monofilament Suture, 213, 216

**N**

Nasal Endotracheal Intubation, 110
Nasal Intubation, 93, 96-97, 99, 110
Nasopalatine, 66, 70-71
Nausea And Vomiting, 18, 23, 38, 46, 53, 89, 103, 106, 113, 202, 235-236, 241, 247

**O**

Office-based Anesthesia, 77, 83, 85, 89-90
Oliguria, 241-242
Oncology, 5, 198, 245
Opiods, 34, 38, 41
Oral And Maxillofacial Surgery, 1, 3-4, 6-7, 12, 18, 22-24, 48, 60, 71, 77-78, 83, 85, 91, 113, 206, 208-210, 212, 214, 231, 246-247
Organ Transplant, 194, 199, 208
Oropharynx, 17, 105, 231, 238
Orthognathic Surgery, 4, 10, 36, 43, 108, 114, 130, 194-197, 200, 204, 206-209, 237, 245

**P**

Parameters of Care, 22, 83, 91
Patient-controlled Analgesia, 21, 204, 208-209, 235, 246
Pediatric Patient, 15, 74

Polybutester, 215
Polypropylene, 213, 215
Postoperative Bleeding, 44, 106, 244
Postoperative Period, 10, 20, 36, 106, 108, 145, 197-198, 209, 231-232, 234-238, 240, 245
Preanesthetic Evaluation, 10, 15, 86
Preoperative Assessment, 12, 15, 17, 20, 44, 92
Preoperative Evaluation, 10-11, 22, 86, 139
Prevent Contamination, 196, 210
Prophylactic Antibiotics, 188, 194, 197, 199, 207, 247

**R**
Radiotherapy, 6, 13, 25, 44-45, 93

**S**
Salivation, 35
Sedation, 10, 18-19, 33, 35, 66, 77-79, 83-85, 87-91, 98, 111, 122, 187
Sedation Techniques, 85, 89
Seroma, 244
Simple Interrupted Suture, 218-219, 221, 225
Specialist Consultation, 11, 93
Sphenopalatine Ganglion Block, 73-74, 76
Stroke, 11, 13-14, 20, 24, 31-35, 46, 55, 113, 120, 234, 240
Subcuticular Suture, 222-223, 228
Surgical Drain, 242
Suture Thread, 211, 213, 217, 220, 223, 226

**T**
Temporomandibular Joint, 17, 33, 119, 126, 130, 144, 150, 154, 193
Throat Pack, 103, 109, 231
Toxic Airway, 93
Trauma Patients, 22, 93, 237, 245

**V**
Vasoconstrictors, 27, 34, 62-63, 103
Vertical Mattress Suture, 220, 226

**W**
Wound Closure, 210-211, 215-216, 218, 224-225, 228-230

**X**
Xerostomia, 34-35, 44

www.ingramcontent.com/pod-product-compliance
Lightning Source LLC
LaVergne TN
LVHW082124200926
848484LV00008B/2005